Relations between Language and Memory

Fachrichtung Angewandte Sprachwissenschaft
sowie Übersetzen und Dolmetschen
der Universität des Saarlandes

Alberto Gil – Johann Haller – Erich Steiner – Elke Teich
(Hrsg.)

Sabest

Saarbrücker Beiträge zur Sprach- und Translationswissenschaft

Band 23

PETER LANG
Frankfurt am Main · Berlin · Bern · Bruxelles · New York · Oxford · Wien

Cornelia Zelinsky-Wibbelt (ed.)

Relations between Language and Memory

Organization, Representation, and Processing

PETER LANG
Internationaler Verlag der Wissenschaften

Bibliographic Information published by the Deutsche Nationalbibliothek
The Deutsche Nationalbibliothek lists this publication in the Deutsche Nationalbibliografie; detailed bibliographic data is available in the internet at http://dnb.d-nb.de.

Cover illustration:
imprint with kind permission
of Peggy Daut.

ISSN 1436-0268
ISBN 978-3-631-57753-0

www.peterlang.de

Preface

I wish to express my thanks to all authors who contributed to this volume. The relation between a theory of grammar and the language user's representation and processing of linguistic experience in human memory is an old topic in cognitive linguistics. The idea of this book originates from a small-scale project on lexicalization patterns, more specifically from the second cycle of LexiKurs funded by the German Research Foundation ("Deutsche Forschungsgemeinschaft", DFG, reference number ZE 345/5-3). This funding enabled a rigorous verification of linguistic theory through experimental methods (cf. Zeschel and Deppert, Zelinsky-Wibbelt, this volume) which gave rise to the invitation of further such projects for testing grammatical claims. Cognitive linguistics is currently busily engaged in coming up to the demands and challenges of an empirical science, most notably through the development of corpus-linguistic and experimental-linguistic methodologies. The current volume is equally engaged in putting cognitive linguistics on a solid empirical footing in that the majority of the contributions are devoted to experimental (Marian and Kaushanskaya, Novak and Lamb, Rummer and Engelkamp, Garnham and Cowles, Zeschel and Deppert) or corpus-linguistic (Zelinsky-Wibbelt, Morales and Taylor) investigations.

The edition of this volume has been enabled by the series editors of Sabest (*Saarbrücker Beiträge zur Sprach- und Translationswissenschaft*), in particular Johann Haller, who became first interested in the idea of this publication, and to whom many thanks are due.

Finally, thanks go to my husband, Hans-Bernd Wibbelt and to my former student assistant Florian Petran, for assisting me with the type setting of the book in LaTeX and TeX.

Saarbrücken, May 2011 Cornelia Zelinsky-Wibbelt

Contents

Introduction

Cornelia Zelinsky-Wibbelt

1 Human language and memory

Memory is commonly assumed to accomplish the encoding, the storage, and the retrieval of information (Anderson, 1995). It is thus prerequisite of all types of cognitive processing. Human memory exceeds the memory capacity of any other animate being. This is not only due to the huge storage capacities and the specialization of the human brain but follows necessarily from language as the medium through which information processing is communicated and in terms of which information becomes encoded, stored, and retrieved. It follows from this that language plays a central role in all memory processes. Language permeates the speakers' memory, in that linguistic structures provide organizing principles of human knowledge. More recently, language comprehension and production become investigated in terms of the organization and entrenchment of language in long-term memory and the corresponding retrieval in working memory (Bybee and Hopper, 2001; Gentner and Goldin-Meadow, 2003; Assink and Sandra, 2003). By taking different perspective points, speakers may express the same situation by different grammatical and lexical choices which in turn influences the organization and retrieval in human memory. Thereby whole situations may be remembered in different ways (Clark and Clark 1968; Bransford et al. 1972; Levinson 2003). Vice versa, linguistic input could not be processed without speakers retrieving their long-term store of knowledge in working memory. Language comprehension heavily depends on how the speakers' knowledge representation drives their inferential reconstruction of information (Barsalou, 2005).

The present book addresses these interactions between language and memory from the interdisciplinary perspective of cognitive science.

2 The architecture of language and memory

2.1 The container metaphor of language and memory

Traditionally, the architecture of human memory is conceived of in terms of the container metaphor. According to this image, human memory is compared to a box where everything humans have learned may be safely stored in order to search through this container whenever any content needs to be unpacked and used. Originally, distinct modules have been assumed to be responsible for the acquisition and storage, as well as for the retrieval of different types of information (Broadbent, 1971). The assumption of clearly distinguished memory systems due to storage-specific coding differences (Baddeley, 1986; Atkinson and Shiffrin, 1968) had to be revised in favour of elaborateness of processing and interactivity between levels. In the same vein, Tulving's distinction (1972) between semantic and episodic memory as the distinction between the more stable store of intersubjective knowledge on the one hand and the more variable store of personal, contingent experiences on the other has come under scrutiny more recently from a more dynamic perspective on the genetic relationship between the two.

The container metaphor has equally been applied to the organization of the linguistic system as conceived of by generative linguistics (Chomsky, 1986). From this mentalist stance, a distinction is made between meaning and reference, between the steady state of linguistic competence as the strictly rule-governed content of the human mind and the corresponding dynamic application of rules in linguistic performance by taking them out of the human mind. This naive view on the relation between competence and performance is caricatured by the CONDUIT METAPHOR of communication (Reddy 1993; Langacker 1987, 161f; Lakoff 1987, 449). Linguistic forms are seen as stable containers of meanings which the speaker pumps through a channel to a receiver who takes the meanings out of the container. Epistemologically, the distinction between the recursive rules of the linguistic system and the declarative facts of world knowledge reflects this dichotomy between knowledge and behaviour. The container metaphor equally comprises the distinction and correspondence between different linguistic (sub)systems (this volume, Rummer and Engelkamp, Zelinsky-Wibbelt, Zeschel and Deppert).

The contributions to this volume point out that the integration of these dichotomies becomes inevitable in the explanation of higher-order functions of human language and memory, such as the representation, organization, and communication of concepts (Garnham and Cowles, Schwarz-Friesel, Zeschel and Deppert). The processing of linguistic constructions in language comprehension and production (Rummer and Engelkamp, Tuggy, Zelinsky-Wibbelt, Zeschel and Deppert) establishes another case in point. Linguistic creativity and iconicity come into play when linguistic input which is not part of the speakers' conventionalized store in long-term memory (cf. Fortescue, Schwarz-Friesel, Garnham and Cowles, Bartsch, Novak and Lamb, Zelinsky-Wibbelt, Rummer and Engelkamp, Zeschel and Deppert) becomes processed through inferential and recursive reasoning. Vice versa, the organization and functioning of human memory is assumed to depend on the linguistic system (Marian and Kaushanskaya). As an integral part of the mind human memory is in turn represented through its connectionist neural basis in the brain (Bartsch, Novak and Lamb, Morales and Taylor, Fortescue, Zeschel and Deppert).

2.2 Storage vs. computation

A major issue of the book is how human memory is organized in order to manage the acquisition, the storage, and the retrieval of language so seemingly easily. Roughly, we may discern three ways of explanation which have been pursued in the study of language in linguistics (Beaugrande, 1980).

From the traditional view of prescriptive grammar, all complexities are organized in storage, this allowing for a cheap retrieval. As this model restricts linguistic processing to what is encoded, creative and inferential reasoning are impossible. No account is given of associative learning by analogy, contiguity, and abstraction. Hence the linguistic encoding of knowledge is seen as an arbitrary result of its function, and no explanation of the relation between storage and retrieval is provided.

According to the structuralist view of the lexicon as a store of irregularities, storage is cheap and retrieval is expensive. This view conforms to the "lexicon as waste-basket" metaphor which denies many low-level, not fully productive structures. Langacker refers to this model as the rule-list fallacy, the exclusion of the paradigmatic from the syntagmatic dimension of language (Langacker, 1987, 42). Only fully productive lexical relationships were originally accounted for by lexical redundancy rules (Chomsky, 1965, 168), partially productive patterns were listed. This dichotomy is still reflected in more recent generative models of the mental lexicon. Rule-based approaches generate all and only fully productive word formations, thereby not distinguishing between full and partial compositionality (Halle and Mohanan, 1985; Yang, 2000). Complex units which are not fully productive are taken to be memorized as unanalyzed wholes. Clearly, this approach does not account for how speakers acquire, store and retrieve the conjugation patterns of verbs in inflecting languages. These verb classes have to be learned paradigmatically while they are applied syntagmatically on different levels of schematicity.

Within the generative morphological tradition, dual systems distinguish a rule-based syntagmatic system which operates fully productively from an associative paradigmatic system which as a result of frequency and similarity produces semi-regular distributions of paradigmatic clusters (Chialant and Caramazza, 1995; Clahsen, 1999; Pinker, 1999; Alegre and Gordon, 1999). While full productivity remains an ideal, the relation between paradigmatic and syntagmatic processes is not accounted for by this approach. Yet, generative grammar books generally abound with exceptions to the rule.

By abandoning the container metaphor, cognitive linguistics rejects the distinction between rule-based syntagmatic structures as part of the linguistic system and paradigmatically organized facts as part of world knowledge in favour of associative networks achieving a compromise between storage and retrieval due to frequency of activation. Associative networks represent and process fully and partially productive relationships in a single system (Bybee, 1995; Bybee and Scheibman, 1999; Sereno and Jongman, 1997; Hare et al., 1995; Schreuder and Baayen, 1995). Syntagmatically complex units are integrated into paradigms to different degrees, due to similarity between substructures and frequency of activation. The more substructures become integrated into a paradigm, the more tightly their constituents become associated with the common schema of the paradigm, and the more liable speakers are to memorize the complex unit as an instance of this regular association pattern. By contrast, the less interconnected a syntagmatically complex complex unit is, the more liable speakers are to memorize the complex pattern in terms of an unanalyzed idiosyncratic whole.

In this probabilistic network model the syntagmatic structure of an instance is represented as a function of its degree of integration into different paradigms of association schemas. Efficiency is not enabled by economy of storage. Instead redundancy of storage becomes the key to how language is processed (cf. Zeschel and Deppert, Zelinsky-Wibbelt, this volume). The grammar of a language is organized at different levels of schematicity, ranging from full specifications of lexical units, over low-level, semi-regular schemas, to high-level fully regular abstract schemas (cf. ibd. and Fortescue, this volume), where the trade-off between storage and computation becomes represented as a result of activation frequency. Fully specified lexical networks (Quillian, 1968; Collins and Loftus, 1975) grow through the speakers' ability to categorize lexical meanings in terms of abstract schemas, their specialization by instantiation and the extension thereof to contiguous and analogous concepts (Langacker 1987; Zeschel and Deppert, this volume). Grammatical networks result from the speakers' integration of lower-level into higher-level constructions (cf. Goldberg 1995; Croft 2001; cf. this volume Zeschel and Deppert).

From the cognitive grammar perspective taken by Tuggy (this volume) the traditional dichotomy between static storage and dynamic retrieval evaporates in favour of the activation of computational pathways between the original and the to-be-conventionalized linguistic unit. While the activation of these pathways is initially highly salient, it decreases with frequent computation when retrieval becomes more automatic and hence less dependent on the pathway, and may possibly fade with the full conventionalization of a linguistic unit.

As the result of a quantitative corpus-linguistic experiment, the traditional trade-off between storage and computation is abandoned by Zelinsky-Wibbelt (this volume). At the lexicon-syntax interface, the hybrid role of compounds represents the continuum of compositionality both by the asymmetry between autonomous and dependent predications along the syntagmatic dimension and the asymmetry between high-level and low-level schemas along the paradigmatic dimension. Along the paradigmatic dimension, the productivity values verify a competition among construction schemas. Along the syntagmatic dimension, this competition turns out to be a symbolically unified process (Langacker, 1991, 532), in that the derivation pattern of the ground is diagnostic of the compound meaning. The productivity of the PURPOSIVE relation of the $V - ing_N N$ construction provides evidence of a high activation level leaving strong memory traces, thereby facilitating retrieval in terms of a routinized and semantically transparent word formation process.

2.3 Episodic vs. semantic memory

By turning against the partitioning of different linguistic subsystems, cognitive linguistics claims a single hierarchically organized knowledge base as being encyclopedic in nature (Miller and Johnson-Laird, 1976; Langacker, 1987; Lakoff, 1987; Beaugrande, 1980). Cognitive linguistics is thus consonant with the psychological relaxation of the corresponding storage capacity distinctions. The distinction between episodic and semantic memory calls for a theoretical and empirical account of how categorization induces the latter from the former, since the archetypical form of human knowledge acquisition obviously starts from episodes (Beaugrande, 1980, 72). The problems with which this distinction is fraught, become obvious in the contribution of Marian and Kaushanskaya (this volume). They work within the paradigm of context-dependent memory. Proceeding from the weak version of the Sapir-Whorf hypothesis, they extend Tulving's (1979) encoding specificity principle[1] to the language-dependent memory hypothesis (Marian and Neisser, 2000). This hypothesis implies that the language of encoding influences how speakers are capable of retrieving the respective experiences. In an investigation with bilingual speakers the authors point out that retrieval in both episodic and semantic memory is not only a function of the context of encoding but also a function of the particular linguistic disposition at encoding and retrieval. The authors mention the same phenomenon to arise in a monolingual environment. This context-dependence of both episodic and semantic memory is clear evidence of the continuous development of semantic from episodic memory in the process of categorization (Anderson and Conway 1997, 240; Posner and Keele 1968; Dagenbach et al. 1990; Hintzman 1986).

3 Conceptual representations in semantic memory

3.1 The experiential basis of categorization

The process of categorization, that is the origin of lexical concepts, their representation in memory and their use in the speakers' categorization of novel concepts (Hampton, 1997) is investigated as the mental lexicon (Glenberg, 1997).

The role of lexical meanings in the speakers' knowledge representation is a matter of theoretical controversy. If meanings correspond to mental representations, do word meanings correspond to concepts or are they comprised by concepts? Or else, are word meanings related to, but distinct from concepts? The first option is counterargued by the claim that humans may engender concepts which lack a corresponding encoding in some languages (Murphy, 1991). Yet, although there may be lexical gaps in a language, in principle, every language is disposed of the expressive power to encode any thought whatsoever. At least this would follow from the weak version of the linguistic rela-

[1] With this principle, Tulving demonstrated the principled context-dependence of episodic memory. Semantic associates presented to the learner with to-be-remembered words improved their performance if they were also presented during recall.

tivity hypothesis. While the strong version posits cognitive processing to be dependent on the abstract language-specific system, the weak version postulates this dependence on the behavioural level, in that cognitive processing is influenced by linguistic performance (Billman and Krych 1998; Slobin 1996; Gentner and Loewenstein 2002). This is the thinking-for-speaking hypothesis, according to which the speakers' language-specific encoding of their experiences influences their memory (Slobin, 2003, 159), as evidenced by Marian and Kaushanskaya (this volume).

The assumption of linguistic relativity occurring on the behavioural level is corroborated by a long history of ultimately successful translations between typologically different languages. These language-specific forms could not be related if, in the spirit of generative linguistics, semantic representations were distinct from conceptual representations, if they were subjective and thus immune to intersubjective communication, as propagated by the strong version of linguistic relativity.

If we consider categorization as being theoretically and empirically constrained, both by the ontology of reality and by the conventional behaviour of the speech community, then meanings establish the interface between what Fodor has defined as "narrow" and "broad content" of mental representations (1987, 51). The ontological qualia of Fodor's broad content will remain inscrutable to the language user (Quine, 1960, 206) and are excluded from mental representations by Putnam (1988, 124).

Yet, through our theories our concepts are made coherent both across different speech situations and across different members of the speech community. Most importantly, through language the concepts of Fodor's narrow content are evaluated to meet the similarity standards across situations and speakers, as well as against the ontological constraints imposed by reality. By communicating our theories linguistically, this narrow content of concepts does no longer remain inscrutable to the language user. Meaning thus conceived corresponds to the communication of concepts in accordance with the experiential and epistemic constraints on the one hand and with the speakers' intentions on the other. This excludes the objectivity of conceptual representations with a strict type-token inheritance.[2]

The classical theory, which had reduced human memory to the skeletal representation of homogeneous categories, has turned out to be descriptively inadequate because it is incommensurable with the speakers' flexible negotiation between form and meaning which exceeds a definition for category membership. The experientially based communication of concepts clearly cannot cope with a priori ontological qualia.

3.2 The categorization of prototypes

By overcoming the descriptive rigidity of the Aristotelean model of categorization, prototype semantics accounts for the multitude of experiences as resulting in the graded structure of categories (Rosch and Lloyd, 1978). Within this model, categories are not defined in terms of necessary and sufficient attributes. Instead, different instances of a category are organized in terms of their typicality, depending on how many attributes are shared with the typical instance representing the centre of the category. "Good" members of a category share many attributes with the prototype. By contrast, towards the periphery of a category, members will share less attributes with the prototype and possibly attributes with neighbouring categories. Categorization thus occurs by comparing a stimulus with the prototype of the category via the number, the salience, and the interconnectedness of attributes (Langacker, 1987, 369ff).

Furthermore, the salience of attributes determines the typicality of instances and the stability of concepts. For one thing, this salience of attributes is experientially grounded, in that more frequently occurring attributes become more characteristic or typical in the representation of a category. For another thing, salience is epistemically

[2] Truthconditionally, speakers are assumed to represent meanings intensionally by conjunctions of necessary and sufficient conditions which should then unambiguously define the extension as the set of members falling under the respective intension (Frege, 1975).

defined, in that for instance the attribute CAN-FLY causally depends on birds which HAVE-WINGS (Hampton 1997, 101; Rogers and McClelland 2004, 232ff).

Focussing on the cognitive and social framing of human memory (this volume), Tuggy takes speakers to communicate their conceptual representations along a multitude of dimensions which clearly surmount the constraints of a reality-bound ontology. Dependent on the speakers' social status, the CONSUMER sense of the noun *ham sandwich* and the CREATOR sense of the proper noun LAKOFF may be either stored and retrieved en bloc or generated compositionally, bottom-up from conventionalized usage patterns, or else inferred top-down (cf. Tuggy, this volume), by integrating the conceptual components into frames or mental models through which speakers categorize their experiences in terms of analogous representations of the perceived situation (Garnham, this volume).

3.3 Exemplar-based categorization

Exemplar models do not abstract categories but instead assume similar exemplars to converge into clusters which are stored in memory. An implicit organization between exemplars of a cluster comes in through similarity. In the same way as in prototype models, similarity is measured via the sharing of attributes. A stimulus would be evaluated as an instance of a cluster if its overall similarity to all stored exemplars exceeds the overall similarity to the stored exemplars of contrast clusters. This similarity metric could equally well explain the observed prototype effects. The instance which has the highest overall similarity to the within-category exemplars is logically equivalent to the prototype while instances with an equal similarity to members of contrast clusters are logically equivalent to peripheral members of prototype models (Medin and Schaffer, 1978; Nosofsky, 1986).

By following the empiricist philosophical tradition (cf. Wittgenstein, 1977; Quine, 1960), Bartsch (this volume) proceeds from the ability of concept formation on the experiential level, thereby denying the notion of a concept as a mental representation altogether. Experientially, concepts are constructed exemplar-based, in that exemplars are organized in equivalent classes through similarities and contrasts. When series of exemplars preserve their internal similarity, this results in the stabilization of quasi-concepts. A quasi-concept thus conforms to a theoretical construct which through spatial, temporal, causal and other contiguity relations becomes organized in semantic networks. Linguistically, this semantic organization of theoretical concepts is supported by characteristic usage patterns represented in terms of syntactico-semantic frames. Thus concept formation becomes intersubjective through the norms of language which enable speakers to share their conceptualizations, that is to understand situations in the same way. From the nominalist view Bartsch pursues, to understand something in the same way means that the experienced situation is integrated into the same similarity set of previous experiences. Intersubjectivity is reflected in the degree to which the experienced and the to-be-remembered situation(s) form sufficiently similar sets across different speakers. If an experienced situation is not sufficiently similar to a remembered situation, this results in understanding by similarity under a new perspective which leads to the creation of a new metaphorical concept.

3.4 The neural basis of concepts

Connectionist networks implement the categorization processes of exemplar models physically, through training the connections between nodes conceived as behaviourally equivalent to neurons and neural patterns in the brain. These neural networks equally develop an implicit organization in terms of clusters around attractors which through a high activation-level due to a large number of connections represent a category implicitly and thereby simulate an abstract prototype (Shanks 1997, 130f; McClelland and Rumelhart 1985).

Connectionist models of memory are well compatible with prototype models of categorization as emerging from frequent usage events (cf. above, p. 4) and conforming to the similarity metric of exemplar models. Through their dense interconnections between neurons simulating clusters of similar exemplars, connectionist networks enable the representation of every degree of regularity and thus impose structure on only partially productive patterns which are listed in the traditional account. By the same token, through its parallel processing of information, a neural network may perfectly cope with incomplete or even inappropriate input, thus perfectly complementing and adjusting defective activation patterns. While one concept emerges from an activation pattern distributed over a large number of nodes, the same nodes may participate in many different activation patterns and thereby may give rise to the emergence of many different concepts. Due to the massively parallel processing of connectionist networks, they exhibit retrieval parsimony in spite of their exhaustiveness. Retrieval parsimony resides in the fact that the learning algorithm consists solely in excitatory and inhibitory transmissions of information between nodes. Firstly, there is no principled distinction between representation and computation in that a representation is implicit in similar responses to similar inputs. Secondly, as a connectionist system, human memory is capable of transcending the representation of perceived similarities between training exemplars, in that it is from individual, interconnected neurons in lower-level subconceptual networks in the brain, that higher-level, conceptual networks emerge at the level of the mind by being made meaningful through the whole pattern of interconnected neurons (cf. McClelland 1986, cf. Bartsch, this volume).

Bartsch's experientially based model of concept formation proceeds from a connectionist neural basis in which recursive activation circuits result in the strengthening of connections between nodes. This unconscious strengthening ultimately results in the conscious reconstruction of quasi-concepts. Semantic memory thus conceived develops as a stabilized system of conceptual indicators, which, due to its physical basis, is the unconscious disposition to consciously reconstruct remembrances through the formation of concepts. In order to prevent an infinite regress of recursive activation circuits, Bartsch views these circuits as interacting with primary, e.g. sensorial and motor fields. These primary fields of the mind, such as perception, concept formation, emotion, motor activities, proprioception, and linguistic representations are localized in specialized brain areas.

Fortescue follows the same path by assuming universal form-meaning correlations to be constrained through inherent sensory and sensorimotor schemas embodied in specific brain regions. Bartsch's and Fortescue's rescue in subsymbolic and pre-linguistic representations circumvents the circularity involved in defining the meta-language in terms of the object language. On the other hand, the recursive nature of representations as conceived by Bartsch and the mutual overlap between object- and meta-language as assumed by Fortescue imply a holistic view of the cognitive system in which linguistic meaning is inextricably integrated. Thus memory of language is memory. In Fortescue's metasemiological methodology clusters of form-meaning relations in the memory of the individual speaker approximate semi-universal relations represented at the community level which surface in diachronic change.

By implicitly representing similarities between training exemplars and stimuli, parallel processing systems are capable to learn (cf. Hofstadter, 1996, 205), i.e. to entrench their knowledge incrementally whenever the processed information is sufficiently compatible with the knowledge of the system (cf. Morales and Taylor, this volume).

Morales and Taylor verify experimentally that categories represented at different hierarchical levels are not experienced with equal frequency. By training artificial neural networks with data from MacWhinney's (2000) CHILDES database[3], they point out that unequal type-token ratios enhance the memorizability of the respective categories and hence their learnability. The more variable, yet cheaper type-token ratios, i.e. types with a lower number of tokens, obviously achieve better encoding and consequently retrieval results than the more uniform, yet more expensive distributions of type-token ratios (cf. also Zelinsky-Wibbelt, this volume), this improving learning and language acquisition in particular. The authors conclude that such frequency effects provide evidence about the entrenchment of linguistic association patterns originating in the connectionist architecture of the human brain.

---

[3] This database includes the thirty most frequent content words which caretakers have directed at the infants under three years of age.

3.5 Modality-specific and localized categorization

Within the neural basis of the human brain, linguistic categories are assumed to be localized and processed in modality-specific regions. According to Simmons and Barsalou (2003), the assumption that particular sensorimotor areas of the brain become active in the processing of particular categories is well reconcilable with a distributed neural basis of the brain, represented in terms of converging clusters of association patterns in a connectionist network (Damasio, 1989). Lamb's (1999) relational network model provides an account of how the processing of grammatical information is specialized in different areas of the human brain. Novak and Lamb (this volume) corroborate this model experimentally with aphasic patients. The results consistently evidence the syntactic, morphological, phonological and semantic-conceptual representations of verbs and nouns to be widely distributed over specialized regions of the brain. By contrast, the lemma is the central access node located in the posterior regions of the left hemisphere with nouns, whereas the access nodes of verbs are located in the anterior regions of the left hemisphere. Another result consistent with the model is the modality-specific functioning of the grammatical categories of verbs and nouns.

4 Language comprehension in working memory

Language comprehension is information retrieval which goes beyond the matching of signs with stored information. The bulk of comprehension consists in making signs meaningful through inferring implicit information not explicitly conveyed. These inferences arise from the connections which speakers can draw between explicit signs on the basis of their stored knowledge in long-term memory. Kintsch's construction-integration model simulates spreading activation processes in huge associative networks which are ultimately assumed to evolve into the speakers' combination of lexical concepts into meaningful texts (Kintsch 1998; Zeschel and Deppert, this volume). Johnson-Laird's (1983) theory of mental models explains how speakers may access implicit information by a combined linguistic-propositional and analogous representation of the situation presented in the text (cf. Garnham and Cowles, Schwarz-Friesel). In particular, the construction of mental models enables speakers to render an underspecified text coherent, whereby they may resolve anaphoric and implicit referents.

Relevance theory accounts for how speakers communicate linguistic information (Sperber and Wilson 1995; Zeschel and Deppert, this volume) on the background of different knowledge stores. Thereby superficially analogous sentences may give rise to different inferences and hence may receive drastically different interpretations.

4.1 Sentence comprehension

Rummer and Engelkamp provide a model of verbal working memory by investigating how short-term sentence recall is enabled through the generation of conceptual information. In their view, working memory does not correspond to a separate cognitive system, but to the currently activated linguistic information, while acoustic-sensory, phonological, morpho-syntactic, syntactic, and lexico-semantic representations become activated in modality-specific cognitive processes. By assuming a multimodal model of verbal short-term memory, short-term sentence recall is assumed to take place in a conceptual regeneration process (Potter and Lombardi, 1990). In this process a conceptual-propositional representation of the sentence is generated in accordance with Friederici's serial approach to sentence comprehension (2002), activating the same types of information but taking place in the reverse order (Levelt 1989, 1999).

4.2 Text comprehension

The failure of mentalist approaches to make the relation between language and memory explicit is most conclusively overcome by explaining mind-internal processes in terms of external behaviour through the speakers' interaction with the environment. These interactions become necessary, because the propositional information explicitly given in the text is insufficient for its coherent interpretation. In addition, readers seek to elaborate the explicitly conveyed information in order to make the referentially underspecified text coherent. By activating semantically related information from long-term memory readers select the implicit referents to be inserted into the mental model of the text.

Garnham and Cowles provide psycholinguistic evidence of the speakers' resolution of indirect anaphoric referents through the representation of mental models (Johnson-Laird, 1983; Garnham, 1981, 1987). The constraints which working memory imposes on the form of anaphoric expressions are investigated with the discourse function of focussing. By focussing on the semantic characteristics of the intended referents, speakers keep these in the centre of attention in working memory (Sidner, 1983; Grosz and Sidner, 1986). The authors thereby set themselves off from purely referential accounts of anaphoric resolution, in particular Almor's Informational Load Hypothesis (1999) according to which the form of an anaphoric expression is constrained by an interference effect in working memory, due to a semantic overlap between the anaphor and its antecedent. By complementing Almor's inverse typicality effect by an inverse semantic distance effect for focussed antecedents, Garnham and Cowles extend Almor's purely referential account of local focus by a more global conception capable of explaining the speakers' partitioning of mental models, as for instance achieved by the signalling of a thematic shift or a perspective change (Grosz and Sidner, 1986).

By analyzing three indirect anaphoric reference types, Schwarz-Friesel equally sets herself off from purely referential accounts of anaphoric reference. In particular, she provides an alternative to the commonly accepted distinction between bottom-up oriented, data-driven and top-down oriented, knowledge-based text comprehension. In this alternative, the strict distinction between linguistic storage and computation is overcome in favour of activation strength fostering inferential processing. On a par with this, she analyses indirect anaphora both as grammatical means providing processing instructions, in that their definiteness signals the accessibility of the implied referent in the text, and as inferential problem-solving devices providing access to new referents in the text-world model. She concludes that implicitly coherent texts are processed with the same ease as explicitly coherent texts.

Investigating the interpretation of poems experimentally, Zeschel and Deppert rely on Kintsch's construction-integration (C-I) model in order to explain their observations of the retrieval of idioms both as wholes and by way of their decomposed constituents. In line with this model, the authors proceed from an associative organization of the mental lexicon according to which the most frequently co-activated and thus most deeply entrenched lexical units turn out to be primed first in the construction phase which basically works in a bottom-up fashion. By contrast, during the contextually, i.e. top-down determined integration phase only the most strongly interconnected units are correctly explained to survive. Yet, the CI-model may not explain the observed poetic effect of the rhyme word, which the poet has deliberately avoided. The authors succeed in explaining the inferential processes involved in reconstructing the pun by Sperber and Wilson's Relevance Theory (1995). Still their modular account, which predicts the activation though not the phonological decoding of the rhyme word, is inadequate for explaining its comprehension. Allport's theory of "distributed memory" (Allport, 1985) is consistent with the authors' original hypothesis of the mental lexicon as a huge and massively redundant associative network of overlapping usage patterns. The converging retrieval cues of the rhyme word may be explained in terms of global coherence through top-down inheritance. The compositional path of the multi-word unit, by contrast, is explained as being inherited locally, through integrating its substructures into potentially multiple grammatical construction schemas, represented at different levels of the hierarchically organized network.

5 Conclusion

It is the particular intention of the editor to point out that an explanatory account of language is intrinsically related to psychological models of the human mind. In this volume different models of human memory are shown to be isomorphic with certain theoretical assumptions about language as a cognitive system. Many linguistic phenomena may thus be explained as a memory effect. The authors pursue this explanation by investigating the architecture of language and memory, the representation of concepts and their linguistic structures in the mental lexicon as well as their neural basis, and, finally, the role of memory in language comprehension.

References

Alegre, Maria and Peter Gordon. 1999. Rule-based versus associative processes in derivational morphology. *Brain and Language* 68(347–357).

Allport, D. A. 1985. Distributed memory, modular subsystems and dysphasia. In: S. Newman and R. Epstein (eds.), *Current Perspectives in Dysphasia*. Edinburgh: Churchill Livingstone, 207–244.

Almor, Amit. 1999. Noun-phrase anaphora and focus: The informational load hypothesis. *Psychological Review* 106: 748–765.

Anderson, John R. 1995. *Learning and Memory*. New York: Wiley.

Anderson, Stephen J. and Martin A. Conway. 1997. Representations of autobiographical memories. In: Martin A. Conway (ed.), *Cognitive Models of Memory*. Hove East Sussex: Psycology Press, 217–246.

Assink, Egbert M. H. and Dominiek Sandra. 2003. *Reading Complex Words*. Dordrecht: Kluwer.

Atkinson, R.C. and R.M. Shiffrin. 1968. Human memory: A proposed system and its control processes. In: K.W. Spence and J.T Spence (eds.), *The Psychology of Learning and Motivation*. New York: Academic Press, 89–195.

Baddeley, Alan D. 1986. *Working Memory*. Oxford: University Press.

Barsalou, Lawrence. 2005. Situated conceptualization. In: *Handbook of Categorization in Cognitive Science*, chapter 28. Oxford: Elsevier, 619–649.

Beaugrande, Robert de. 1980. *Text, Discourse, and Process*. London: Longman.

Billman, Dorrit and Meredyth Krych. 1998. Path and Manner verbs in action: Effects of "skipping" and "exciting" on event memory. In: *Proceedings of the 10th Annual Conference of the Cognitive Science Society*. Hillsdale, NJ: Lawrence Erlbaum, 156–161.

Bransford, J. D., J. R. Barceley and J. Franks. 1972. Sentence memory: A constructive versus interpretive approach. *Cognitive Psychology* 3: 193–209.

Broadbent, D. E. 1971. *Decision and Stress*. London: Academic Press.

Bybee, Joan. 1995. Regular morphology and the lexicon. *Language and Cognitive Processes* 10: 425–455.

Bybee, Joan and Paul Hopper (eds.). 2001. *Frequency and the Emergence of Linguistic Structure*. Amsterdam: John Benjamins.

Bybee, Joan and Joanne Scheibman. 1999. The effect of usage on degrees of constituency: The reduction of *don't* in English. *Linguistics* 37: 575–596.

Chialant, Doriana and Alfonso Caramazza. 1995. Where is morphology and how is it processed? The case of written word recognition. In: Laurie Beth Feldman (ed.), *Morphological Aspects of Language Processing*. Hillsdale: Lawrence Erlbaum, 55–76.

Chomsky, Noam Avram. 1965. *Aspects of the Theory of Syntax*. Cambridge, Mass.: MIT Press.

Chomsky, Noam Avram. 1986. *Knowledge of Language*. New York: Praeger.

Clahsen, Harald. 1999. Lexical entries and rules of language: A multi-disciplinary study of German inflection. *Behavioral and Brain Sciences* 22: 991–1060.

Clark, Herbert H. and Eve V. Clark. 1968. Semantic distinctions and memory for complex sentences. *Quarterly Journal of Experimental Psychology* 20: 129–138.

Collins, A. M. and E. F. Loftus. 1975. A spreading-activation theory of semantic processing. *Psychological Review* 82: 407–428.

Croft, William. 2001. *Radical Construction Grammar*. Oxford: Oxford University Press.

Dagenbach, D., S. Horst and T. H. Carr. 1990. Adding new information to semantic memory: How much learning is enough to produce automatic priming? *Journal of Experimental Psychology: Leraning, Memory and Cognition* 16: 581–591.

Damasio, Antonio R. 1989. Concepts in the brain. *Mind and Language: Forum, What is a Concept* 4(1/2): 25–27.

Fodor, Jerry. 1987. *Psychosemantics: The Problem of Meaning in the Philosophy of Mind*. Cambridge, MA.: MIT Press.

Frege, Gottlob. 1975. Über Begriff und Gegenstand. In: Gottlob Frege (ed.), *Funktion, Begriff, Bedeutung*. Göttingen: Vandenhoek and Ruprecht, 66–80. (Original: *Vierteljahresschrift für wissenschaftl. Philosophie*, 1892, NF, pp. 192–205).

Friederici, A. D. 2002. Towards a neural basis of auditory sentence processing. *Trends in Cognitive Sciences* 6: 78–84.

Garnham, Alan. 1981. Mental models as representations of texts. *Memory & Cognition* 9: 560–565.

Garnham, Alan. 1987. *Mental Models as Representations of Discourse and Text*. Chichester: Ellis Horwood.

Gentner, Dedre and Susan Goldin-Meadow. 2003. *Language in Mind. Advances in the Study of Language and Thought*. Cambridge, Mass.: MIT Press.

Gentner, Dedre and J. Loewenstein. 2002. Relational language and relational thought. In: J. Byrnes and E. Amsel (eds.), *Language, Literacy, and Cognitive Development*. Mahwah: Lawrence Erlbaum, 87–120.

Glenberg, Arthur M. 1997. Mental models, space, and embodied cognition. In: Thomas B. Ward, Steven M. Smith and Jyotsna Vaid (eds.), *Creative Thought: An Investigation of Conceptual Structures and Processes*. Washington, D.C.: American Psychological Association, 495–522.

Goldberg, Adele. 1995. *Constructions. A Construction Grammar Approach to Argument Structure*. Chicago: University of Chicago Press.

Grosz, Barbara J. and Candace L. Sidner. 1986. Attention, intentions and the structure of discourse. *Computational Linguistics* 12: 175–204.

Halle, Morris and K. Mohanan. 1985. Segmental phonology of Modern English. *Linguistic Inquiry* 16: 57–116.

Hampton, James E. 1997. Emergent attributes in combined concepts. In: Thomas B. Ward (ed.), *Creative Thought: An Investigation of Conceptual Structures and Processes*. Washington, D.C.: American Psychological Association, 83–110.

Hare, Mary, Jeffrey L. Elman and Kim G. Daugherty. 1995. Default generalization in connectionist networks. *Language and Cognitive Processes* 10(6): 601–630.

Hintzman, D. L. 1986. 'Schema abstraction' in a multiple-trace memory model. *Psychological Review* 93: 411–428.

Hofstadter, Douglas R. 1996. Analogy-making, fluid concepts, and brain mechanisms. In: A. Clark and P. J. R. Millican (eds.), *Connectionism, Concepts, and Folk Psychology. The Legacy of Alan Turing. Volume 2*, chapter 11. Oxford: Clarendon Press, 195–248.

Johnson-Laird, Philip N. 1983. *Mental Models. Towards a Cognitive Science of Language, Inference, and Consciousness*. Cambridge, Mass.: Cambridge University Press.

Kintsch, Walter. 1998. *Comprehension: A Paradigm for Cognition*. Cambridge: Cambridge University Press.

Lakoff, George. 1987. *Women, Fire and Dangerous Things: What Categories Reveal about the Mind*. Chicago: University of Chicago Press.

Lamb, Sydney. 1999. *Pathways of the Brain: The Neurocognitive Basis of Language*. Amsterdam: John Benjamins.

Langacker, Ronald. 1987. *Foundations of Cognitive Grammar. Theoretical Prerequisites*, volume 1. Stanford: Stanford University Press.

Langacker, Ronald. 1991. *Foundations of Cognitive Grammar. Practical Applications*, volume 2. Stanford: Stanford University Press.

Levelt, Willem J. M. 1989. *Speaking: From Intention to Articulation*. Cambridge, MA: MIT Press.

Levelt, Willem J. M. 1999. Models of word production. *Trends in Cognitive Sciences* 3: 223–232.

Levinson, S. C. 2003. Language and mind: Let's get the issues straight! In: D. Gentner and S. Goldin-Meadow (eds.), *Language in Mind. Advances in the Study of Language and Cognition*. Boston: MIT Press, 25–46.

MacWhinney, Brian. 2000. *The CHILDES Database: Tools for Analyzing Talk*, volume 2. 3rd edition. Mahwah, NJ: Lawrence Associates.

Marian, Viorica and Ulric Neisser. 2000. Language-dependent recall of autobiographical memories. *Journal of Experimental Psychology: General* 129: 361–368.

McClelland, James L. and David E. Rumelhart. 1985. Distributed memory and the representation of general and specific information. *Journal of Experimental Psychology* 114: 159–188.

McClelland, James L. and David E.. Rumelhart. 1986. *Parallel Distributed Processing. Explorations in the Microstructure of Cognition*, volume 2: Psychological and Biolgical Models. Cambridge, Mass.: MIT Press.

Medin, Douglas L. and Schaffer. 1978. Context theory of classification learning. *Psychological Review* 85(3): 207–238.

Miller, George A. and Philip N. Johnson-Laird. 1976. *Language and Perception.* Cambridge: Cambridge University Press.

Murphy, Gregory L. 1991. Meaning and concepts. In: Paula J. Schwanenflugel (ed.), *The Psychology of Word Meanings: A Publication of the Cognitive Studies Group and the Institute for Behavioral Research at the University of Georgia*. Hillsdale, N.J.: Erlbaum, 11–35. Psychology of Word Meaning Conference, University of Georgia.

Nosofsky, Robert M. 1986. Attention, similarity, and identification-categorization relationship. *Journal of Experimental Psychology* 115(1): 39–57.

Pinker, Steven. 1999. *Words and Rules*. New York: Basic Books.

Posner, M. I. and S. W. Keele. 1968. On the genesis of abstract ideas. *Journal of Experimental Psychology* 77: 353–363.

Potter, M. C. and L. Lombardi. 1990. Regeneration in the short-term recall of sentences. *Journal of Memory and Language* 29: 633–654.

Putnam, Hilary. 1988. *Representation and Reality*. Cambridge, Mass.: MIT Press.

Quillian, Ross M. 1968. Semantic memory. In: Marvin Minsky (ed.), *Semantic Information Processing*. Cambridge, Mass.: MIT Press, 227–270.

Quine, Willard van Orman. 1960. *Word and Object*. Cambridge: Cambridge University Press.

Reddy, Michael J. 1993. The conduit metaphor: A case of frame conflict in our language about language. In: Andrew Ortony (ed.), *Metaphor and Thought*. Cambridge: Cambidge University Press, 164–201.

Rogers, Timothy T. and James L. McClelland. 2004. *Semantic Cognition. A Parallel Distributed Processing Account*. Cambridge, Mass.: MIT Press.

Rosch, Eleanor and Barbara B. Lloyd. 1978. *Cognition and Categorization*. Hillsdale, N.J.: Erlbaum.

Schreuder, Robert and R. Harald Baayen. 1995. Modeling morphological processing. In: L. B. Feldman (ed.), *Morphological Aspects of Language Processing*. Hillsdale: Lawrence Erlbaum, 345–364.

Sereno, J. A. and A. Jongman. 1997. Processing of English inflectional morphology. *Memory and Cognition* 25: 425–437.

Shanks, David R. 1997. Representation of categories and concepts in memory. In: Martin A. Conway (ed.), *Cognitive Models of Memory*. Cambridge, Mass.: MIT Press, 111–146.

Sidner, Candace L. 1983. Focusing in comprehension of definite anaphora. In: M. Brady and R. C. Berwick (eds.), *Computational Models of Discourse*. Cambridge, MA: MIT Press, 267–330.

Simmons, K. and Lawrence W. Barsalou. 2003. The similarity-in-topography principle: Reconciling theories of conceptual deficits. *Cognitive Neuropsychology* 20: 451–486.

Slobin, Dan I. 1996. Two ways of travel: Verbs of motion in english and spanish. In: M. Shibatini and Sandra A. Thompson (eds.), *Grammatical Constructions: Their Form and Meaning*. Oxford: Oxford University Press, 195–217.

Slobin, Dan Isaac. 2003. Language and thought online: Cognitive consequences of linguistic relativity. In: D. Gentner and S. Goldin-Meadow (eds.), *Language in Mind: Advances in the Study of Language and Thought*. Cambridge, MA: MIT Press, 157–191.

Sperber, Dan and Deidre Wilson. 1995. *Relevance: Communication and Cognition*. Oxford: Blackwell.

Tulving, E. 1972. Episodic and semantic memory. In: E. Tulving and M. Roberts (eds.), *Organization of Memory*. New York: Academic Press, 381–403.

Tulving, Endel. 1979. Relation between encoding specificity and levels of processing. In: L.S. Cermack and F.I.M. Craik (eds.), *Levels of Processing in Human Memory*. Hillsdale, N.J.: Lawrence Erlbaum, 401–428.

Wittgenstein, Ludwig. 1977. *Philosophische Untersuchungen*. Frankfurt/Main: Suhrkamp.

Yang, C. D. 2000. Knowledge and learning in natural language. Unpublished doctoral dissertation, MIT, Cambridge, MA.

On the storage vs. computation of complex linguistic structures

David Tuggy

1 Introduction

It would be difficult to find a distinction more basic to the linguistic thought of the 20th century than the distinction between what is regular in language and what is irregular or arbitrary. Archetypically the irregular or arbitrary has been equated with the idiosyncratic and the regular with the predictable and with the systematic, and it is assumed that the systematic / predictable / regular aspects of language are to be accounted for by a system of general rules. It is further assumed that language speakers must learn separately or memorize what is idiosyncratic / arbitrary, while the systematic / predictable / regular aspects are not learned, but rather produced by the psycho-cognitive analogue of linguists' rules. It is often taken for granted that these two kinds of linguistic structures should be separated out from each other. Typically the idiosyncratic is localized to a lexical component or module, and what is rule-governed to a grammatical module or modules.[1,2] This traditional conception of

1 Thus the immensely influential Chomsky (1965, 87) states: "In general, all properties of a formative that are essentially idiosyncratic will be specified in the lexicon," and he notes that this is in accordance with the scarcely less influential Bloomfield's (1933, 274) characterization of the lexicon as "really an appendix of the grammar, a list of basic irregularities", and Sweet's (1913, 31) dictum that "grammar deals with the general facts of language, lexicology with the special facts."

2 The idiosyncratic/lexical was often considered basically uninteresting if it was not actually excluded from the natural subject-matter of linguistics. This was doubtless connected with the view that Science is only concerned with regular and predictable phenomena. For instance, Akmajian and Heny (1975, 1) say that "In general, the existence and meaning of individual words are somewhat isolated facts that have to be specially acquired, and it is not at all surprising that individual speakers have never learned many of them." This contrasts

the composite distinction we will call the *Predictability Distinction*, reflecting my feeling that many linguists have viewed predictability / arbitrariness as the central issue in the distinction. The Predictability Distinction is represented graphically in Figure 1: what is regular is equated with what is systematic, predictable, and produced by rule, and all such phenomena are included in the Grammar, which does not overlap at all with the Lexicon, wherein are included all phenomena which are irregular, arbitrary, and idiosyncratic, and must be learned.

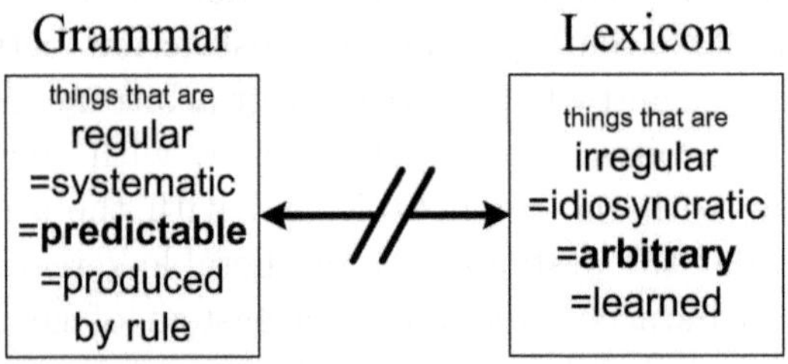

Figure 1. The Predictability Distinction

The absolute identification with each other of the sub-distinctions of the Predictability Distinction, and their modularization, are closely connected with a view of them as as binary, dichotomous, all-or-nothing distinctions. Much argumentation assumes the stance "Phenomenon X is not (i.e. not totally) arbitrary, therefore it is predictable"; other argumentation maintains that "Phenomenon X is not (i.e. not totally) predictable, therefore it is arbitrary." Ruhl (1989) is an extended example of the first type; Chomsky (1967/70) is an example of the second. Of course if this is a strict dichotomy, both modes of argumentation would be legitimate.

One of the distinctives of Cognitive Linguistics (Geeraerts and Cuyckens, 2007) has been its rejection of the dichotomous view of

with "...a systematic way of relating ...a precise rule..." (1975, 3). In the rest of the 400-odd pages of their book, they never again evince more than the slightest interest in the non-regular matters, beyond what is necessary to make the syntactic machinery run.

the predictability distinction. Rather than taking the totally arbitrary and the inevitable or fully predictable as strict alternatives; it views them as end-points of a continuum of reasonableness or motivatedness. Similarly regularity and systematicity are viewed as gradual or scalar rather than binary properties. Dichotomies can certainly obtain locally for particular phenomena, but they cannot be expected for every phenomenon. And when the data of linguistics are looked at in this light, it seems clear that much that was originally considered arbitrary is in fact motivated to some degree, and much that was considered rule-governed is in fact far from inevitable or fully predictable. Other linguistic frameworks seem to be moving in the same direction as well: the introduction in virtually every linguistic model of rules into the lexical component and the widespread recognition of exceptionality in syntactic phenomena are cases in point.

If we reject the dichotomous nature of the sub-distinctions it becomes difficult to maintain their absolute identification. It seems reasonable, for instance, that whatever is not predictable, yet is part of the language, must be learned by the speakers of the language. But it need not follow that whatever is motivated in some degree, even fully predictable, is therefore not learned but rather generated. Nor need it follow that all that is learned is non-systematic: in fact systematicity may be among the factors increasing the ease (and therefore the probability) of our learning a structure.

The sub-distinction between what is learned and what is productively formed is of especial interest in that it is a directly cognitive distinction (as e.g. the predictable/arbitrary cline may not be). I wish to discuss this distinction as viewed in Langacker's (1987; 1991; 2000; 2007), (Taylor, 2002), Cognitive Grammar model (CG). I will be especially interested to point out certain implications of that model which are not widely understood, sometimes even among those who are sympathetic with it.

2 Storage versus computation: the computer analogy

As befits its name, CG claims that language is a matter of cognition, and thus the cognitive phenomena involved in our traditional

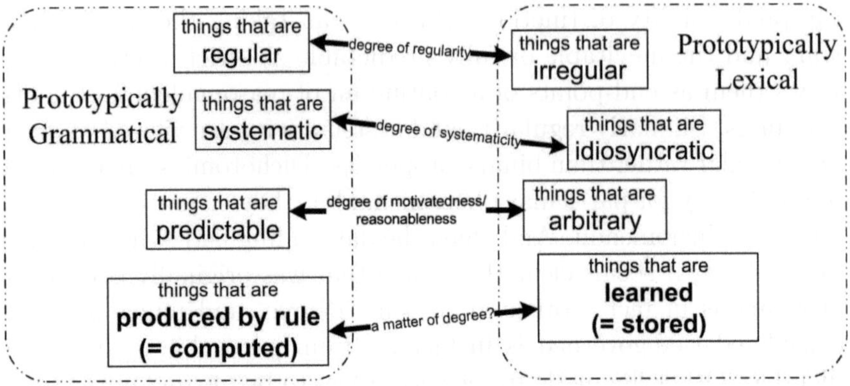

Figure 2. The same distinctions under Cognitive Grammar

distinction are basic. The cognitive distinction between learned and productively generated linguistic structures is a basic fact: correlations of that distinction, whether absolute or partial, with the arbitrary/predictable distinction, or the regular/irregular distinction, are quite interesting, but may well be less basic to what language is.

The cognitive distinction between what is learned and what is productively generated is also of interest in that it is less immediately or intuitively obvious, to my mind at least, that it is a gradual distinction. It looks, on the face of it, like it might really be a non-gradual difference in kind.

It seems indisputable that there are some things in language that are learned by all speakers and some that are not learned by any speakers but which might be produced by any speaker on particular occasions and will certainly be understood by hearers. I know no one who would argue, for instance, that *chalk* or *bask* means what it does as a result of general cognitive patterns of English coming together in people's minds as the word is used to make this happen. Those who speak the language had to learn the particular associations of a sound and its meaning. Similarly, no one would claim that any of the sentences in this paragraph is likely to be learned by any English speakers, much less by many or all of them: clearly there are multiple patterns of the language that enable us to produce and understand such sentences without ever learning them.

A standard, and in many ways a useful, way of conceptualizing this cognitive difference is on the analogy of a computer. The computer has long-term storage media such as a hard disk, and certain information patterns are stored on those media. It also has programs (also typically kept in long-term storage), and information patterns can be computed by executing those programs, generally using input from the stored information. So on a computer, and by analogy in the mind, we may speak of a difference between *stored* and *computed* information. Stored information is, by definition, learned information: computed information is accessed without having to be learned.

Construed in this way, is not this a difference in kind, a real plus-or-minus distinction? What gradation is there between information permanently residing on disk and information temporarily brought into existence by computation but not stored? Doesn't the distinction even correspond to real, physical, modules within the computer?

The computer analogy can take us several steps further than this, however. Besides the long-term *storage* the computer also has short-term, volatile *working memory* where information may exist briefly. (In the computer it will last there until it is replaced or until the computer is switched off. In the mind such information is even more volatile: it will degrade spontaneously if it is not periodically refreshed.) Working memory is where the information produced by computation shows up, but information may also be brought there directly from long-term storage. Thus a given information pattern in working memory may have come from storage or it may be the result of a programmed calculation. This is the distinction, whether on a computer or in the mind, which we will refer to as "storage" vs. "computation".

This begins to erode what perhaps seemed at first an absolute distinction between storage and computation. Yes, there is a physical, modular distinction between a pattern of bits in storage and a similar information pattern in working memory, just as there is a physical, modular, if you like, distinction between the word "the" written on one page, with one bit of ink, and the same word written on another, with other ink. But no one speaking of a linguistic form is referring to anything that concrete. Rather the pattern is the thing, no matter where it occurs, even if it occurs on a completely different computer, we still think of it as the same word, or morpheme, or phrasal construction, etc. And this is quite purely practical and right. Information, to be utilized, has to go into working memory. The information itself is of the same type no matter whether it comes from storage or is computed, and which way it got into working memory is, for most practical purposes, irrelevant from that point on.

What is more, such information can be, and constantly is, transferred between storage and working memory. There is nothing that prohibits the same information pattern from being in both places at once. In fact the original data, the program that massages it, and the resulting computed data can all exist together in long-term memory, or in working memory, or in both, at the same time. There is not going to be a clear, fixed, easy-to-determine boundary between *kinds* of information that are stored and kinds that are computed. Certainly it would be perverse to insist *a priori* that, because of the demands of theoretical simplicity, a particular piece of information must always be processed in one way and never in the other.[3]

This ties in reasonably with our own experience of non-linguistic cognition. What is 9 x 8? How do we know? We might figure, or remember, that 10 x 8 is 80 and subtract 8. We might remember that 9 x 10 is 90 and subtract 9 x 2 (=18). We might remember that 8 x 8 is 64 and add 8. Those are all different computational pathways. Or we might, having memorized it, just remember that 9 x 8 is 72. That would be retrieval from storage. Similarly, consider how we might bring to mind a particular date, say a birthdate of a family member. We might "just remember" it: i.e. it might be directly accessible from long-term storage. We might compute it in a number of different ways. E.g. my brother's birthday, which happens

---

[3] Computer gurus tell me that, despite the physical modularities, there are related fuzzinesses of the category borders between working memory and long-term storage, and between data and programs.

to be April 14th, could be remembered as generally near Eastertime (with various methods of zeroing in from there), or as two weeks after April Fools' Day, or as being the same day of the year that Abraham Lincoln was shot, as being two months after St. Valentine's day, as being the day before U.S. income taxes are due, etc. There is no one way that this information must be processed for it to appear usefully and accurately in our minds.

The human cognitive apparatus differs from the computer in a couple of well-established ways which further blur any category lines. (1) On a computer, data, whether in working memory or long-term storage, is either completely "there", or completely absent. In the mind there seem rather to be differences of the energy level or *salience* with which the information patterns occur. Information of low salience is not as clearly "there" as information of high salience. (2) When information is to go from a computer's working memory to its long-term storage, the information must be, and can be, explicitly transferred, and the effects are instantaneous and complete. In the mind, this kind of transfer happens automatically but is not so easy to make happen at will. Nor is it, typically, instantaneous. It seems rather to depend on the salience with which the pattern occurred in working memory, on how well it connects in to already existing patterns, and especially on how often (and how recently) it is repeated. Thus when we need to commit a pattern to long-term memory we cannot just choose to have it there: we must repeat it, try to link it with other patterns, and try to emphasize it to ourselves. In this way, as a pattern occurs repeatedly, energetically, and coheringly in working memory, it becomes more and more thoroughly *entrenched* in long-term memory (storage).

To return to the example of a birthdate, it could conceivably occur so energetically in its first occurrence that it is immediately stored long-term: otherwise it will usually take several short-term occurrences before a long-term version of it begins to be accessible. These short-term occurrences might be computed, repeatedly in the same way or in different ways; alternatively, once the information is ensconced even tentatively in long-term memory, it may be accessed directly from that storage. With repeated activation it becomes more and more thoroughly entrenched in long-term storage, thus easier to access and likely to occur more saliently when it is.

A further well known difference is that computers are better at computing, and humans are better at understanding and nuanced learning, and at recognition, which involves highly sophisticated retrieval from storage. "The human cognitive system capitalizes tremendously on complex storage."[4] Both computers and humans can both store and compute, but humans are able (and therefore apt) to store much more fully detailed and intricately interconnected information, and to activate that information when and where it is relevant.

Another fact that complicates matters is that language is a social phenomenon. To extend our analogy, we should think of many computers linked in a sort of inefficient network, one which lets them pass messages in a sort of awkward code, but does not allow direct replication of most kinds of information, much less provide direct access to the long-term storage or working memory of the other computers. Furthermore, there is no big server on the net, accessible to all the computers, on which Language resides. Rather, in each computer's storage, a complex model of the other computers' stored information is gradually built up, on the basis of the messages exchanged, including especially that information common to most if not all the other computers.

Sometimes whole individual messages are stored; more often, given the fact that storage requires repetition, recurrent bits and their patterns of combination are stored. These are reinforced and further

4 In particular, "the evidence overwhelmingly supports [models which suggest that] the human cognitive system is not very good at abstraction, so it opts for simple learning computations ... This further suggests that human storage and retrieval are powerful, ... the human cognitive system seems capable of storing much detailed information and retrieving it during categorization (as well as matching it to the item to be categorized)." (Larry Barsalou, email posted on the FunkNet list on 10/11/98). Barsalou links this to evidence from studies on problem-solving (e.g. Kolodner 1993), and theories of skill (e.g. Anderson's ACT* (1993), Logan's exemplar-based skill model (1985), Newell's SOAR (1990)), "each [of which] includes two ways of producing a behavior – computation vs. retrieval – and assumes that novices mostly compute but increasin[g]ly retrieve as they become expert.")

entrenched every time they are used in a message, which is of course far more often than any particular large-scale structures incorporating them are used.

Think again of my brother's birthdate. Another of my siblings and I might come up with such an exchange as "Fred's birthday is April 14th, isn't it?" "That's right." One of us might be retrieving the date from storage, another calculating it as two months after Valentine's, or both retrieving it or both computing it in different ways, without it affecting the messages. And the effect of those messages would be to confirm or entrench the information, regardless of how it was arrived at.

This, I think, fits the picture of how language works pretty well. It is at least pretty close to the picture CG assumes as true. And it has certain implications for the distinction between stored and computed information.

3 Maxims arising from the CG model

If CG is right, whether or not something is stored or computed is in the last resort an empirical issue. It may not be an easy one to determine, however.[5] I present below five Maxims which either are overt parts of the CG model or logically follow from what is stated. (A sixth Maxim is presented in section 5.) If they are true, every usage must (in principle) be investigated individually to get a truly definitive answer.

[5] A further issue is what can be admitted as empirical evidence in the matter. Reported intuitions or introspective conclusions (e.g. "I'd never heard that before", or "Of course I know that word", or "everybody says that"), especially as they are coincident across numerous speakers, should be given considerable weight. Statistical and distributional studies are important; psycholinguistic tests and experiments, where practicable, are also important. It is generally not possible, especially for field linguists, to arrive at unquestionable, rock-solid conclusions, but quite reliable probabilistic statements are feasible, as long as one is not hampered from the outset by question-begging theoretical presuppositions of the sort the Maxims address.

3.1 What happens to one form doesn't have to happen to all of them

Not infrequently a plausible case is made that a certain member of a category is computed (or equivalently, under the traditional archetype, predictable, or produced by rule)—perhaps it is unproblematically understood even though novel. Perhaps a few other examples in the category are shown to be similar It is then assumed (often, no doubt, on grounds of simplicity) that all other members of that category are also computed (predictable, generated by rule). It is clear that many noun phrases are computed. For instance, the eminently forgettable NP from the preceding paragraph, *five Maxims ... what is stated*, is unlikely ever to be stored as a whole in anyone's mind. So, it seems reasonable to assume that all NP's must be computed. In a parallel argument, a case may be made that certain forms are stored (arbitrary, idiosyncratic, lexical), and thus all members of their category must be treated in the same way. Thus Newmeyer (1980) summarizes one of Chomsky's (1967/70) arguments for the Lexicalist hypothesis, as that "a transformational rule should capture a regular productive relationship. But the relationship between D[erived] N[ominal]s and their corresponding verbs is highly IRREGULAR.[6] A lexical treatment of DN's is the natural way to capture this irregular behavior – the lexicon, after all, is the repository of what is idiosyncratic in language." Clearly a crucial assumption underlying this argument is that the category of DN's is homogenous in this regard: if some DN's are irregular and therefore lexical, then all DN's must be. Cognitive Grammar denies the underlying premise of such arguments. Rather:

> **Maxim #1:**
> Computation or storage of some members of a category does not guarantee computation or storage of all its members. Or,
> *What happens to one form doesn't have to happen to all of them.*

[6] particular examples follow

Langacker (1987,297–298, 2000,127–128) cites the example of nominalizations in *-er*. *Sidler* or *flinger* are presumably novel or near-novel formations: they did not show up in my computer's spell-checking dictionary, for instance. Probably most readers will have had to compute them upon encountering them just now. *Shouter* or *screamer* are quite possibly established forms (they are in the computer dictionary), but one might well compute them any time one uses or hears them. *Swimmer*, *runner* (in the sense "person who runs") and *diver* are certainly established for most English speakers, but they are easily computable if they should happen not to be stored. *Speaker*, *hearer*, and *reader* are quite certainly established for English speaking linguists and doubtless virtually all other English speakers as well.[7] *Computer*: well, if there are any contemporary English speakers in whose minds that form is not stored and well-entrenched, they are highly exceptional. In fact, we all have very definite specifications attached to it which go well beyond what mere computation would yield. Not everything that computes can easily be called a computer. *Propeller* and *rocker* are certainly established for most speakers, in fact many speakers are surprised to realize that they are *-er* nominalizations. Even more than with computers, not everything that propels or rocks can be called a propeller or a rocker. A *ruler* is more saliently for most English speakers a device for measuring rather than for ruling lines. *Drawer* or *prayer* are probably never computed except perhaps by a tiny minority of speakers. So: are *-er* nominalizations computed, or stored? The answer is, it depends. Some are computed, some are stored. You have to check each case: it is an empirical issue.

The standard argument against this sort of treatment has been that it violates simplicity. It permits massive redundancy. Why should we posit that people are learning things when there's a per-

---

7 They are also established in several less-than-fully-predictable versions: e.g. a *speaker* in many contexts is a machine that turns electric signals into sounds, and a *reader* one that senses electronic pulses on a storage medium, or (in other contexts) a Christian Science practitioner, or a book used by those learning to read. Similarly a *runner* can be a long piece of carpet or floor-protecting matting as well as a person who runs.

fectly good way to figure them? And the answer is, Yes, there is redundancy. This is good because it is true. To argue otherwise is like arguing that the computer cannot have any information in its long-term storage that a program could have produced from other stored information, because that would be redundant. Whether or not it would be redundant, it can and does happen.[8]

In sum: *It is ultimately an empirical issue whether a particular linguistic form is stored in language speakers' minds or whether it is computed from other information.*

The phrase "it is an empirical issue" does not mean that there is necessarily an easy empirical test that will let one find out. It does mean that in principle it could be either way, and to settle the issue definitively one must examine relevant data.

3.2 Your doing it doesn't mean everybody has to

The next three Maxims address issues that much linguistics never even allows you to raise. Traditional modern linguistics assumes that its object of study is an ideal grammar, a matter of competence not performance, a static system not affected by individual differences in how (be it well or poorly or just differently) users may handle their language from time to time. The assumptions stated by Chomsky in *Aspects* (1965, 3-4) were for many years almost universally and

8 It is also fair to point out that there is a trade-off of complexities. An economic metaphor (related to that underlying the word "trade-off") is sometimes used, according to which computation is said to economize on storage, but do so at the cost of expensive calculations every time a structure is used. Massive and redundant storage, though relatively expensive in its own right, and entailing expensive routines for accessing the stored data, economizes on computation at the time of usage (when time may be at a premium). It is not a priori clear which wins out in terms of cost vs. benefit. But the evidence indicates that the human cognitive system typically opts for maximizing the storage and economizing on the computation (Barsalou and Hale, 1993). Yet, of course, this does not mean humans cannot and do not compute. The main contention of this article is that, regardless of how the possibilities are weighted in different systems (human or electronic), there is nothing in principle that says it must only be done in one way. It thus is an empirical issue which way it is in fact done in a given case.

often unquestioningly adopted, and allowed to shape much linguistic thought:

> Linguistic theory is concerned primarily with an ideal speaker-listener, in a completely homogenous speech-community, who knows its language perfectly, and is unaffected by such grammatically irrelevant conditions as memory limitations, distractions, shifts of attention and interest, and errors (random or characteristic) in applying his knowledge of the language in actual performance.

"Primarily" tended to mean, in practice, "only", and the phrase "grammatically irrelevant" embodies a crucial assumption. Chomsky is no doubt correct in assessing this as "the position of the founders of modern general linguistics." The fact that these are explicitly admitted to be idealizations does not alter the fact that assuming them removes certain possibilities from consideration. Speech communities are not completely homogenous, however. And this fact is relevant to the storage/computation distinction.

> **Maxim #2:**
> Computation or storage of a form by some speakers does not guarantee its computation or storage by all speakers.
> Or,
> *Your doing it doesn't mean everybody has to.*

Recall the earlier discussion of how to "get" (compute or retrieve) 8 x 9. Different people prefer to do it in different ways, and that is not a problem. The same is true with calculating or remembering dates. And I think we all are aware of instances of language use where we know that the same thing is happening. I remember laughing in surprise when I first heard the phrase *That was all she wrote*, with the contextually clear meaning 'it was all over with.' I of course had had to compute the phrase and its metaphorical extension, and was very aware of the fact. But the one who said it was surprised at my surprise, and made it clear that for him it had been perfectly ordinary, a cliché pulled out of storage and thrown in to the discourse. This sort of thing is not a terribly unusual occurrence, and, of course, it is to be expected that in most cases the matter will not be explicitly discussed or otherwise clarified. The cases where we are highly aware of such mismatches are just the tip of the iceberg of their actual occurrence.

Relatedly, one type of computation by one speaker does not guarantee the same kind of computation by another. One speaker might build the word *unbelievably* out of *un* and *believably*, and *believably* out of *believe* and *-ably*, while another might build it out of (or analyze it into) *unbelievable* and *ly*, then *un-* and *believable*, then *believe* and *-able*, while another might pull the word off the shelf as a whole, *unbelievably* (but quite believably). The meanings and the phonological structures will add up to near enough the same thing in any case, so that the speakers can communicate perfectly well. What matters most is *how* the pieces are combined (or analyzed out) and *what is the result* of their combination, not *when* or *in what order* or even precisely *which pieces* get combined (or analyzed). Similarly, one person might think of a *hangman* as a *man who hangs* people (as a *cutworm* is a *worm that cuts* plants), while another thinks of him (or, as the case might be, her) as a person who *hangs a man* (as a *pickpocket* is a person who will *pick a pocket*). These differences are unlikely to cause any communication problem, and CG would have us expect to find such, or at least to be unsurprised if we do.

In sum: *It is ultimately an empirical issue whether a particular form is stored in a particular individual speaker's mind or whether he (or she) computes it in one way or another from other information.*

3.3 You can change the way you do it

Most if not all of us have had the clear experience of "tumbling to" an analysis of what had been previously monomorphemic to us. I grew up calling a papaya (in Spanish) a *lechosa* and butter *mantequilla.* It was not until I was in college that it dawned on me that *lechosa* was *lech-osa* (*milk-ous*, referring to the milky sap of the *lechosa* tree), and that *mantequilla* was the diminutive *-illa* on the stem *manteca* 'lard'. Similarly it was not until middle adulthood that it hit me that the verb *heft* was clearly derived from the same root as *heavy*, or that *ruth(less)* was related to *rue* much as *truth* is related to *true*. What I had, previously, simply retrieved from storage I began to compute.

Similarly as derivedness fades what was previously computed is simply retrieved from storage. In my youth I often computed the word *awesome*, and was very aware of its derivation from the noun *awe*. Now, under the influence of my children's generation's use of the word to describe virtually anything that excites their fancy, regardless of whether it instills anything even close to awe in the beholder, I am sure I often hear and even speak the word without particularly activating *awe* or *-some*. I simply retrieve it from storage.

> **Maxim #3:**
> A form which has been exclusively computed or accessed from storage may begin to be processed in the other way as well. Or,
> *You can change the way you do it*

In sum: *It is ultimately an empirical issue whether a form that has always been stored or computed in a given speaker's mind will be accessed exclusively in that same way in the future.*

3.4 You don't have to do the next time what you did this time

Having computed *heft* or *lechosa* today, I very likely won't run through the computation the next time I use it. But I might well the time after that.

> **Maxim #4:**
> Computation or access from storage of a form by a speaker on one occasion does not guarantee computation or access from storage of that form by the same speaker on another occasion. Or,
> *You don't have to do the next time what you did this time.*

In sum: *It is ultimately an empirical issue, for a particular form, whether a particular individual speaker accesses it from storage on a particular occasion or whether he (or she) computes it from other information on that occasion.*

3.5 You can do both at the same time

It is quite possible to bring a form up from memory, then check it by computation. Or to compute it, then think, in essence, "Yes, that's right, I remember that". The mind clearly has enough parallel processing capacity to do both simultaneously.

> **Maxim #5:**
> A single speaker can both compute a form and access it from storage, or compute it in more than one way, sequentially or perhaps even simultaneously, on the same occasion. Or,
> *You can do both at the same time.*

In sum: *It is ultimately an empirical issue, for a particular form on a particular occasion, whether a particular individual speaker accesses it exclusively from storage or whether he (or she) exclusively computes it in any one particular way from other information, or whether he (or she) accesses it in more than one way simultaneously or successively.*

4 The storage/computation distinction in perspective

If the CG perspective, including these Maxims, is accepted, the distinction between storage and computation of linguistic structures looks rather different from the traditional archetype's view. To begin with, it is not just an appendage or effect of the composite Predictability Distinction, it must be assayed separately from the arbitrary/predictable and idiosyncratic/systematic distinctions. And, while it may rest on two discrete modes of cognitive operation, it cannot be used to dichotomously categorize linguistic structures as they are normally conceived.

Some linguistic structures are always accessed from storage, never computed, and others, equally clearly, are always computed and are never stored. But you cannot tell in principle which these will be, and there are many structures whose status with respect to the distinction cannot be described so simply. A structure may be almost always computed, or computed by almost all speakers, or always computed but stored as well; in any case it cannot be unequivocally considered to be computed. Or a structure may be almost always retrieved from storage, or retrieved from storage by almost all speakers, or always retrieved from storage but occasionally computed as well, without being unequivocally considered to be stored. And there can be all degrees in between. Besides this is the matter of salience, which implies degrees of "being there" in storage or not.

From this perspective it is clearly wrong to think of computation vs. storage as a dichotomy dividing linguistic structures into separate categories. It makes a lot more sense to talk about these as two modes by which the same structures can be accessed. They form a two-dimensioned gradation with respect to which linguistic structures can be positioned. They might allow for precise localization within that gradation for particular individuals' usages of a form on particular occasions, but if multiple usages are considered—still more the usages of multiple individuals, even more the usages of whole categories of structures by multiple individuals—we can only expect to find tendencies at best.

This has implications for our analyses of complex structures in all of the basic areas of linguistics, including the lexicon, phonology, semantics, and grammar. The general implication, of which we will see a number of particular applications, is this: regular and predictable forms can be and often are learned. Idiosyncratic or unpredictable forms, to be sure, must be stored, though they may be computed in some degree as well.[9] But people learn (store) regular forms also.

In all areas of language,
more is likely to be stored than must be stored.

9 As Langacker (1987, 448–466) shows, they may be, and often in fact are, born with irregularities already in them, so irregularity need not follow storage chronologically. But by the time they are established as acceptable with those irregularities, they (or something to account for the irregularity) must be in storage. It is a very important point that the mechanisms of computation are not irrelevant to such stored forms, but it will not be emphasized as much as the balancing point stated in the text, that even if the mechanisms of computation are able to account for a form, it still may be stored.

4.1 Storage vs. computation in the lexicon

The lexicon, perhaps by definition, consists of structures which have been learned and are stored. But as we have seen in a number of examples given above, this does not preclude their being computed as well. Thus, if a definition is followed whereby the lexicon is composed of fixed, learned, uncomputed expressions,[10] then the Maxims clearly imply that this will not be a crisply defined, clearly bounded set. Rather what is fixed and not computed for one speaker on one occasion may not be so for the same speaker on other occasions, or for other speakers, and certainly placing one structure in the lexicon will not mean that all structures of its type will be in the lexicon.

If the lexicon is conceived of as the domain of words (whether or not the patterns of their formation are included there as well), then clearly there are unstored, computed words as well as stored (and perhaps uncomputed) structures above the word level, such as phrases and clauses.

However it is defined, the lexicon will be seen to grade into (other aspects of) the grammar, rather than being a separate, self-contained module. This constrains the analysis of those other aspects of the grammar in important ways: they must be of such a nature that forms do not have to suddenly change their character or suddenly function according to a completely different set of rules from how they are or act when treated lexically by speakers.[11]

4.2 Storage vs. computation of phonological structures

Phonological alternations attributable to retrieval from storage of the related forms, rather than to computation of one from the other, have traditionally been called "suppletive". Suppletive morphology has often been considered "totally irrelevant to phonology" (Somerstein, 1977, 42, 71), and typically handled by completely separate mecha-

[10] Cf. Langacker (1987, 456) 'If the notion "lexicon" has any content, it refers to fixed expressions, and primarily those that are less than fully compositional.'

[11] The seamlessness of CG in these regards is a seemly feature of the model.

nisms from those of regular phonology (e.g. by special spell-out rules preceding the input stage to the phonological component.)[12]

Thus the past participial form [*sin*] 'seen' will typically be produced by rule from the combination of [*si*] 'see' and [*ən*] '-en', since it follows a pattern like that of [*thro*^{w}*n*] 'thrown' and other verbs ending in a 'long' vowel, but [*wəz*] 'was' and [*bɪn*] or [*bɛn*] 'been' will be treated as a suppletive forms of [*bi*] 'be', and not handled by the phonology, since they are idiosyncratic.

Our Maxims, however, would lead us to consider that forms like [*sin*] (and [*thro*^{w}*n*], [*bro*^{w}*kən*], etc.), despite being in some degree predictable by rule, are likely also to be learned and may be retrieved from storage rather than computed. Such alternating forms can, in principle, be accessed both ways. There is evidence that this is, in fact, often enough the case. Rule-governed allomorphy notoriously persists after its conditioning environment has disappeared. For example, in Mösiehuali̠ (Tetelcingo Nahuatl) a well-established epenthesis, ø → i / {C,#}C__C, explains a k-/ki- '3rd person object' alternation. So the form *nenkineki* 'you all want it' would be derived from **nen-k-neki* (you.pl-it-want), cf. *nikneki* 'I want it'. When the subject prefix changed to *ne-* the alternation persisted: the form pronounced today is *nekineki*, not the predicted **nekneki*. This makes sense if the very common 3rd person object prefix is learned (stored) as *ki-* when following a 2nd person plural subject prefix and preceding a consonant (a quite common environment.) Thus the evidence indicates that the form was "suppletive" as well as (or instead of) "rule-governed" at least by the time that, and probably even before, the subject prefix changed (Tuggy, 1981, 1997).

All common "rule-governed" phonological forms will tend to be learned (stored) in this way.

---

[12] In the usage of some linguists, suppletion is limited to cases where there is no historical or plausible current phonological connection between two alternating forms, or where it can be shown that historically part of one paradigm was recruited to fill a missing part of another. Thus the alternation of [*go*] vs. [*wɛnt*] is considered suppletive (*went* being originally the past tense of *wend*), but the alternations of [*bi*] 'be' vs. [*bɪn*] or [*bɛn*] 'been', though idiosyncratic and doubtless learned (stored) are not.

4.3 Storage vs. computation of morphological and syntactic constructions

The *-er*-nominalization pattern discussed in section 3.1, running the gamut from *flinger* to *drawer*, is typical of derivational morphology in general. It may in fact be nearly definitional for the category—derived forms are generally understood to be less predictable, less systematic, more likely learned and not computed, than inflected forms. Yet derivational morphology may be productive, and when it is used to produce novel forms the forms are clearly computed, not (yet) stored.

It can certainly be argued (cf. Bybee 1985, 81–110, Payne 1986) that the inflectional category itself is not really homogenous with respect to predictability, productivity, etc. Yet even for prototypical inflectional morphology, highly predictable and highly productive, it need not be the case that it is never stored. Few would deny that the English noun plural is inflectional. But many, perhaps most English-speaking children learn plural forms such as *shoes* or *socks* before they learn the pluralization pattern. It is quite unreasonable to suppose that they forthwith forget these structures that they have learned and thenceforth always compute them. Rather we should expect that they remain in these children's mental lexicons, now enriched by their participation in the productive pattern. *Sock* may be, for such speakers, more a back-formation from *socks* than *socks* a pluralized form of *sock.*

Inflectional morphology is not immune to irregularity or idiosyncrasy. For instance, the plural form *dishes* has meaning beyond what is computable (in *wash/do the dishes*, or *the dishes are draining next to the sink*, many non-*dish* items are included); and *annals* has no singular form. It should not follow either that (a) this is non-linguistic "pragmatic" meaning – it is certainly language-dependent –, or that (b) *-(e)s* and the pluralization pattern are not relevant to the words. But whether there is such irregularity or not, inflected forms may well be learned and then retrieved from storage, instead of or besides being computed.

Whether they exemplify derivational or inflectional morphological patterns, then, thousands of complex words, in any language, may be expected to be stored even though they fit more-or-less regular word-formation patterns of the language. (Taylor 2002, 307–320 argues, and summarizes evidence, that this is in fact often the case.)

A related matter is the issue of larger conventional expressions. Thousands of such expressions are stored, even if they are quite regular and fully computable, and in fact likely sometimes computed. Irregularity of such phrases is often discussed under the rubric of idiomaticity. But the phenomenon goes far beyond idiomaticity, and is almost totally ignored by traditional syntax.

> This dichotomous perspective [of syntax vs. lexicon] made it inevitable that a large body of data belonging to neither category would be mostly ignored. I refer here to the huge set of stock phrases, familiar collocations, formulaic expressions, and standard usages that can be found in any language and thoroughly permeate its use. ...This is why a seemingly perfect knowledge of the grammar of a language (in the narrow sense) does not guarantee fluency in it; learning its full complement of conventional expressions is probably by far the largest task involved in mastering it. Yet conventional expressions have received so little attention that I found it necessary to invent this term for the class as a whole. ...The grammar [i.e. the linguistic description] of a language is responsible for listing its full set of conventional expressions (such as *go for a walk, absolutely incredible, have a good time, ...cheap imitation, the seconds are ticking away, and so on*, and so on). To furnish such a list would obviously be a vast undertaking, for there are many thousands of such expressions, and new ones are always forming. ...The issue of whether conventional expressions should be included in a grammar is factual rather than methodological in a framework taking seriously the goal of psychological reality in linguistic description. If a speaker does in fact learn a large set of conventional expressions as fixed units, it is incumbent on the grammar to represent this fact by providing an inventory of these expressions. The simplest description that accurately accommodates all the data must by definition include such a list.* (Langacker, 1987, 35–36)
>
> *Footnote: With apologies to Sapir, we can say that not only do all grammars leak, they also list (massively).

Of course, as structures get longer and more complex, the probability that they will be stored as wholes decreases. Nevertheless, even quite long and complex syntactic structures may be stored in speakers' long-term memory. For former generations of Americans long passages from such documents as Shakespeare's plays, the Bible, the Constitution and the Gettysburg Address, were memorized by many speakers, and much language use depended on that fact (e.g. paraphrases and parodies on these memorized passages were easily recognized and appreciated.) For modern Americans advertising slogans and the lyrics of popular songs function similarly. The awareness of where these phrases come from is a relatively idiosyncratic part of their meaning which goes beyond what could be computed from their parts, but this need not deny that multiple layers of computation may be going on together with retrieval from storage of these structures.

4.4 Storage vs. computation of polysemy

Many want to reduce polysemy by showing that certain extended senses are systematically related to other senses, perhaps even to the point of being predictable. The Maxims say that will not guarantee non-polysemy, i.e. non-storage of the multiple senses.[13].

An example of this kind of argumentation is the following:

(1) [One waiter to another:]
The ham sandwich *in the corner wants some more coffee.*

(2) ***Plato*** *is on the top shelf next to* ***Lakoff***.

(3) ***John*** *got a dent in his left fender.*

> [Such cases are] uncontroversial ... I think everyone agrees that they derive their reference by a general process: no one thinks that the mental lexicon lists ham sandwich as potentially referring to a person, or Lakoff as referring to a book, or John as referring to a car. (Jackendoff, 1996, 111)

It is true that these cases are transparently derivable, in fact virtually if not absolutely predictable given the appropriate productive rules, and that they need not be stored to be usable.

[13] Much polysemy is not even nearly so predictable that such explaining away is plausible, but that is in some degree a different issue

Jackendoff's phrase "the mental lexicon" is problematic from the point of view I am espousing. The assumption is that there is only one for English, and it is homogeneous in this regard: all metonymies from order to customer, or from author to book, or from driver to vehicle, will always be computed only by all speakers and hearers, and not stored. I would expect, to the contrary, that for waiters or waitresses who often refer to customers by naming what they have ordered, *ham sandwich* (with the required meaning) may very well come to be stored in their lexicons.

I suspect that I am not the only linguist to have read enough discussions of the phenomenon that this sense of *ham sandwich* (and not parallel senses of, e.g., *zucchini casserole* or *liver-and-onions*) is in long-term storage in our minds. Those who have read cognitive linguistics or linguistics-related political commentary may indeed have learned to put *Lakoff* on the storage shelf along with *Plato* and *Shakespeare* and other books, but non-linguists are less likely to have done so. *Shakespeare* and *Plato* themselves were clearly there for virtually all educated English speakers of a few generations ago, and, although their place is somewhat less secure nowadays, it is still generally more firm than that of *Lakoff* or (for instance) *Harry Smith.* Most of us have not had many occasions to talk or hear talk of John specifically as a car, so we probably do not have his name stored with that meaning, but those who do might; for many fans of stock-car racing such meanings for names like *Bobby* or *Donnie Allison*, *Dale Earnhardt* (Jr. or Sr.) are very likely well-entrenched in their mental storage. Many of us who often drive automobiles have stored versions of pronouns like *he, she, him, his* or *her* which involve reference not to body parts but to car-body parts.[14] The same is less likely to be

[14] This is not contradictory to but rather complementary with an account that would claim that the car-part terms also have as part of their meaning a construal whereby they are a sort of bodyparts of their drivers. It is also complementary rather than contradictory to a generalized account of the sort Jackendoff presumably has in mind, whereby a rule (schematic pattern) would state something like "a person may be equated with a vehicle he or she is (skillfully) controlling" or at an even higher level of generality (schematicity), "a person may be equated with a thing with which he or she is associated in some way".

true, for instance, of parts of a tricycle or a hammock. Thus one can easily say *He hit her on the left front fender*, but not ?*She hit him on the [hammock] strings.*

The fact that one could and perhaps often would compute those extended meanings does not mean the meanings cannot exist in one's mental storage as well. Jackendoff is correct that they need not be already stored to be usable. The empirical question remains: *are* they stored?

5 A final issue: storage of a computation vs. storage of its result

A distinction in some ways parallel to the distinction between storage and computation (if it is not indeed the same distinction in another form) is this: An information pattern may itself be learned or routines for constructing or accessing it may be learned and automatized. Another way to put the distinction would be to say that a computation pattern may be stored or its result may be stored.

This raises a host of issues regarding the form in which information is stored and accessed in the brain or mind. CG assumes that all such "structures" or "information patterns" are dynamic patterns of cognitive activations rather than static physical configurations.[15] Storing an information pattern is thus by nature a matter of entrenching a set of cognitive routines that result in its activation as a whole. In other words, what is stored, and the process of its retrieval from storage, are themselves kinds of stored computational pathways. It is

[15] Thus Langacker (2007): "Viewed as a mental phenomenon, a language resides in organized processing activity (patterns of neural activation). The convenient use of terms like 'linguistic knowledge', 'linguistic system', and 'internalized grammar' should not be allowed to obscure its essential dynamicity or to suggest a discretely bounded module. Knowing a language is having mastered a set of skills: a vast number of perceptual, motor, and cognitive operations that can be recruited and executed along with many others in speaking and understanding.' Cf. also Langacker's constant and conscious use of the term *conceptualization* in preference to *concept*: "meaning is not identified with concepts but with conceptualization, the term being chosen precisely to highlight its dynamic nature" (in preparation, see also 2000, 361-376).

thus not only possible but likely that many of the questions that tend to be raised in one's thinking by this putative distinction —between storing a computation and storing its result— are pseudo-issues. For many purposes and in many instances the two ways of talking about a pattern may be notational variants.

Nevertheless, in some applications of the distinction, the two are not equivalent. Rather the distinction discriminates between two alternative computational pathways. This is particularly clear in talking of figurative extensions of meaning. Consider, for instance, the metonymic extension, mentioned in section 4.4 above, from author to literary oeuvre. Let us take it as given that there is an established meaning of *Shakespeare* which refers to his writings. This would be in contrast to *Harry Smith*, which does not have such a meaning for most English speakers – aficionados of the history of the Peninsular Campaign or of the War of 1812-1814 likely excepted. As Jackendoff indicates, there is "a general process" that can be recruited to allow anyone who hears of Sir Harry Smith's autobiography to refer to that work, in a novel usage, not yet established for him or her, as *Harry Smith.* But in the case of Shakespeare the parallel usage is already established.

The question before us is, what exactly is established? Is it (a) an established cognitive pathway from the meaning SHAKESPEARE_p (our conceptualization of the person named Shakespeare) leading to activation of SHAKESPEARE_w (our conceptualization of the written work[s] called *Shakespeare*), or is it (b) SHAKESPEARE_w itself? The first would be storing the computation, and the second storing its result. The two are not equivalent. If option (a) alone is posited, the implication would be that you cannot activate SHAKESPEARE_w without activating SHAKESPEARE_p also, probably in fact first.[16] SHAKE-

[16] I equivocate on the temporal priority of the "literal" sense SHAKESPEARE_p because of the way the influence of context works. The point may be clearer with a novel instance in mind, such as the putative case of HARRY SMITH_w mentioned in the next paragraph. Suppose A says to B, *Where could I find a description of the Battle of New Orleans from a British soldier's point of view?*, and B replies: *Why don't you look in Harry Smith?* By the time the words *Harry Smith* are pronounced, the context would have strongly activated the

SPEARE$_w$ will be effectively computed every time. What is stored is (i) the "rule" for deriving NAME$_w$ from NAME$_p$ and (ii) the fact that this rule is standardly applied to SHAKESPEARE$_p$. Another way to say it might be that SHAKESPEARE$_p$ is lexically marked to undergo the metonymy rule, and that lexical marking constitutes the relevant difference between *Shakespeare* and *Harry Smith.* Under option (b) SHAKESPEARE$_w$ could be activated without necessarily activating either SHAKESPEARE$_p$ or the connection between the two concepts at all.

The position of CG on this issue should come as no surprise. Both (a) and (b) are, in principle, possible. They are neither incompatible nor equivalent. Presumably one should expect that early in the process of establishing a new meaning the computational pathway which prompted its conceptualization in the first place will be highly salient and perhaps invariably activated when it is activated. Thus activating HARRY SMITH$_w$ will inevitably entail activating HARRY SMITH$_p$ and the metonymic computational path. But as HARRY SMITH$_w$ is activated repeatedly, it can with increasing ease be activated in its own right whether or not HARRY SMITH$_p$ is activated before or along with it. Nevertheless it is highly likely that, long after direct activation of HARRY SMITH$_w$ is well established, activation of HARRY SMITH$_p$ and the computational pathway between the two will often or even usually, or at least contingently, occur as well.

Applications of this to such matters as the fading of metaphors should be obvious. When the metaphor is novel, the "literal" sense

---

expectation of a book being named, and the metonymical link may in effect be run "backwards" from the novel sense HARRY SMITH$_w$ to the "literal" sense HARRY SMITH$_p$ instead of (or besides) the other way around. In fact, HARRY SMITH$_p$ may well not be yet established for A at that point, but the storage process will immediately begin, as A realizes, and thus starts to learn, that "OK, there must be someone named Harry Smith who wrote a book that has the sort of thing I'm asking about."

Nevertheless there is a sense in which the "literal" sense is the natural "starting point" (MacWhinney 1977, Langacker 2000, 363) for the metonymic pathway, and one of the outworkings of that fact will be a "naturalness" in activating the literal sense first in processing time. It is in that sense that I speak in Maxim #6 below of "a process beginning with another meaning".

and the computational pathway to the metaphorical sense are perforce activated. As long as the metaphor is still a live metaphor, the literal sense and computational pathway are activated, though the metaphorical sense may be activated in its own right as well. As the metaphor fades, activation of the literal sense and any computational pathway becomes less salient, more contingent and perhaps more sporadic, and in a dead metaphor they will be activated only rarely if at all. For many of us, for instance, the metaphor of death in the phrase *dead metaphor* is faded to the point of near death: despite the transparency of the phrase (the ready activability of the "literal" meaning of *dead* to enrich the meaning) we typically do not think of physical death at all when we say or understand the phrase.[17] In principle any degree of these possibilities may obtain. We might state, then, a final Maxim:

> **Maxim #6**
> A speaker can access a meaning as the endpoint of a computational process beginning with another meaning, or access it independently of such a computational process, or both. Or,
> *You can go the long way to get to a meaning or go to it directly.*

In sum: *It is ultimately an empirical issue whether a meaning is activated only as a result of a computational process starting with another meaning, or activated in other ways which do not involve that particular process, or both.*

6 Summary

It has traditionally been assumed in linguistics that what is regular, systematic and predictable is not learned but rather produced by rule,

[17] The studies summarized in chapter 3 of Gibbs (1994) indicate that hearers can access figurative meanings more quickly than literal meanings. This suggests, obviously, that they are in such cases not first activating the literal meaning before arriving at the figurative meanings.

while what is irregular, idiosyncratic and arbitrary is learned. It is normally assumed as well that these distinctions are binary and coincide with each other so exactly as to be practically equivalent. Important aspects of the architecture of many theoretical models depend on these assumptions, notably the modular distinction between lexicon (where the irregular, idiosyncratic, arbitrary and learned structures reside) and grammar (the domain of rules for producing the unlearned, regular, systematic, and predictable phenomena of language).

CG maintains, on the contrary, that the distinctions are all gradual rather than binary, and that they do not coincide exactly. In particular, while what is irregular, idiosyncratic or arbitrary must be learned, much that is regular, systematic and in some degree predictable may also be learned. This has important implications for the structure of the CG framework, notably for the ways lexicon and other aspects of grammar grade into each other.

We have considered six Maxims that are relevant to the issue of what is learned (cognitively stored) vs. what is computed without having been learned. They are as follows:

1. *What happens to one form doesn't have to happen to all of them.* Showing that one member of a class is learned or computed does not show that all members of the class are treated the same way.
2. *Your doing it doesn't mean everybody has to.* What is stored or computed for one speaker of a language may not be for another. This includes —and in fact all the Maxims include—the possibility of computing the form in different ways.
3. *You can change the way you do it.* A speaker who has always computed or always stored a form may change the way he or she accesses it in the future.
4. *You don't have to do next time what you did this time.* A speaker can compute a form one time and retrieve it from storage the next, or vice versa.
5. *You can do both at the same time.* A speaker can both retrieve a form from storage and compute it, or compute it in different ways, on the same occasion.

6. *You can go the long way to get to a meaning or go to it directly, or both.* A speaker may activate one meaning and then compute another from it, or can compute the second meaning without going through the first (including retrieving the second meaning directly from storage), or do both.

These Maxims have obvious applications to the way the lexicon is conceived, but also to phonology, syntax, and semantics. If CG is right on these points, the architecture of language must look rather different than what many other theories have portrayed it to be.

References

Akmajian, Adrian and Frank Heny. 1975. *An Introduction to the Principles of Transformational Syntax*. Cambridge, Mass. and London: MIT Press.

Anderson, John R. 1993. *Rules of the Mind*. Hillsdale, NJ: Erlbaum.

Barsalou, Larry W. and C. R. Hale. 1993. Components of conceptual representation: From feature lists to recursive frames. In: I. Van Mechelen, J. Hampton, R. Michalski and P. Theuns (eds.), *Categories and Concepts: Theoretical Views and Inductive Data Analysis*. San Diego, CA: Academic Press, 97–144.

Bloomfield, Leonard. 1933. *Language*. New York: Holt.

Bybee, Joan. 1985. *Morphology: A Study of the Relation between Meaning and Form*. Amsterdam and Philadelphia: John Benjamins.

Chomsky, Noam. 1965. *Aspects of the Theory of Syntax*. Cambridge, Mass: MIT Press.

Chomsky, Noam. 1967/70. Remarks on nominalization. In: Roderick Jacobs and Peter Rosenbaum (eds.), *Readings in English Transformational Grammar*. Waltham, Mass: Ginn and Co, 184–221. reprinted.

Geeraerts, Dirk and Hubert Cuyckens (eds.). 2007. *Handbook of Cognitive Linguistics*. Oxford: Oxford University Press.

Gibbs, Ray. 1994. *The Poetics of Mind: Figurative Thought, Language, and Understanding*. Cambridge: Cambridge University Press.

Jackendoff, Ray. 1996. Conceptual semantics and cognitive linguistics. *Cognitive Linguistics* 7: 93–129.

Kolodner, Janet. 1993. *Case-based Reasoning*. San Mateo CA: Morgan Kaufmann.

Langacker, Ronald L. 1987. *Foundations of Cognitive Grammar. Theoretical prerequisites*, volume 1. Stanford, CA: Stanford University Press.

Langacker, Ronald L. 1991. *Foundations of Cognitive Grammar. Descriptive application*, volume 2. Stanford, CA: Stanford University Press.

Langacker, Ronald L. 2000. *Grammar and Conceptualization*, volume 14 of *Cognitive Linguistics Research*. Berlin: Mouton de Gruyter.

Langacker, Ronald L. 2007. Cognitive Grammar. In: Dirk Geeraerts and Hubert Cuyckens (eds.), *Handbook of Cognitive Linguistics*. Oxford: Oxford University Press, 421–462.

Langacker, Ronald L. in preparation. A course in Cognitive Grammar.

Logan, Gordon D. 1985. Skill and automaticity: Relations, implications, and future directions. *Canadian Journal of Psychology* 39: 367–386.

MacWhinney, Brian. 1977. Starting points. *Language* 53: 152–168.

Newell, Allen. 1990. *Unified Theories of Cognition*. Cambridge, MA: Harvard University Press.

Newmeyer, Frederick J. 1980. *Linguistic Theory in America: The First Quarter-century of Transformational Generative Grammar*. New York: Harcourt Brace Jovanovich.

Payne, Doris. 1986. Inflection versus derivation: is there a difference? *Proceedings of the First Annual Pacific Linguistics Conference* 5.

Ruhl, Charles. 1989. *On Monosemy: A Study in Linguistic Semantics*. Albany: State University of New York.

Somerstein, Alan H. 1977. *Modern Phonology*. London and Baltimore: Edward Arnold and University Park Press.

Sweet, Henry. 1913. *Collected Papers*. Oxford: Clarendon Press.

Taylor, John R. 2002. *Cognitive Grammar*. Oxford: Oxford University Press.

Tuggy, David. 1981. Epenthesis of *i* in Classical and Tetelcingo Náhuatl: Evidence for multiple analyses. *Texas Linguistic Forum* 18: 223–277. On line (2003): http://www.sil.org/~tuggyd/1981Epenthesis/epenth.htm.

Tuggy, David. 1997. Rule-governed allomorphy can be suppletive also. *Work Papers of the SIL at UND* 41. On line: http://www.und.nodak.edu/dept/linguistics/wp/1997Tuggy.PDF.

Resolving the dichotomy between storage and computation: The analysability of compound meanings

Cornelia Zelinsky-Wibbelt

1 Storage vs. computation in the mental lexicon

During the last decades linguists have put the traditional concept of the lexicon onto a new footing. A major reason for this revision are new psychological insights into the organization of the mental lexicon as part of human memory. Through these insights the waste-basket metaphor of the lexicon as a repository of all irregular "primitives" (Bloomfield 1933; Di Sciullo and Williams 1987, 3) has largely been overcome. Instead, much as the grammar of a language, the mental lexicon is conceived of as improving its memory capacities through an intelligent organisation. From this dynamic view, words are not contained in storage-expensive lists, but are continuously chunked into clusters of similar lexical items retrieved via their commonalities. Thus it is a truism in second language acquisition that learners do not stop short with acquiring the vocabulary of a language in terms of a piecemeal storage of words. An efficient long-term memory rather benefits from the acquisition of words within their typical contextual relationships. This observation confirms that the most frequent paradigmatic and syntagmatic relations within which words are used are reflected in the organisation of the mental lexicon. We may imagine the mental lexicon to be organized like a vast thesaurus similar to the index of a library (Aitchison, 1993, 32). Recent developments in the archiving of books give rise to the debate of whether readers should be supported in their search for ready-made books or whether an intelligent indexation should enable them to compose their books chapter-wise on demand. By analogy to this image, the lexicologist may ask whether the intelligent organization of the mental lexicon permeates and thereby supports the speakers' retrieval, e.g. of polysemy or word formation patterns. Alternatively, this organization may represent the result of their computation. This metaphor of the mental lexicon as a high-tech library reflects the theoretical dispute about the trade-off between two memory functions: the dispute about whether and how the morphological structure of a language impinges on the storage and retrieval of lexical information in language comprehension and production.

Traditionally, this trade-off is conceived of in terms of the container metaphor. According to this image, the morphological structure of a language is parsimoniously stored in a container to be used on demand in accordance with the prescriptive device of the grammar. In these terms the offspring of generative grammar is seeking for a non-redundant storage capacity, from which different morphological structures may be retrieved through an intelligent computational algorithm. The cognitivist view, by contrast, claims redundancy of storage to provide the key to an efficient grammatical computation.

From this cognitivist view, different structures are stored in vast networks and interconnected paradigmatically through the sharing of similar substructures. Through their syntagmatic similarities, the instances of a paradigm are motivating each other and thereby converging towards a prototype organisation (Croft and Cruse, 2004, 302) while contrasting with syntagmatically dissimilar members of alternate paradigms. Instead of inducing a single ideal representation underlying alternate linguistic realizations of putatively the same state of affairs, this view asks for how speakers experience a situation which may linguistically be expressed in alternate ways and vice versa, why different situations may be expressed by the same form.

It is clear that these radically opposing views conceive differently of the trade-off. By undermining the storage capacities of human memory, the generative view puts the main burden on the computation of morphological structures. In this way storage is kept cheap and retrieval becomes expensive. The cognitive view grants human memory huge storage capacities. Yet, this does not give rise to a cost-benefit-ratio between storage and retrieval, as the cognitive view rejects the framing of human memory in terms of these separate devices. As an alternative, particular linguistic structures are weighted in terms of activation strength as a result of frequency of activation. Activation strength in turn is assumed as determining processing ease.

2 Compounds as multi-word units

2.1 The idiomaticity of compounds

Compounds establish a paradigm case for dealing with the trade-off of the mental lexicon due to their hybrid role in natural language systems. Formally, compounds as multi-word units are complex in being composed of more than one lexeme. Syntactically, the lexicalization of nominal compounds results from noun phrases in which a nominal head is modified by an adjective or noun. Semantically however, many compounds are not composed according to regular relations between their component lexemes. Let us consider this point with the fairly idiosyncratic compound *sheepsfoot roller.*

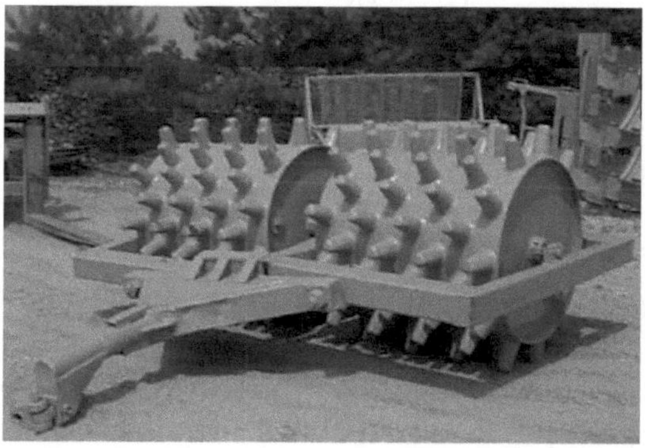

Figure 1. Sheepsfoot roller

Even if we make reference to the picture in Figure 1, it is not clear how the meaning of the noun *sheepsfoot* contributes to the meaning of the noun *roller* by combining with it in a compound. The modifier *sheepsfoot* may refer to the company which produces the roller or to the form of the spikes as parts of the roller, or even to the result which the spikes are intended to produce on the ground. It becomes obvious from this special language term that context-independently, its meaning does not derive straightforwardly from the meanings of its components. And this idiomatic and domain-dependent behaviour is observable with many compounds: their meanings are not fully predictable from a productive word formation rule. On the other hand, the principled listing of compounds as unanalysable wholes in traditional lexicons does not do justice to their formal and semantic behaviour either (Langacker, 1987, 298).

2.2 The composition of compounds

Let us consider how the composition of compounds works with some more regular examples built with the same head noun *roller* (Haspelmath 2002, 223ff; Plag 2003, 148ff; Rickheit 1993, 76ff; Meyer 1993; Ryder 1993):

(1)	a.	*garden*	*roll -er*
		N	V -er$_N$
		THEME	INSTRUMENT
	b.	*road-*	*roll -er*
		N	V -er$_N$
		THEME	INSTRUMENT

In contrast to the idiosyncratic compound *sheepsfoot roller* the compounds *garden roller* and *road-roller* are composed in a fairly regular way. This is captured by the common construction schema underneath. Both compounds are instances of the compound type NN, by being composed of two nouns. The second noun is formally derived from the verbal base *roll* through the suffix *-er*. Semantically therefore, this nominalization profiles one participant of the process designated by the verbal base *roll*, the INSTRUMENT, which is metonymically extended from the prototypical AGENT who uses the INSTRUMENT. Thereby the process meaning of the verbal base remains unprofiled, representing the schematic background of the nominal concept, according to which an INSTRUMENT is conceptualized as exerting a force on a THEME. The analysability of compounds (Langacker, 1987, 292ff), such as *garden roller* and *road roller*, may be motivated historically through their origin as reduced propositions still recoverable in syntactic paraphrases, such as *a roller which rolls the garden.*[1] Many inflectional remnants, as for instance the possessive inflection of the first component in the compound *sheepsfoot roller*, are still reminiscent of the syntactic origin of compounds. On the other hand, due to their general lack of inflections compounds represent the final stage of lexicalization which multi-word units run through on their path from syntax to lexicon.[2]

2.2.1 The lexicon-syntax continuum

Construction grammar represents this continuum between lexicon and syntax, which compounds instantiate, through a hierarchy of constructions, ranging from top-level, i.e. fully compositional, schematic-syntactic schemas to low-level, completely idiosyncratic, specific lexical schemas (Goldberg, 1995, 67). The superficially complex noun *sheepsfoot roller* would have to be located at the lower end of this hierarchy, due to a lack of substructures shared with similar compounds. That is, the meaning of this compound does not follow a productive construction schema in terms of which it is composed as a transparent form-meaning relationship and accordingly analysable in the speakers' comprehension process. Full compositionality represents the ideal case in which the meaning of a complex form derives in a regular way from the meanings of its components. Complete idiosyncracy represents the other end of the continuum of compositionality. At this end we find archaic or obsolete form-meaning relationships

1 Strictly speaking it is not the garden but the ground of the garden which is rolled. That is, the noun *garden* is also used metonymically in this compound, in that it does not make reference to the whole garden but to a geometrically related part, its horizontal surface.

2 This characteristic of compounds becomes more obvious in an inflecting language, such as German, where the adjective has to agree morphologically with the noun in terms of gender, case and number. In the process of lexicalization, the feminine noun phrase *die süße Kartoffel* ("the sweet potato") has thus become reduced to the uninflected compound *Süßkartoffel.*

of multi-word units which are semantically opaque in that speakers are incapable of decoding a transparent semantic relation between their components without heavily relying on the original situational context.[3]

By organizing compounds as instances of constructional schemas, we can account for the degree to which their components are composed according to regular formal and semantic relations.

2.2.2 The productivity of constructions

The analysability of multi-word units in the speakers' process of comprehension and production comprises their creation of new compounds. Along the dimension of *productivity* we may observe newly coined compounds to be sanctioned by existing construction schemas to different degrees. A construction schema is productive to the degree that speakers apply it to produce formally and semantically analogous compounds. The more productive a constructional schema is, the higher its strength of activation is in the speakers' memory. Hence the more readily the components of the schema may be instantiated in the speakers' manipulation of new compounds.

By framing productivity in terms of the activation of schemas, cognitive linguistics refrains from hard-wired rules applying in a deterministic fashion, predicting the continuum of compositionality as an alternative.

---

[3] It was indeed the particular situation which gave rise to the creation of the compound *sheepsfoot roller.* Much in the same way as sheep were trained to use their feet for stamping the ground of dikes flat in former times, the spikes of this machine are intended to be used today in the domain of highway engineering. Through inheriting this information from the larger discourse context, the compound *sheepsfoot roller* became an instance of partial compositionality, semantically once on a par with compounds such as *waffle iron, zigzag machine,* in which an INSTRUMENT designated by the head noun produces a particular pattern referred to by the modifying component. As we have noted, neither this semantic relationship nor the original model is necessarily transparent to the expert users today.

2.2.3 Inheritance between constructions

Within the hierarchy of constructions, each instantiation embodies redundancy relative to its constructional schema. This is captured by normal mode inheritance which allows for subregularities, in that information is inherited transitively from the dominating to the dominated node, except for the more specific information of the latter conflicting with the more general information of the former (Goldberg, 1995, 67, 73f). In this case, conflict resolution rules take care of the more specific construction schema to be included in more than one general construction schema in a semantically motivated operation (Goldberg, 1995, 97f). For instance, the particular compounds we have analysed under (1) inherit the properties of the more general NN compound construction, which in turn inherits the properties of the most general compound construction, the only constraint on which is that it combines two or more bases which are semantically associated. In the case of conflicts between the more specific and the more general representation, the former may inherit partial information from two or more dominating, conflicting nodes. This is multiple inheritance which we have illustrated in section 2.2 above. The compound *garden roller* inherits from more than one constructional schema. On the most general level, the compound *garden roller* given under (1) has been pointed out to instantiate the NV-er$_N$ construction corresponding to the semantic schema THEME AGENT. On a structurally more finegrained level we have seen both constituents to instantiate alternate semantic representations, the metonymic schema INSTRUMENT OF AGENT represents the second constituent and the metonymic schema PART OF WHOLE the first constituent. In this way, metonymic and metaphorical inferences may be drawn in accordance with more encompassing knowledge systems evolving in the larger discourse context.

3 The word-formation trade-off

Along the dimension of *analysability* we have pointed out the degree to which a meaning may be recognized through explicit symbolization (Langacker 1987, 292ff; Goldberg 1995, 136ff; Croft 2001, 181ff; Croft and Cruse 2004, 251ff; Langacker 1991, 532f). In contrast to semantically opaque compounds like *sheepsfoot roller*, explicit symbolization enhances memorizability, as has been illustrated with the compounds *garden roller* and *road roller*. The more compositionally compounds behave, the more speakers would retrieve them on the basis of their components, while towards the lower end of the compositionality hierarchy compounds would be represented as holistic, unanalysable wholes.

Due to their hybrid nature, compounds establish an ideal battle ground for competing theoretical explorations into the trade-off between storage and retrieval in the mental lexicon. To account for the generative capacity of morphologically complex words, the generative paradigm assumes them to be lexically stored and accessed in terms of their decomposed morphemes. As a consequence, morphological parsing takes place prior to lexical access (Marslen-Wilson et al., 1994; Halle and Mohanan, 1985; Yang, 2000) and is dedicated to different components of the linguistic system in different specifications of this theory. Arguing for the non-generativity of language, the other extreme assumes all morphologically complex words to be stored as wholes (Butterworth, 1983; Lukatela et al., 1980). Denying the competence-performance distinction in view of the continuum of compositionality, compromise positions favour exemplar-based models over the storage-retrieval dichotomy.

3.1 The rule-based position

Taft and Forster (1975) have introduced the assumption that speakers attempt morphological decomposition, independently of any evidence about the internal semantic transparency of the putative compound. On this view, even semantically opaque compounds as well as pseudo-compounds and -derivations are initially stripped off their stems and affixes (*part/ partridge, prime/ primrose, past/ pasty*) in order to be lexically accessed through their alleged base forms.

This hypothesis results from the generativist image of an extremely limited word store so that multi-morphemic words would have to be economically organized through an alphabetical order and in terms of their abstract modality-independent morphemes to which all modality-specific realizations are linked (Marslen-Wilson et al., 1994). By taking novel word formations to be comprehended and produced on the basis of their decomposed morphemes, this procedure is equally assumed for existing word formations because initially, speakers have to evaluate the input as existing or novel. On a par with this decompositional view, form and meaning are represented independently of each other in autonomous modules and processed strictly sequentially (Zwitserlood, 1994, 364). This position is weakened by the existence of less transparent, less compositional and even idiosyncratic word formations which lack (fully) compositional procedures for their interpretation. Empirical evidence against the decompositional procedure is provided by lexical gaps, as well as by opaque and pseudo-compounds (Sandra, 1990; Marslen-Wilson et al., 1994), which are synchronically akin to monomorphemic forms. The decompositional view, however, rejects this evidence by claiming that speakers may only discard opaque or pseudo-compounds as non-decomposable on semantic grounds which is achieved at later processing stages where the morphological activations have already decayed (Zwitserlood, 1994, 363).

3.2 The full-listing approach

By taking word formations to be primarily idiosyncratic, whole-word models deny morphological structure to play any role in lexical representation and access (Lukatela et al., 1980; Butterworth, 1983). Yet, empirical evidence in recognition and manipulation tasks with morphologically complex words does not seem to support the assumption of an "a-morphous" mental lexicon (Stolz and Feldman, 1995). In fact, most of these whole-word models incorporate a "back-up store" and "fall-back procedures" on phonological, orthographic, and semantic structures as access codes for the processing of novel and infrequent words (Butterworth, 1983; Aitchison, 1993; Seidenberg, 1987; Rumelhart et al., 1986) and thereby come near to compromise positions.

3.3 Compromise positions

As a strict defense of the full-listing approach is as difficult as a principled purport of the decompositional model, hybrid models consider frequency of activation in order to induce the degree of unithood.

3.3.1 The Dual System Model

Within the generative tradition, the Dual System Model distinguishes between two systems in both storage and retrieval. While fully compositional word-formations are rule-generated from their decomposed, lexically stored morphemes, irregular words are stored as wholes associated via their common schemas weighted according to their frequency of activation (Clahsen, 1999; Pinker, 1999; Pinker and Ullman, 2002).

As is generally the case with the assumption of different subsystems, a relative threshold or quality which gives rise to the distinction is not defined as the frequency measures remain absolute token counts. The dual-system model thus cannot explain how speakers would switch from the processing of schemas to the processing of rules, which is nevertheless tacitly implied. In this way, processes such as language acquisition and language development cannot be accounted for (Bybee, 1995, 449f).

3.3.2 The Morphological Race Model

By contrast, morphological race models assume a redundant representation of multi-morphemic words both in terms of whole words and their decomposed morphemes to be accessed equally in a competition procedure. The more productive and semantically transparent a word formation pattern is, the higher the activation level of its constituent morphemes becomes in the mental lexicon and accordingly the more prone the complex word is to be parsed on the basis of a transparent word formation pattern (Plag, 2003, 177). Vice versa, less productive and less transparent forms leave very poor memory traces and hence are more liable to be accessed as wholes. This unit status may be measured in terms of the notion of relative frequency (Frauenfelder and

Schreuder, 1992; Schreuder and Baayen, 1995; Baayen, 1992; Baayen and Dijkstra, 2003; Hay, 2001). If the whole word is more frequent than its base, whole-word access wins out. By contrast, if, as is usually the case, the complex word-formation is less frequent than its base, access to the decomposed constituents applies in a productive word-formation process. This ratio is measured in terms of the division of the token frequency of the complex word by token frequency of its base. We may apply this formula to compounds by dividing the frequency of the compound by that of its head.

Bien et al. (2005) investigate unit strength in compounds by comparing the effects of constituent token frequency on reaction times to those of compound frequency. The results of their study point out that processing is eased slightly more significantly by the token frequency of the modifier, i.e. the summed frequencies of the same modifier in other compounds. Not only is the positional frequency effect lower for the head, a high root frequency of the head, i.e. its summed frequency of occurrence in all inflected and derived forms, independently of their position, has an inhibitory effect on processing, whereas the reverse is evidenced for the modifier. On the other hand, a high frequency of the head in monomorphemic words is verified to ease processing.

We presume that these results reflect the meaning-bearing function, which the head of the compound shares with mono-morphemic words. In contrast to this, the position-independent root-frequency effect of the modifier may be explained, not in terms of incremental processing (Levelt, 1993), as has already been partly rejected by Bien et al. (2005), but in terms of the relation-linking function of the modifier, which varies substantially across different word-formation contexts. From a cognitive view, this high root frequency effect of the modifier results from its associations with a whole lot of constructions in which its form occurs with different meanings. The more frequently different but similar compound types become activated in the speakers' memory, the more densely their similar substructures become associated and the more readily the activation spreads through the network, thereby facilitating the processing of the respective instances. The inhibitory effect of high root frequency on processing provides evidence for the non-decompositional route, i.e. whole-word storage of the respective compounds.

Jong (2002) has compared type and token frequency effects of modifier and head. The results point out a token frequency effect of both modifier and head with concatenated compounds. Again, this is taken as evidence for the non-decompositional route since token frequency is not coupled with semantic activation. According to this model, high token frequency is taken as evidence for only the phonological access of a word being facilitated. Instead of inhibited semantic access, though, as presumed by Jong's sequential processing model, it is rather a loss of semantic transparency which has generally been attested to result from high token frequency coupled with low type frequency. That is, a decrease in productivity, due to semantic opacity would predict whole-word storage (Bybee, 1995; Hay, 2001). By contrast, a type frequency effect would be evidence of a productive word formation process due to semantic transparency.

Baayen (2000) measures the productivity of a derivative in the narrow sense through its type-token ratio, by dividing the number n_1 of types derived by an affix only once in the corpus, the hapax legomena through the token frequency N of an affix.

$$P = \frac{n_1}{N}$$

We may apply this model to the modifying components and their interaction with specific heads in compounds.

3.3.3 Associative Models

The distinction between whole-word storage and decomposition is abandoned entirely by purely associative morphological systems (Bybee, 1985, 1995; Seidenberg, 1987; Sereno and Jongman, 1997; Seidenberg and Gonnerman, 2000) in favour of usage-based models in which a prototype organisation emerges from product-oriented generalizations. Clusters of exemplars result from similarities between phonological, orthographic, morphological, and semantic patterns. More specifically, the formation of transparent paradigms results from frequency of activation. The more relations a word formation entertains to formally and semantically analogous forms, the stronger its internal structure becomes represented within a network of lexical connections. By contrast, the more frequently a complex form is experienced without formal and semantic similarities to other word formations, the stronger its lexical representation becomes and the more easily it is accessed as an autonomous unanalysed unit which is resistant to change and does not contribute to productivity. An essential ingredient of this network model is its symbolic motivation. Weaker semantic relations could be attested to correlate with a greater degree of formal variation (Bybee, 1995, 429). This model has the advantage that an input which is not fully compatible with a stored representation, may be computed through lexical connections between partially unified types. An input would be evaluated as participating in a cluster if its overall similarity to all stored exemplars exceeds the overall similarity to the stored exemplars of neighbouring clusters. The more exemplars would share a particular substructure, the stronger the connections between them. As a consequence, the more saliently their substructure would be represented in terms of activation strength and the more easily it would be accessed. This access model would also entail novel word formations whereby these substructures gain in productivity without any types being abstracted.

In this organisation, high-level schemas correspond to heavily entrenched representations due to strong commonalities between the substructures which they interconnect. By contrast, low-level schemas correspond to poor representations resting on weak correspondences between interconnected substructures. They may thus equally be associated with instances of neighbouring constructions. This hierarchy reflects the position of a complex form on the scale of productivity. At the weakly productive pole, low-level schemas represent opaque and semi-regular, complex forms with many constraints on a high number of tokens while at the strongly productive pole, high-level schemas represent strong lexical connections within transparent paradigms relating many types with few tokens. This probabilistic model is well in keeping with the cline of compositionality which compounds represent.

4 Concept combination models

In the preceding sections we have analysed the meaning of compounds to exhibit a prototype organization, in that their concept combination does not constitute a genuine hyponymy of the head concept. The investigation of weak compositionality in compounds is the particular intention of the psychological paradigm of concept combination (Murphy, 1988; Medin and Shoben, 1988; Shoben, 1991; Hampton, 1991; Costello and Keane, 2000; Wisniewski, 1997; Gentner and Gunn, 2001; Estes and Glucksberg, 2000; Gagné and Shoben, 1997). Basically, the paradigm makes assumptions compatible with associative morphological models. Neither hard-wired rules, nor a purely instance-based processing can explain the speakers' memory capacities (Shoben, 1991, 132). Instead, the composition of compounds is assumed to be controlled by the head noun's schema to be specified or changed through the meaning of the modifying constituent.

4.1 Schema-based theories

Alignment theory (Wisniewski, 1997) is particularly concerned with how speakers compare the attribute-value structures of the concepts to be combined. Normally this means that speakers apply a property or attribute of the modifier to the concept of the head. The comparison results in *commonalities* if modifier and head share the same values of the specified attributes. In the case of *non-alignable* differences, the head normally lacks an attribute which the modifier adds to its structure. In comparison to this one-step addition of attributes, *alignable* differences are computationally more expensive. In this case the conflicting values of a common attribute have to be changed, which would normally apply to the attribute-value structure of the head. For instance in the compound *hovercraft car* the head noun *car* would have to be modified as not moving in the prototypical manner by rolling on its wheels. Instead, the wheels as part of the car are overridden by the cushion of air, designated by the modifying component *hovercraft*, on which the vehicle is capable of moving over land or water.

Alignment theory rests solely on a mechanical matching of arbitrary attribute-value structures, without explaining the origin of the coercion effects. Without motivating the alignment, the theory is incapable of constraining these effects. By not considering the degree of alignment, the cline of compositionality represented by these concept combinations cannot be accounted for.

As an extension of alignment theory, the *interactive property attribution* model explains the matching of attribute-value structures within the compound-internal context. If a *non-alignable* attribute is particularly diagnostic of the head concept, the concept combination may be impeded, if this attribute is inconceivable in the modifying concept, such as the attribute THORNS in the combination of *violet roses* (Estes and Hasson, 2004, 1084). Vice versa, we may conclude that the diagnosticity of an alignable attribute may ease the coercion if the constituents' semantic representations are closely associated in terms of the sharing of weighted attribute-value structures.

4.2 The Constraint Theory

Being equally concerned with a compound-internal computation of matches, the *Constraint Theory* (Costello and Keane, 2000) generates all combinations of attribute-value structures syntactically possible between the constituents' concepts in a first step. In a second step, three constraints filter the acceptable compound interpretations.

1. The combination must inherit *diagnostic* attributes from both components. Diagnostic attributes are particularly characteristic of a category and distinguish them clearly from contrast categories. As an example, Costello and Keane (2000) mention the form attribute PRICKLY which figures as more diagnostic in characterizing the concept of the noun *cactus* in comparison to the colour attribute GREEN and thereby is inherited by the combination *cactus fish*. This notion of diagnosticity is consonant with the assumption of weak compositionality pursued by cognitive linguistics. Diagnostic attributes cannot be inherited from the constituents in isolation but are constrained by the combination.

2. The *plausibility* of an interpretation derives from the frequency by which speakers have experienced a combination of attributes with other compositions. This amounts to the productivity of attribute-value structures resulting from activation strength in purely associative systems.
3. A compound is *informative* to the degree that the concepts are combined in a non-redundant manner. This applies to a modifying constituent which semantically restricts the polysemy of the head. Vice versa, a modifier is semantically redundant, if it predicates a typical attribute of the head. By this communicative motivation, the tautological combination * *wheel car* does not follow a lexicalization pattern as the modifier predicates a typical property of the head. This constraint corresponds to the assumption of pragmatic motivation in construction grammar. Still, it has to be admitted that the notion of informativeness purported by Costello and Keane (2000) remains a purely formal device without any content.

We may conclude that Costello and Keane (2000) use pragmatic constraints in order to reduce syntactically possible combinations to semantically possible ones, without though, explaining the pragmatic origin of these constraints.

4.3 The Competition-Among-Relations-In-Nominals Theory

Gagné and Shoben (1997) set themselves off from the schema-based model of concept combination which, much in accordance with generative models, attributes priority to the meaning-bearing function of the head noun. In claiming speakers to select from an experientially based preference order of semantic relations, the CARIN model defended by Gagné (2002, 556f) is in conformity with associative models of exemplar-based morphological processing. According to her usage-based experiments, speakers select the semantic relation from the meaning of the modifier as this further differentiates the meaning of the head noun. More specifically, the preference order of semantic relations is derived from:

1. the frequency with which the modifier occurs with a semantic relation
2. the modifier's relational distribution as consisting in the number of relations with which it occurs
3. competitive strengthening which predicts the relative frequency of the to-be-selected relation as resulting from the most probable alternative selections. This probability is calculated from the three most frequent alternative relations with which the modifier occurs by dividing the frequency of the to-be-selected relation by the sum of the frequency of the to-be-selected relation and the frequency of the three most likely alternative relations.
4. the frequency of recently created combinations with semantically similar or synonymous modifiers. This may be compared to high type-frequency relations embodying a low token frequency in associative morphological systems, in which the increase and decay of activation through time is taken to influence schematic transparency and thereby the ease of retrieval. The more recently a type has been created, the less tokens it will subsume and the more productive it will be, that is, the more speakers will rely on an attribute-value structure shared by modifier and head in the novel creation.

The slightly more significant token frequency effects of the modifier reported by Bien et al. (2005) are evidence of the relation being induced from the modifier. Gangnés prediction of the selection on the basis of the token frequency of the to-be-selected relation in comparison with competing relations is well in keeping with the productivity measure in the narrow sense (Baayen, 2000; Jong, 2002). While Baayen's productivity measure is intended to indicate unit strength on the basis of a simplified type-token ratio, we favour the prediction of unit strength in accordance with exemplar-based prototype models (Bybee, 1995), in that a whole lot of schemas are competing with each other via the sharing of substructures.

5 Unifying figure and ground in construction schemas

Construction grammar compares the substructures of autonomous and dependent predications within constructions (Fillmore, 1999). Computationally, the attributes of different substructures unify, if they share the same values (Covington, 1994, 293).[4] Semantically, the unification of modifier and head is analysed in terms of their valency structure, the gestalt-psychological asymmetry between figure and ground. Cognitive linguistics claims this asymmetry to arise in the perceiver's distribution of attention on the one hand and to frame the speaker's grammatical organization on the other. In gestaltpsychological terms the figure attracts the perceivers' focus of attention (Talmy 2000a, 320; Langacker 1987, 187f; Polinsky 1996). In the compound *touring car*, the head noun *car* provides the primary information bearing unit (Croft, 2001, 257ff), which is thus the conceptually more autonomous figure and hence the profile determinant from which the compound inherits its meaning (Langacker, 1987, 290, 333ff): context-independently, the figure *car* is specified by the larger number of attributes (Murphy and Medin, 1985; Murphy, 1988) and context-dependently it elaborates a salient substructure of the dependent predication, the ground *touring* (Langacker, 1991, 6) which is only represented with minimal cognitive effort.

5.1 Unifying figure and ground in the V-ing$_N$N construction

The compound *touring car* instantiates the $V - ing_N N$ construction. This construction is claimed to designate unambiguously what we have introduced as the PURPOSIVE construction of composition by Bauer (1978, 170f) if the first constituent is derived from a verb and bears primary stress. Bauer's claim establishes an ideal candidate for calling into question the generative status of rules. This is particularly interesting with the phenomenon of morphological derivations, as their hybrid character has split up the generative community into

4 Unification is a procedure which has been introduced for Natural Language Processing systems in computational linguistics by Martin Kay (1985).

the defenders of lexically generated morphological derivations and those who banish this process to other linguistic modules.

From a cognitive perspective, the semi-compositional relation between figure and ground in the $V - ing_N N$ construction rests on an implicit secondary predication through which the ground semantically modifies the figure.

In the composite term *touring car*, the ACTION nominalization of the ground *touring* explicitly designates such a predication. In the construction $V - ing_N$, the *-ing* suffix formally derives a noun from the verbal base.[5] Semantically, the nominalization through *-ing* achieves two things. Firstly, *-ing* imposes a perspectivization on the scene designated by the verb. The sequentially scanned MOTION event expressed by the verbal base implies a change-of-state through time. The nominalization shifts this event to a region, in which the component states of the MOTION are scanned in summary (Langacker, 1987, 144ff). The relations between the participants are still contained in the concept of the nominalization. This is the concept of the verbal base *tour*, where an agent moves around a location without a distinctive goal, that is the ACTIVITY concept. Yet, this event structure is not in profile, it is schematically reduced to a region, and this region is profiled by the nominalization. In accordance

5 In this term, the noun *car* cannot be modified by an adjectival derivation, as it is the function of the attributive adjective to characterize the modified figure in terms of the properties which are part of its meaning. The adjectival ground *touring* would thereby characterize the figure *car* by the concept of its verbal base, i.e. by the intentional motion of *to tour*. Yet, image-schematically, the car represents an INSTRUMENT of a HUMAN PRODUCER as the volitional agent. It is thus an extension of the human body (Langacker, 1991, 296), on whom it is conceptually and functionally dependent. As only the human body is capable of volitionally controlling the car's motion (Talmy, 2000b, 38), the adjectival function of *touring* may only be dependent on the metonymic use of the figure *car*. By the same token, the adjectival derivation *touring* inherits the dependence on a volitional and intentional figure from the verbal base. By contrast, the special-language term *car* has a non-volitional function. Hence semantically, the adjective *touring* cannot unify with the the INSTRUMENTAL sense of the noun *car*. This analysis is in conformity with Simpson and Weiner (1989). It is therefore surprising how willingly Messinger (2000) is nevertheless inclined to assume *touring* as fulfilling an adjectival function in this compound.

with Langacker (Langacker, 1991, 215), these alternate ways of profiling the same situation are represented through the heavy-line time axis corresponding to the sequentially scanned concept of the verbal base *tour* in Figure 2 in contrast to the heavy-line circle which indicates the summary-scanned region designated by the nominalization *touring* in Figure 3.

tour -	*ing*
SEQUENTIAL	SUMMARY-SCANNED
MOTION	

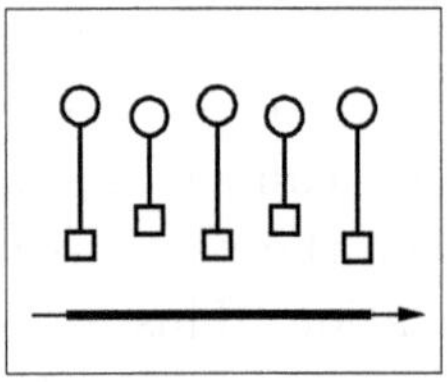

Figure 2. *tour*, V – sequential scanning of MOTION through TIME

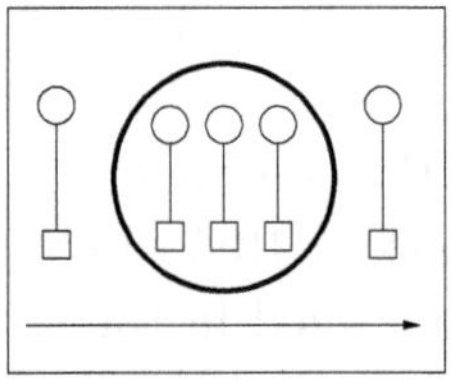

Figure 3. *touring*, N – summary scanning of HOMOGENEOUS & UNBOUNDED REGION

In Figure 3 the nonprofiled relations between the participants are indicated by the thin lines between a thing represented by the encircled region and the more abstract conceptualization of an entity represented by the box.

Secondly, the nominalization through *-ing* achieves the unboundedness of this region. In this region, the potential occurrences of MOTION events designated by the verb stem are construed as equally representative states which extend indefinitely beyond the conceived situation (Langacker, 1991, 26). That is, the *-ing* derivation achieves a cumulation of MOTION events which is internally homogeneous and externally unbounded in the same way as the event expressed by the corresponding progressive construction. This conceptualization of an ACTION nominal is consonant with a type specification, since its reification does not yield in an instantiation (Langacker, 1991, 33). In compounds, such as *touring car* and *racing car*, the construal of a type corresponds to the PURPOSIVE predication of *touring* and *racing* for all potential occurrences in the past, present, and future.

We may conclude that the ground of a V-ing$_N$N construction is particularly diagnostic of a generic purpose. Moreover, the ACTION nominalization is also informative (Costello and Keane, 2000) in constraining the polysemy of the figure *car* vis-à-vis the alternative $V - ing_{Adj}N$ construction. As we have seen, this constraint is imposed in dependence of the domain knowledge. By the same token, the informativeness of this figure-ground relationship becomes more plausible, the more semantically similar figures become constrained in this way, that is, the higher its type frequency.

The figure *car* is intrinsically specified by the attribute INSTRUMENT which entails a PURPOSE, meaning "in oder to perform action X". This entailment unifies with the concept of the ACTION nominalization of the ground *touring* (Langacker, 1991, 26). On account of this conceptualization, the ground is prerequisite for selecting the PURPOSIVE relation which has motivated the composition evidenced by the ground's primary stress (Olson, 2000, 898). The attribute-value structure of the more general PURPOSIVE construction in Figure 4 is meant to provide for the unification of the figure *car* and the ground *touring* in a simplified form. This figure represents the PURPOSIVE construction by a complex attribute-value structure. At each level the attribute-value structure consists of an attribute representing a variable on the left-hand side to be specified by a value on the right-hand side. Values may be simplex or again consist of complex attribute-value structures. The PURPOSIVE construction represents the semantic dependency between figure and ground as arguments of the implicit relational predicate PURPOSIVE. The INSTRUMENTAL figure entails a PURPOSE, that is an ACTION performed in order to enable another state of affairs (Valin and Lapolla, 1997, 383). This is elaborated through the ground's ACTION nominalization which along with the primary stress corroborates the lexicalization of a compound.

$$\begin{bmatrix} \text{composition} & \begin{bmatrix} \text{syn} & \text{NN} \\ \text{sem} & \textsc{Purposive} \end{bmatrix} \\ \text{figure} & \begin{bmatrix} \text{syn} & \text{N} \\ \text{phon} & \text{secondary stress} \\ \text{sem} & \begin{bmatrix} \textsc{Instrument} & \begin{bmatrix} \textsc{Purposive} & \textsc{Action} \end{bmatrix} \end{bmatrix} \end{bmatrix} \\ \text{ground} & \begin{bmatrix} \text{syn} & \text{N} \\ \text{phon} & \text{primary stress} \\ \text{morph} & \begin{bmatrix} \text{figure} & \begin{bmatrix} \text{syn} & \text{V} \end{bmatrix} \\ \text{ground} & \begin{bmatrix} \text{syn} & \text{N} \\ \text{sem} & \textsc{Action} \end{bmatrix} \end{bmatrix} \end{bmatrix} \end{bmatrix}$$

Figure 4. Unifying attribute-value structures in constructions

5.2 Coercion

When two or more dependent predications become unified by a grammatical construction, numerous construction schemas compete with one another on the basis of the specificity and entrenchment which their attribute-value matrices embody vis-à-vis the lexicalized instances. As the result of this competition procedure the semantic specification of the unified instance should be properly included in the semantic specification of that constructional schema with which it shares a relevant semantic substructure (Michaelis, 2004, 16). This result is computed in terms of elaborative distance between schema and instance, that is the degree of the schema's underspecification relative to its instantiation (Langacker 1987, 69; Taylor 2002, 301f).[6] If the attribute-value structures of figure and ground do not unify in accordance with the agreement specifications of a construction, the override principle ensures that those constructional schemas augment the valence structure of the conflicting instances that provide

[6] In order to ensure an efficient computation, the elaborative distance criterion calls for low-level schemas accounting for subregularities, which in the extreme case may collapse with an idiosyncratic instance.

the nearest possible match in terms of the number and specification of attributes (Michaelis, 2004, 25f.). Instead of coercion effects arising in an autonomous semantic module from agreement constraints of the head (Jackendoff, 1997, 50), these effects originate from the symbolic unity of constructions in a semantically motivated, partially compositional process.

6 A corpus-linguistic experiment

In order to evaluate the unification of figure and ground within the valency structure of the PURPOSIVE construction, we conducted a corpus-linguistic experiment.

6.1 Constructing the experiment

Following Gagné (2002), we predicted the selection of the modifier's semantic relation by calculating the following frequencies.

1. The strength of a construction was calculated on the basis of its morphological ambiguity. We evaluated the significance of a particular morphological construction against alternate constructions of the same orthographic string, by considering the overall number of bigram candidates as instantiations (Bien et al., 2005). The formulas

   $strength_{construction} = \frac{f(xy)}{f(xy)+f(\overline{x}y)_n}$ and

   $strength_{construction} = \frac{f(xy)}{f(xy)+f(x\overline{y})_n}$

   were to measure the relative frequency of a construction's instances against all linguistically predicted constructions of figure-ground relationships.
2. In conformity with the plausibility constraint of the Constraint Theory (Costello and Keane, 2000; Lynott, 2003), the probability of a bigram's figure-ground relationship was calculated against the polysemy of a morphological construction (Gagné 2002, 555; Bien et al. 2005; Aerts and Gabora 2005). The formula

$strength_{relation} = \frac{f(xy)}{f(xy)+f(\overline{x}y)_n}$

was to divide the frequency of the to-be-selected relation by the sum of the frequency of a construction's semantic relations. In this formula X and Y provide slots for semantic categories represented in terms of attribute-value matrices.

3. In order to determine unit strength as a result of the increase and decrease of activation through time which is set equal to ease of retrieval in associative morphological systems, we measured low-frequency types in terms of the type-token ratio of the productivity measure given in section 3.3.2.

6.2 Selecting the data

206 instances of the $V - ing_N N$ construction were extracted from the ReSIST[7] corpus. The extraction was done by the AUTINDEX system developed at the IAI (Gindiyeh et al. 2008; Haller and Schmidt 2006). More specifically, the core system MPRO[8] annotated each lexeme with a morpho-syntactically derived attribute-value tag set (Maas, 1996; Maas et al., 2009), subsequently disambiguated by a shallow syntactic analysis of the KURD system (Carl and Schmidt-Wigger, 1998). The output of this analysis provided the input to the identification of multi-word units. The resulting nominal compound candidates were additionally narrowed down to established lexical units by comparison with special language thesauri[9].

[7] Resilience for Survivability in IST

[8] The MPRO system has been developed at the *Institute for Applied Information Processing at the University of the Saarland* ("Institut für Angewandte Informationsforschung an der Universität des Saarlandes"). Due to an exhaustive lexicon, it is capable of analysing morphologically complex word formations.

[9] TEMA (*Fachinformationszentrum Technik*, http://www.fiz-technik.de/fiz/thesaurus.htm) and MeSH (*Medical Subject Headings thesauri*, http://www.nlm.nih.gov/mesh/)

6.3 Interpreting the data

Of the 203 remaining candidates both figure and ground underwent a manual semantic categorization. The data divided into eight grammaticalized meanings (Langacker, 1987, 1991; Valin and Lapolla, 1997; Talmy, 2000b; Bybee et al., 1994): ACTION nominalizations derived from DYNAMIC (change-of-state) verbs (Langacker 1991, 31ff; Valin and Lapolla 1997, 82ff) are materialized in both figure and ground of the compound *packaging automation.* In fact, all grounds of the investigated $V - ing_N N$ construction consistently instantiated this category. INSTRUMENT nominals bear the syntactic potential of shifting to an INSTRUMENTAL-SUBJECT function (Dowty, 1991, 2000), as e.g. the figure in *testing machine.* The category of MODALITY serves to relate other nominal meanings to reality either by the speakers' will or by their belief (Palmer, 2001; Bybee et al., 1994), as e.g. accomplished by the figure of the compound *blocking probability.* LOCATION nominals are virtual grounds of locative prepositions (Langacker, 1987, 214ff, 277ff), as for instance the figures in the compounds *nesting level, computing centre.* MANNER typically expresses the supporting or co-event of a motion (Talmy, 2000b, 27), as the figure in *timing behaviour.* MEASURE nominals have a classifying function with respect to other nominals by quantifying them in terms of a numerically defined scale (Lyons, 1977, 463), as e.g. the figure nominal in *sampling frequency.* The category of MEDIUM is taken to comprise nominals designating an abstract instrument serving to transfer information, e.g. the figure in *warning signal.* The category COLLECTIVE was associated with only one type vis-à-vis seven tokens and was discarded as insignificant.

Two alternative constructions were sorted out as their composed meanings were not in a metonymic or metaphorical relation to the valency relations between figure and ground in the PURPOSIVE construction. One of them is morphologically marked on the figure which is derived from a verb:

(2) *building renovation, marketing manager*

The semantic relations of these compounds are still recoverable in the argument structure of their verbal bases, in that the THEME expressed by the dependent ground undergoes a change-of-state as a consequence of being controlled by the INSTRUMENT or ACTION designated by the figure. In this derivation, the IMPERFECTIVE EVENT structure of the verbal base of the THEMATIC ground is not in focus but rather shifts towards the nominal concept of an UNBOUNDED OBJECT, perfectly consonant with the generic reference condition of the ground in compounds. This construction is also instantiated by types in which the figure is realized by a zero derivation:

(3) *walking test, positioning test, timing control, processing control*

Due to their deverbal figures, these compounds are likely candidates of synthetic constructions, though not reliably so. The lexical meaning of the figure helps to sort out a number of compounds instantiating the PURPOSIVE construction through the figure's metonymic shift to an INSTITUTION performing the ACTION:

(4) *motoring organisation, training association, broadcasting corporation*

A counter-example of the synthetic construction which is more difficult to explain in terms of grammatical relations is the compound *screwdriving application.* It is part of domain knowledge whether there is some specified context in which the screwdriving activity might conform to a norm like a rule or system, a law, a method, or an idea (Brown, 1996; Cowie, 1989; Quirk et al., 1985) to be operated on or controlled by an application. Rather, the application is a facility intended for screwdriving, meaning that the PURPOSIVE relation is being expressed. The compound *viewing monitor* provides an analogous example.

Other instances which Bauer would unwarrentedly subsume under the PURPOSIVE construction can be analysed as instances of the CAUSE-RESULT construction on account of the lexical meaning of the figure expressing a RESULT of the ACTIVITY designated by the ground:

(5) *shipping history, ageing effect, drug-taking experiences, manufacturing faults*

Dependent on the domain knowledge, figures expressing a MEASURE may also implicate a RESULT and therefore form part of the CAUSE-RESULT construction:

(6) *scanning rate, sorting time, manufacturing costs, switching delay*

Again, this is only half of the story. The majority of compounds with figures expressing a MEASURE instantiate the PURPOSIVE construction:

(7) *operating frequency, processing capacity, operating voltage, nesting level*

Whether the MEASURE implicates a RESULT or a CONDITION is not constrained semantically but by the domain-specific communicative purpose which imposes a particular intention on the ACTION designated by the ground nominal in relation to an implicated background nominal. As can be seen from Table 1 in the next section, with 699 tokens the number of figures conceptualized as MEASURE which generate the PURPOSIVE relation clearly surpasses the number of MEASURE nouns which compose the CAUSE-RESULT relation (256 tokens). With 0.01 their productivity ranges on the penultimate position of the PURPOSIVE relation, whereas the figures of the CAUSE-RESULT relation conceptualized as MEASURE are outright non-productive (0.00). These productivity measures are consonant with the reverse relative frequencies: with 0.655 the figures of the CAUSE-RESULT relation conceptualized as MEASURE clearly surpass the value of 0.194 calculated for the figures conceptualized as MEASURE in the PURPOSIVE relation. Within the PURPOSIVE construction the productivity of figure-ground relations increases to the degree that their relative frequency decreases. Both this inverse relationship within the PURPOSIVE construction and the comparison with the figures of the CAUSE-RESULT construction clearly evidence that the ground's derivation pattern is diagnostic of the compound's meaning in dependence of particular semantic and pragmatic configurations of figure and ground.

A comparison with German corroborates our radical analysis of a continuum of grammatical constructions (Croft, 2001, 6) in that the CAUSE-RESULT construction is in fact represented by a more encompassing valency structure. In the German compound *Herstellungsfehler* ("manufacturing defects") the so-called linking-*s* establishes a remnant of the genitive inflection (Krott et al., 2007, 27). This may be included as a dependent predication of the CAUSE-RESULT construction in order to augment the valency and thereby to shift the semantic type of language-specific lexical units, e.g. of English *manufacturing defects/ faults.* This higher-level cross-linguistic semantic analysis distinguishes the alternative meanings of superficially equivalent forms as instances of different constructions. In fact, both constructions establish near-antonyms as the respective constituent meanings generate a reversed asymmetry between figure and ground.

This analysis clearly verifies the meaning of the compound to result from the figure-ground asymmetry of the construction (Langacker, 1987, 306f). Although the morphological $V - ing_N$ structure of the ground is highly indicative of the compound's meaning, we also need to analyse the morpho-semantic structure of the figure, though not in the sense of schema theory as head-centred property matching, but in terms of the coded dependency between figure and ground, which in the less obvious cases would have to involve recourse to domain-specific knowledge. Categorizations on the level of domain-specific knowledge would require low-level schemas within the hierarchy of constructions which thus remain consonant with a purely associative model.

6.4 Results and discussion of the experiment

The results of the experiment clearly corroborate our hypothesis that the attribute-value structure of the ground is highly diagnostic of the relational meaning of the compound construction. As the figures in Table 1 indicate, the high productivity of the PURPOSIVE meaning of the $V - ing_N$N construction clearly correlates with the consistent ACTION nominalization of the ground.

Table 1. Productivity of figure-ground relations in the PURPOSIVE construction

Ground $V - ing_N$	$Figure_N$	Types	Tokens	Relative Frequency	Hapaxes	Productivity
Action	$\sum$	175	3611	1.000	51	0.014
Action	Medium	40	1691	0.468	9	0.005
Action	Measure	36	699	0.194	7	0.010
Action	Action	24	331	0.092	6	0.018
Action	Modality	19	270	0.075	6	0.022
Action	Instrument	11	221	0.061	5	0.023
Action	Manner	22	183	0.051	6	0.033
Action	Location	23	216	0.060	12	0.056

Table 2. Productivity of the CAUSE-RESULT construction

Ground $V - ing_N$	$Figure_N$	Types	Tokens	Relative Frequency	Hapaxes	Productivity
Action	$\sum$	21	391	1.000	3	0.008
Action	Measure	12	256	0.655	0	0.00
Action	Result	7	126	0.322	2	0.016
Action	State	2	9	0.023	1	0.111

Table 3. Productivity of figure-ground relations in the THEME-ACTION construction

Ground $V - ing_N$	Figure $V - suff_N$	Types	Tokens	Relative Frequency	Hapaxes	Productivity
Action	Action	6	15	1	2	0.133

Since the degree of activation results from the unification of the attribute-value structures of figure and ground, speakers need to store both construction schemas and the instances' decomposed constituents. As the number and diagnosticity of attributes represent the degree of unification between instance and schema, redundancy becomes the key to compositionality. The continuum of compositionality is represented in terms of the degree to which the attribute-value structure of the instance is included in the attribute-value structure of the construction. The figures in Table 1 and 2 represent the continuum of compositionality, in that the productivity of an attribute-value structure increases to the degree that its token frequency decreases. Thereby activation strength overcomes the dichotomy between whole-word storage and decomposition.

Our results thus replicate the findings of psycholinguistic studies (Bybee and Hopper, 2001; Bybee and Scheibman, 1999; Bush, 2001; Jurafsky et al., 2001; Hare et al., 2001). Accordingly, human memory has to be attributed huge storage capacities enabling this redundancy between grammar and lexicon (cf. Novak and Lamb, Tuggy, this volume). At the same time, this full-entry model minimizes computing time by lexicon and grammar converging towards a prototype organization (Croft and Cruse, 2004, 278). Speakers seem to memorize as much information as possible in a symbolically organized hierarchy of type-instance constructions, in order to minimize processing effort (Barsalou, 1992, 180f).

6.5 The ACTION *nominalizations in the conversion*

The symbolic unity of the $V - ing_N$ construction of the ground was furthermore corroborated by conducting a complementary experiment with 202 NN compounds in which a conversion derives the ground from a verb. Morphologically, the $V - \emptyset_N$ construction of the ground establishes a proper subpart of the $V - ing_N$ construction (Goldberg, 1995, 78f). Thereby the more specific attribute-value structure entails the more schematic attribute-value structure as a subpart. Through this subpart link the dominated construction is an instance of the dominating construction and thereby is motivated to the degree that it inherits the properties of the latter. Semantically, the conversion may denote an event schema, such as the ACHIEVEMENT and ACTIVITY concepts of the grounds in the compounds *trade-in car, combat car* and *patrol car*. By lacking the imperfectivizing -

ing derivation, the nominal conversions of these grounds do not code their dependency on the HABITUAL PURPOSE relation of the compound. In fact, the event schemas of their verbal bases are incompatible with an imperfectivizing *-ing* derivation. ACHIEVEMENTS, as in the compound *trade-in car*,[10] may not to be imperfectivized through *-ing* (Ryle, 1949, 53). ITERATIVE ACCOMPLISHMENTS, as in the compounds *combat car, patrol car*,[11] already express IMPERFECTIVITY. The ground *patrol* behaves in the same way. Apart from the compound *patrol car* this conversion only occurs in other multi-word units, as for instance in the bare construction of *to be on patrol.*

The same holds for the nominal sense of *prowl* which is not lexicalized independently of the idiom *to be on the prowl* and the compound *prowl car* is likely to have developed from *the police is on the prowl by car.*

We may conclude that in these lexicalization of the $V - \emptyset_N N$ construction the meanings of the ground block an imperfectivization through *-ing*. Due to this lack of symbolic unity, the $V - \emptyset_N$ construction of the ground may be assumed to be less diagnostic of the HABITUAL PURPOSE schema. Accordingly, our corpus-linguistic experiment does not verify a significant productivity of the PURPOSIVE relation for the $V - \emptyset_N N$ construction, as evidenced by the figures in Table 4.

[10] The BOUNDED event structure of the ground *trade-in* is symbolically motivated through the particle *in.* It embodies the transitive usage pattern of the ACHIEVEMENT concept expressing a GOAL to which the car as the THEME is transferred through the agent's force. Once this PATH OF MOTION has been traversed by the car, the MOTION terminates, it may not be reified, i.e. imperfectivized (Ryle, 1949, 53).

[11] In the compound *combat car*, the ITERATIVE manner of a force-dynamic motion event designated by the verb *to combat* is inherited by the nominal conversion. This UNBOUNDED concept likewise cannot additionally undergo imperfectivization through an *-ing* derivation.

Table 4. Productivity of the PURPOSIVE relation in the $V - \emptyset_N N$ construction

Relation	Purposive	Cause-Result	All
tokens	5397	342	6247
types	153	17	202
productivity	0.003	0.009	0,004

7 Conclusions

In this paper we have raised the issue of compositionality with compound meanings. More specifically, the analysability of compound meanings has been investigated with the trade-off between two memory functions: the speakers' storage and retrieval of lexical meanings. As our corpus-linguistic experiment points out, the hybrid role of compounds as multi-word units calls for a revision of the traditional lexicon-syntax distinction.

The meanings of compounds may be compositionally computed to a large extent. However, a significant proportion of compound meanings falls out from fully compositional procedures as their meanings are dependent on experience and domain knowledge in addition to consistently used lexical encodings. These contrasting poles of schematicity and idiosyncracy provide evidence for the process of composition to represent a gradient phenomenon. According to these empirical findings, the process of composition cannot be constrained by abstract principles of universal grammar to become maximally non-redundant. Instead, the continuum of compositionality has to be accounted for by maximally rich lexical representations. Resulting from frequency of activation these lexical representations continuously strive towards a prototype organization. This prototype organization has been shown to correspond to a hierarchy of constructions, ranging from low-level, weakly entrenched or even idiosyncratic schemas to high-level, deeply entrenched, even fully regular schemas. Computationally, these rich representations remain "cheap" by enabling speakers to unify the substructures which figure and ground share within the valency structures of constructions. By quantifying the constituents' unification of attribute-value structures (Langacker, 1987, 280f) we have pointed out the continuum of compositionality both by the asymmetry between autonomous and dependent predications along the syntagmatic dimension and the asymmetry between high-level and low-level schemas along the paradigmatic dimension. This redundancy between grammatical schemas and their lexical instantiations allows speakers to evaluate how well these more specific lexical representations fit into multiply competing more abstract grammatical constructions (Langacker 1987, 42; Goldberg 1995, 72ff). Our quantitative corpus-linguistic experiment has verified this competition among constructions to be symbolically motivated (Langacker, 1991, 532). The figures evidencing the constructions' activation strength indicate that the morphology of the ground is diagnostic of the compound meaning, in that the morphologically explicit $V - ing_N$N construction wins out against the $V - \emptyset_N N$ construction in symbolizing the HABITUAL PURPOSE schema.

Replicating the results of psycholinguistic studies in this way, our computation of a construction's degree of activation on the scale of compositionality may be taken to resolve the dichotomy between whole-word storage and morphological decomposition, i.e. the trade-off between storage and computation.

References

Aerts, Diederik and Liane Gabora. 2005. Quantum physics. A theory of concepts and their combination. *Kybernetes* 34(1/2): 151–175.

Aitchison, Jean. 1993. *Words in the Mind: An Introduction to the Mental Lexicon.* Oxford: Blackwell.

Baayen, R. Harald. 1992. Quantitative aspects of morphological productivity. In: Geert E. Booij and J. van Marle (eds.), *Yearbook of Morphology 1991*. Dordrecht: Kluwer, 227–254.

Baayen, R. Harald. 2000. *Word Frequency Distribution.* Dordrecht: Kluwer Academic Publishers.

Baayen, R. Harald and A. J. F. Dijkstra. 2003. Frequency effects in regular inflectional morphology: Revisiting Dutch plurals. In: R. Harald Baayen and Robert Schreuder (eds.), *Morphological Structure in Language Processing*. Berlin: Mouton de Gruyter, 355–390.

Barsalou, Lawrence W. 1992. *Cognitive Psychology: An Overview for Cogntive Scientists*. Hillsdale: Lawrence Erlbaum.

Bauer, Laurie. 1978. *The Grammar of Nominal Compounding with Special Reference to Danish, English, and French*. Odense: Odense University Press.

Bien, Heidrun, Willem J. M. Levelt and R. Harald Baayen. 2005. Frequency effects in compound production. In: *Proceedings of the National Academy of Sciences*, volume 102(49). 17876–17881.

Bloomfield, Leonard. 1933. *Language*. New York: Holt.

Brown, Cathrene (ed.). 1996. *Collins COBUILD English Learner's Dictionary*. London: Harper Collins Publishers.

Bush, Nathan. 2001. Frequency effects and word-boundary palatalization in English. In: Joan Bybee and Paul Hopper (eds.), *Frequency and the Emergence of Linguistic Structure*. Amsterdam: John Benjamins, 255–280.

Butterworth, B. 1983. Lexical representation. In: B. Butterworth (ed.), *Language Production*, volume 2: Development, Writing and other Language Processes. London: Academic Press, 257–294.

Bybee, Joan. 1995. Regular morphology and the lexicon. *Language and Cognitive Processes* 10: 425–455.

Bybee, Joan and Paul Hopper (eds.). 2001. *Frequency and the Emergence of Linguistic Structure*. Amsterdam: John Benjamins.

Bybee, Joan, Revere Perkins and William Pagliuca. 1994. *The Evolution of Grammar. Tense, Aspect, and Modality in the Languages of the World*. Chicago and London: The University of Chicago Press.

Bybee, Joan and Joanne Scheibman. 1999. The effect of usage on degrees of constituency: The reduction of *don't* in English. *Linguistics* 37: 575–596.

Bybee, Joan L. 1985. *Morphology: A Study of the Relation between Meaning and Form*. Amsterdam: John Benjamins.

Carl, Michael and Antje Schmidt-Wigger. 1998. Shallow post-morphological processing with KURD. In: D.M.W. Powers (ed.), *New Methods in Language Processing and Computational Natural Language Learning*. Conference on Computational Language Learning, Sydney, 257–265.

Clahsen, Harald. 1999. Lexical entries and rules of language: A multi-disciplinary study of German inflection. *Behavioral and Brain Sciences* 22: 991–1060.

Costello, Fintan and Mark T. Keane. 2000. Efficient creativity: Constraint-guided conceptual combination. *Cognitive Science* 24(2): 299–349.

Covington, Michael A. 1994. *Natural Language Processing for Prolog Programmers*. Englewood Cliffs: Prentice Hall.

Cowie, Anthony P. (ed.). 1989. *Oxford Advanced Learner's Dictionary of Current English*. 4th edition. Oxford: Oxford University Press.

Croft, William. 2001. *Radical Construction Grammar*. Oxford: Oxford University Press.

Croft, William and Allan D. Cruse. 2004. *Cognitive Linguistics*. Cambridge: Cambridge University Press.

Di Sciullo, A. and E. Williams. 1987. *On the Definition of Word*. Massachusetts: MIT Press.

Dowty, David. 2000. The garden swarms with bees' and the fallacy of 'argument alternation'. In: Yael Ravin and Claudia Leacock (eds.), *Polysemy. Theoretical and Computational Approaches*. Oxford: Oxford University Press, 111–128.

Dowty, David R. 1991. Thematic proto-roles and argument selection. *Language* 67(3): 547–619.

Estes, Z. and S. Glucksberg. 2000. Interactive property attribution in concept combination. *Memory and Cognition* 28(1): 28–34.

Estes, Zachary and Uri Hasson. 2004. The importance of being nonalignable: A critical test of the structural alignment theory of similarity. *Journal of Experimental Psychology: Learning, Memory, and Cognition* 30: 1082–1092.

Fillmore, Charles J. 1999. Inversion and constructional inheritance. In: Gert Webelhuth, Jean-Pierre Koenig and Andreas Kathol (eds.), *Lexical and Constructional Aspects of Linguistic Explanation*. Stanford, Calif.: CSLI Publications, 113–128.

Frauenfelder, Uli H. and Robert Schreuder. 1992. Constraining psycholinguistic models of morphological processing and representation: The role of productivity. In: Geert Booij and Jaap van Marle (eds.), *Yearbook of Morphology 1991*. Dordrecht: Foris, 165–183.

Gagné, Christina. 2002. The competition-among-relations-in nominals theory of conceptual combination: Implications for stimulus class formation and class expansion. *Journal of the Experimental Analysis of Behavior* 78: 551–565.

Gagné, Christina L. and Edward J. Shoben. 1997. Influence of thematic relations on the comprehension of modifier-noun combinations. *Journal of Experimental Psychology: Learning, Memory and Cognition* 23(1): 71–87.

Gentner, Dedre and V. Gunn. 2001. Structural alignment facilitates the noticing of differences. *Memory and Cognition* 29: 565–577.

Gindiyeh, Mahmoud, Christoph Rösener and Konrad Stockinger. 2008. Automatische Klassifikation von Gerichtsurteilen und juristischen Entscheidungen mit Hilfe von linguistischer Intelligenz. In: Angelika Storrer, Alexander Geyken, Alexander Siebert and Kay-Michael Würzner (eds.), *Text Resources and Lexical Knowledge*. Berlin, New York: Mouton de Gruyter, 97–105.

Goldberg, Adele. 1995. *Constructions. A Construction Grammar Approach to Argument Structure*. Chicago: University of Chicago Press.

Halle, Morris and K. Mohanan. 1985. Segmental phonology of Modern English. *Linguistic Inquiry* 16: 57–116.

Haller, Johann and Paul Schmidt. 2006. AUTINDEX - Automatische Indexierung. *Zeitschrift für Bibliothekswesen und Bibliographie* Sonderheft 89: 104–119.

Hampton, James. 1991. The combination of prototype concepts. In: Paula J. Schwanenflugel (ed.), *The Psychology of Word Meanings: A Publication of the Cognitive Studies Group and the Institute for Behavioral Research at the University of Georgia*. Hillsdale, N.J.: Erlbaum, 91–116. Psychology of Word Meaning Conference, University of Georgia.

Hare, Mary L., Michael Ford and William D. Marslen-Wilson. 2001. Ambiguity and frequency effects in regular verb inflection. In: Joan Bybee and Paul Hopper (eds.), *Frequency and the Emergence of Linguistic Structure*. Amsterdam: John Benjamins, 181–200.

Haspelmath, Martin. 2002. *Understanding Morphology*. London: Arnold.

Hay, Jennifer. 2001. Lexical frequency in morphology: Is everything relative? *Linguistics* 39(6): 1041–1070.

Jackendoff, Ray. 1997. Twistin' the night away. *Language* 73: 534–70.

Jong, Nivja Helena de. 2002. *Morphological Families in the Mental Lexicon*. Nijmegen: Max Planck Institute of Psycholinguistics.

Jurafsky, Daniel, Alan Bell, Michelle Gregory and William Raymond. 2001. Probabilistic relations between words: Evidence from reduction in lexical production. In: Joan Bybee and Paul Hopper (eds.), *Frequency and the Emergence of Linguistic Structure*. Amsterdam: John Benjamins, 229–254.

Kay, Martin. 1985. Parsing in functional unification grammar. In: David R. Dowty, Laury Karttunen and Arnold M. Zwicky (eds.), *Parsing Natural Language*. Cambridge: Cambridge University Press, 251–278.

Krott, Andrea, Robert Schreuder, R. Harald Baayen and Wolfgang U. Dressler. 2007. Analogical effects on linking elements in German compounds. *Language and Cognitive Processes* 22(1): 25–57.

Langacker, Ronald. 1987. *Foundations of Cognitive Grammar. Theoretical Prerequisites*, volume 1. Stanford: Stanford University Press.

Langacker, Ronald. 1991. *Foundations of Cognitive Grammar. Practical Applications*, volume 2. Stanford: Stanford University Press.

Levelt, Willem J. M. 1993. *Speaking : From Intention to Articulation*. Cambridge, Mass: MIT Press.

Lukatela, G., B. Gligorijevic and A. Kostic. 1980. Representation of inflected nouns in the internal lexicon. *Memory and Cognition* 8: 415–423.

Lynott, Dermot. 2003. The role of knowledge support in creating noun-noun compounds. In: *Proceedings of the Twenty-Fifth Conference of the Cognitive Science Society*. Hillsdale N. J.: Erlbaum, 746–751.

Lyons, John. 1977. *Semantics*, volume 2. Cambridge: Cambridge University Press.

Maas, Dieter. 1996. MPRO – Ein System zur Analyse und Synthese deutscher Wörter. In: R. Hausser (ed.), *Linguistische Verifikation, Sprache und Information*. Tübingen: Max Niemeyer, 141–166.

Maas, Heinz Dieter, Christoph Rösener and Axel Theofilidis. 2009. Morphosyntactic and semantic analysis of text: The MPRO tagging procedure. In: Cerstin Mahlow and Michael Piotrowski (eds.), *State of the Art in Computational Morphology*. Workshop on Systems and Frameworks for Computational Morphology, SFCM 2009, Zurich, Berlin: Springer, 76–87.

Marslen-Wilson, William, Lorraine Komisarjevsky Tyler, Rachelle Waksler and Lianne Older. 1994. Morphology and meaning in the English mental lexicon. *Psychological Review* 101(1): 3–33.

Medin, Douglas L. and Edward J. Shoben. 1988. Context and structure in conceptual combination. *Cognitive Psychology* 20: 158–190.

Messinger, Heinz. 2000. *Langenscheidts Handwörterbuch. Teil I Englisch-Deutsch*. Berlin: Langenscheidt.

Meyer, Ralf. 1993. *Compound Comprehension in Isolation and in Context*. Tübingen: Niemeyer.

Michaelis, Laura A. 2004. Type shifting in construction grammar: An integrated approach to aspectual coercion. *Cognitive Linguistics* 15(1): 1–67.

Murphy, Gregory L. 1988. Comprehending complex concepts. *Cognitive Science* 12: 529–562.

Murphy, Gregory L. and Douglas L. Medin. 1985. The role of theories in conceptual coherence. *Psychological Review* 92: 289–316.

Olson, Susan. 2000. Composition. In: Geert Booij, Christian Lehmann and Joachim Mugdan (eds.), *Morphologie. Ein Internationales Handbuch zur Flexion und Wortbildung*. Berlin: Walter de Gruyter, 897–916.

Palmer, F. R. 2001. *Mood and Modality*. Cambridge Textbooks in Linguistics. Cambridge: Cambridge University Press.

Pinker, Steven. 1999. *Words and Rules*. New York: Basic Books.

Pinker, Steven and M. Ullman. 2002. The past and the future of the past tense. *Trends in Cognitive Science* 6: 465–462.

Plag, Ingo. 2003. *Word-formation in English*. Cambridge Textbooks in Linguistics. Cambridge: Cambridge University Press.

Polinsky, Maria. 1996. Situation perspective: On the relations of thematic roles, discourse categories, and grammatical relations to figure and ground. In: Adele Goldberg (ed.), *Conceptual Structure, Discourse and Language*. Stanford: CSLI Publications, 401–419.

Quirk, Randolph, Sidnay Greenbaum, Geoffrey Leech and Jan Svartvik. 1985. *A Comprehensive Grammar of the English Language*. Essex: Longman.

Rickheit, Mechthild. 1993. *Wortbildung. Grundlagen einer Kognitiven Wortgrammatik*. Opladen: Westdeutscher Verlag.

Rumelhart, David E., G. E. Hinton and R. J. Williams. 1986. Learning internal representations by error propagation. In: David E. Rumelhart and James L. McClelland (eds.), *Parallel Distributed Processing*, volume 1. Cambridge, MA.: MIT Press, 318–364.

Ryder, Ellen Mary. 1993. *Ordered Chaos: English Noun-Noun Compounds*. Berkeley and Los Angeles: University of California Press.

Ryle, Gilbert. 1949. *The Concept of Mind*. New York: Barnes and Noble.

Sandra, Dominiek. 1990. On the representation and processing of compound words: Automatic access to constituent morphemes does not occur. *The Quarterly Journal of Experimental Psychology* 42A(3): 529–567.

Schreuder, Robert and R. Harald Baayen. 1995. Modeling morphological processing. In: L. B. Feldman (ed.), *Morphological Aspects of Language Processing.* Hillsdale: Lawrence Erlbaum, 345–364.

Seidenberg, Mark S. 1987. Sublexical structures in visual word recognition: Access units or orthographic redundancy? In: M. Colthaert (ed.), *Attention and Performance*, volume XII. Hove, UK: Lawrence Erlbaum, 245–264.

Seidenberg, Mark S. and Laura M. Gonnerman. 2000. Explaining derivational morphology as the convergence of codes. *Trends in Cognitive Sciences* 4: 353–36.

Sereno, J. A. and A. Jongman. 1997. Processing of English inflectional morphology. *Memory and Cognition* 25: 425–437.

Shoben, Edward J. 1991. Predicating and nonpredicating combinations. In: Paula J. Schwanenflugel (ed.), *The Psychology of Word Meanings: A Publication of the Cognitive Studies Group and the Institute for Behavioral Research at the University of Georgia.* Hillsdale, N.J.: Erlbaum, 117–135. Psychology of Word Meaning Conference, University of Georgia.

Simpson, John A. and E. S. C. Weiner (eds.). 1989. *The Oxford English Dictionary.* 2nd edition. Oxford: Clarendon Press. (Combined with a Supplement to the Oxford English Dictionary, edited by R. W. Buchfield. First edited by James A. H. Murray, Henry Bradley, W. A. Craige and C. T. Onions).

Stolz, Jennifer A. and Laurie Beth Feldman. 1995. The role of orthographic and semantic transparency of the base morpheme in morphological processing. In: Laurie Beth Feldman (ed.), *Morphological Aspects of Language Processing.* Hillsdale: Lawrence Erlbaum, 109–129.

Taft, M. and K. I. Forster. 1975. Lexical storage and retrieval of prefixed words. *Journal of Verbal Learning and Verbal Behaviour* 14: 638–647.

Talmy, Leonard. 2000a. *Toward a Cognitive Semantics, Concept Structuring Systems*, volume 1. Cambridge, Mass.: MIT Press.

Talmy, Leonard. 2000b. *Toward a Cognitive Semantics, Typology and Process in Concept Structuring*, volume 2. Cambridge, Mass.: MIT Press.

Taylor, John R. 2002. *Cognitive Grammar.* Oxford: Oxford University Press.

Valin, Jr., Robert D. van and Randy J. Lapolla. 1997. *Syntax. Structure, Meaning and Function.* Cambridge: Cambridge University Press.

Wisniewski, Edward J. 1997. When concepts combine. *Psychonomic Bulletin and Review* 4(2): 167–183.

Yang, C. D. 2000. Knowledge and learning in natural language. Unpublished doctoral dissertation, MIT, Cambridge, MA.

Zwitserlood, P. 1994. The role of semantic transparency in the processing and representation of dutch compounds. *Language and Cognitive Processes* 9: 341–368.

Language-dependent memory: Insights from bilingualism

Viorica Marian and Margarita Kaushanskaya

1 Language-dependent memory: An introduction

Nabokov, a bilingual Russian-English writer, gives a glimpse of what it is like for a bilingual to transfer memories across languages in this quote from the introduction to his autobiography: "[It] took a long time to write, a particularly agonizing labor, for memory was set in one way – musically under-spoken, Russian – and imposed upon it was a different way, English and thorough." (Nabokov, 1954, 1). Because memory and language are intrinsically intertwined and because the imprint of language on memory runs deep, likely influencing memory's every aspect – the structure, the rhythm, the content, the accessibility – recounting memories in a language other than the one in which they were originally 'set' is a task that is likely to redefine the memory itself. For people who speak two languages, the effect of language on memory can be dramatic. Bilinguals, by their very nature, experience the world around them in two languages, and this may have a profound effect on which events they remember, how well they remember them, and the actual content of these memories. For a bilingual, all the events and experiences that take place in life are marked for language, sometimes in a very vivid way, and sometimes in a more subtle way also experienced by monolinguals (for instance, the events experienced by monolinguals may be marked for dialect, register, or a speaker's voice quality). In this way, language becomes part of the memory trace, colors a bilingual's memory and may influence later recall.

In this chapter, we consider the relationship between language and memory via the prism of bilingualism and focus on the phenomenon of language-dependent memory. We suggest that language serves as a mental frame for encoded information, aiding recall and influencing accessibility and that language may also influence the actual content of memories. Language is a component of the overall environment in which events are taking place, and, just like with other types of contexts (Smith, 1988; Tulving and Thomson, 1973), where memory is improved when retrieval takes place in the same environment in which the material was learned, so is memory facilitated when an event is recalled in the same language in which it originally took place. In the first part of the chapter, the relationship between language and memory is explored in the context of Language-Dependent Memory (Marian and Neisser, 2000). We describe a series of experiments on language-dependent memory in bilinguals, considering both autobiographical and semantic memory. In the second part of the chapter, we center our attention on the influence of language on the content of bilinguals' memories, particularly the effect of language on the expressed self-concept. We suggest that in addition to influencing the accessibility of memory, language may also influence its content, either directly, by imposing linguistic constraints upon the conceptual system, or indirectly, by acting as a cue for the culture in which the particular language is used. In the final part of the chapter, we consider potential mechanisms underlying language-dependent memory, and propose directions for future research.

2 Context-dependent memory

The role of context in cognition has been considered in a number of domains. Gestalt psychologists, for instance, considered the interplay between focal and contextual information in perception, and the role that organizational cues play in encoding visual information (Wertheimer, 1938). It has been proposed that for remembering, context may serve as an organizational cue, triggering clusters of memories (Smith, 1988). For example, one may remember different kinds of information at the supermarket vs. the opera, or when coming down with a cold vs. when going on a date. As early as 1957, Greenspoon and Ranyard showed that a list of items learned in a brightly lit, noisy, and uncomfortable environment is better recalled in that environment than in a dimly lit, quiet, and comfortable environment

– and vice versa. The encoding specificity principle, introduced by Tulving and Thomson (1973), proposed that memories are context-dependent – that is, memory retrieval can be facilitated by putting the participant into the same environment, physical or emotional, in which the encoding originally took place (see Davis and Thomson (1988) for a review). Have you ever gone to get something from another room, forgot what you went to get, and had to return back to the original room to remember what it was you left for in the first place? Such occurrences illustrate the classical context-dependent memory phenomenon.

Experimental manipulation of contextual changes consisted of having participants learn and retrieve stimuli in dramatically different environments, such as underwater or on land (Godden and Baddeley, 1975, 1980), underwater or on a boat (Emmerson, 1986), and inside or outside a sensory deprivation device (Suedfeld and Eich, 1995). Godden and Baddeley (1975), for example, had divers learn lists of words in two natural environments – on dry land and underwater, and recall the words in either the environment of original learning or the alternative environment. Results showed that the lists learned underwater were recalled significantly better under water, and lists learned on dry land were recalled significantly better on dry land. Less drastic manipulations of context consisted of having participants learn stimuli in one room and testing their memory in either the same or a different room (Eich, 1980; Fernandez and Glenberg, 1985), or of manipulating screen color, item color, font, case, or stimulus location on a computer display (Murnane and Phelps, 1993, 1995). Similarly, manipulations of olfactory qualities of the environment have also led to context-dependency effects (Herz, 1997), with a distinctive odor found to be an effective retrieval cue. Such empirical studies are corroborated by anecdotal evidence of cases in which smells and odors evoke memories from days long gone.

Context-dependent memory seems to manifest itself very early in the developmental trajectory with evidence suggesting that the encoding specificity principle applies not only to adults, but also to children and infants. Studies by Rovee-Collier and colleagues, for instance, demonstrated that infants who had previously learned to vigorously kick their legs to activate a mobile attached to their feet with a string failed to generalize this knowledge to circumstances in which environmental differences were as small as the removal of the original bumper sheet from the crib (for reviews, see Rovee-Collier and Hayne (1987); Rovee-Collier and Shyi (1992). Rovee-Collier and colleagues suggested that infant memories are very specific and closely bound to the context in which they were acquired, so that changes to the context in which the infants acquired the memory often resulted in failure to retrieve the memory at testing.

Context may refer to an external environment, such as a room, a field, or a boat, or to an internal state, such as happiness, boredom, or nostalgia. External context, also called environmental context, arises outside the subject, while internal context arises from within the subject (and is also referred to as state-dependency). The distinction between external and internal contexts has long been part of the context-dependent memory discussion. Smith (1988, 31) proposed that the difference between the two is at the operational definition level only, since internal context is manipulated via external forces and external context must be internally represented to cue memory and that both are externally manipulated and internally represented. In a way, Smith expressed the position that almost every memory phenomenon is environmentally context-dependent. On the other hand, Suedfeld and Eich (1995) took the opposing view that almost every memory phenomenon is internally context-dependent. They proposed that environmental state-dependent effects are mediated by alterations in affect or mood and that data that on the surface appear to demonstrate place-dependent memory may, at a deeper level, denote the presence of mood-dependent memory (Suedfeld and Eich, 1995). Most of the time, however, external and internal contexts go hand in hand and different internal contexts accompany different environmental contexts. For example, being at a Hawaiian beach differs from being in a university classroom in environmental context, and it also differs in internal context: relaxed vs. tense, rested vs. tired. Such simultaneous differences in both the environmental and the internal contexts are common occurrences in everyday life.

Multiple underlying mechanisms have been proposed as possible explanations for the effect of context on memory. For instance, *how* the material is encoded may be an important factor. Tulving and Thomson proposed that "Specific encoding operations performed on what is perceived determine what is stored, and what is stored determines what retrievalcues are effective in providing access to what is stored" (1973, 369). McDaniel et al. (1989) conducted a series of experiments in which participants were instructed to use different encoding strategies. They found diminished context-dependency when subjects employed imagery at the time of encoding, organized the input material into sets, used self-referent encoding, and when the input described implausible and bizarre events. These findings suggest that dependence on environmental context cues is partly a function of the degree to which available retrievalcues are provided by the target encoding.

Another factor proposed to explain the effect of context on memory is the relationship between the context at encoding and the information that is being encoded. For example, Fernandez and Glenberg (1985) proposed that whether the events are construed as being causally related to a given environment, rather than simply contiguous with it, will play an important role in finding environmental context-dependent memory. Baddeley and Woodhead (1982), when considering the perceived relationship between context and stimuli in recognition memory, suggested that when stimulus and context bear an arbitrary relationship to each other and are perceived as such by the subject, the addition of the appropriate context or its deletion or substitution by another will have no influence on recognition performance.

These and other hypotheses – the Outshining hypothesis (Smith et al., 1978), the Integration hypothesis (Baddeley and Woodhead, 1982; Godden and Baddeley, 1980; Dalton, 1993), the Experimental Context hypothesis (Fernandez and Glenberg, 1985), the Familiarity hypothesis (Dalton, 1993), the SAM hypothesis (Gillund and Shiffrin, 1984), the Sensitivity hypothesis, the Situational Context hypothesis, and the General Context Model hypothesis (Murnane and Phelps, 1995) – individually and in combination can account for different aspects of context-dependent memory data, but the exact mechanisms driving it remain unclear.

The hypothesis of language-dependent memory is an extension of the encoding specificity principle into the domain of language. It proposes that language is part of the context, and exerts the same effect on memory as other contextual elements. Language is likely to simultaneously include both external and internal components, for language, especially in a bilingual, serves both as part of one's external context (with many memories characterized by linguistic interaction – either a conversation that one took part in during the remembered event, or din of others talking in the background while the event was taking place) and internal context (internal dialogue, linguistic encoding of information, and language as a mental frame).

While linguistic environments at encoding and retrieval may differ for speakers of a single language (e.g., listening to the same vs. different speaker at encoding and retrieval), nowhere is language-dependent memory more evident than in the differences of linguistic environments experienced by bilingual speakers. By studying the language-dependent memory phenomenon through the prism of bilingualism, at least two predictions for the influence of language on memory accessibility can be specified. First, for a bilingual speaker it should be easier to recount events in the same linguistic environment in which they originally took place, and second, a bilingual speaker should remember information better if tested in the same language in which it was learned. These principles are expected to apply both to episodic memories (autobiographical memories of personal nature), and to semantic memories (general memories of everyday knowledge). The distinction between episodic memory and semantic memory refers to the distinction between memory for personal events experienced at a specific time or place, the specific 'episodes' that make up a life, while semantic memory is the internal collection of facts and figures, comprising knowledge of the world (Tulving, 1985, 1993). A series of experiments tested the language-dependent memory hypothesis for both types of memory, episodic and semantic.

3 Episodic memory and language in bilinguals

Although language is likely to always play a role in retrieval of autobiographical memory, a good place to begin the study of language-dependent memory effects is in bilingual contexts, as demonstrated by a study of autobiographical recall in Russian-English bilinguals (Marian and Neisser, 2000). Autobiographical life narratives of Russian-English bilinguals were collected by providing the participants with cue words in either Russian or English, and asking them to recount the first memory that came to mind after hearing the word (Marian and Neisser, 2000). Each memory was then coded for the language in which the events described took place. For instance, if the person, upon hearing the word *summer*, told a story of spending summer vacation visiting his grandmother in a village in the vicinity of Moscow, the memory was coded as Russian at encoding. Results revealed that bilinguals accessed more memories when languages at encoding and retrieval matched than when they mismatched, i.e., Russian-English bilinguals accessed more Russian memories when interviewed in Russian, and more English memories when interviewed in English. Moreover, they were faster accessing Russian memories when interviewed in Russian than when interviewed in English, and faster accessing English memories when interviewed in English than when interviewed in Russian.

In order to localize the effect of language on memory, the experimenters crossed the language of the word prompt with the general language of the interview in a follow-up experiment. For each interview language, half of the prompt words were presented in English and half in Russian, therefore yielding four conditions (Russian interview/Russian prompt words, Russian interview/English prompt words, English interview/English prompt words, and English interview/Russian prompt words). The reasoning behind this manipulation was that, on the one hand, language-dependent memory may be due to the prompt-words, i.e. hearing the word *birthday* evokes a situation in which the word was used, which, in this case, is likely to have taken place during life in the United States, and in English. On the other hand, speaking a particular language may create an overall linguistic context, which exerts influence on memory beyond that of a particular word used to trigger the memory. Results revealed that both variables – word prompt language and the overall linguistic environment – were driving language-dependent memory.

Furthermore, when bilingual autobiographical narratives were analyzed for frequency of code-switches (overt switches to the other language using words from that language), it was found that code-switching behavior was influenced by the match/mismatch between languages of encoding and interview (Marian and Kaushanskaya, 2007a). That is, Russian-English bilinguals interviewed in English code-switched to Russian more for memories that were encoded in Russian than for memories that were encoded in English. It appears, therefore, that the match between language of encoding and language of retrieval influences the accessibility of memories not only by influencing which memories are retrieved, but also the ease with which they are reported.

In a follow-up to Marian and Neisser (2000), autobiographical memories of Russian-English bilinguals were analyzed for emotional intensity (Marian and Kaushanskaya, 2004). Each memory was coded for intensity of the expressed emotion using a Likert scale. Results revealed that memories tended to be higher in emotional intensity when the languages of encoding and retrieval matched than when they did not match. Thus, it appears that emotional expression is strengthened by reinstating the encoding language at the time of speaking. This finding is consistent with the overall hypothesis of language-dependent memory, and extends it to content aspects of episodic memory, in addition to memory accessibility and retrieval efficiency.

The notion that both accessibility and emotional intensity of episodic memories are facilitated by the match between the languages of retrieval and encoding is supported by other studies of autobiographical memories. Otoya (1987) used the word-prompt methodology to examine the effect of cultural transition and language on autobiographical memory in Spanish speakers, who learned English as a second language. She found that, although the effect did not hold for all word-prompts, some Spanish word prompts triggered earlier memories than their English translation equivalents. Other measures, such as internal language of retrieval (i.e., asking bilinguals in which language a memory 'came to them' internally, as in Schrauf and Rubin (1998), also corroborate the Marian and Neisser findings. Schrauf and Rubin (1998) studied the internal language phenomenon in Spanish-English bilinguals, and found that memories recalled internally in Spanish tended to come from the pre-immigration stage of the participants' life, while memories recalled internally in English tended to cluster within the post-immigration age. Evidence for language-dependent memory can also be found in psychoanalytic literature. For instance, Javier et al. (1993) found that memories of bilinguals tend to be richer and more elaborate when retrieved in the language of encoding. Together, these studies of autobiographical memories in bilinguals illustrate the effects of language on episodic memory and provide evidence for language-dependent memory effects in autobiographical remembering.

4 Semantic memory and language in bilinguals

The finding that Russian-English bilinguals retrieved more Russian autobiographical memories when interviewed in Russian, and more English autobiographical memories when interviewed in English Marian and Neisser (2000), demonstrated the language-dependent memory phenomenon experimentally. It also prompted questions about the universal nature of language-dependent memory effects. Is language-dependent memory characteristic of autobiographical retrieval only, or does it extend to other types of memory? To answer this question, Marian and Fausey (2006) and Marian and Kaushanskaya (2007b) tested semantic memories of Spanish-English and Mandarin-English bilinguals in an attempt to generalize the language-dependent memory hypothesis to other types of memory and other groups of bilingual speakers. Marian and Fausey focused on memory for academic-type knowledge, and Marian and Lu focused on memory for real-life semantic information.

4.1 Semantic memory and language in academic learning

Marian and Fausey (2006) tested Chilean Spanish-English bilinguals in an academic setting, and taught them story-form information about History, Biology, Chemistry, and Mythology in two languages, English and Spanish. The stories contained fictitious but reasonable information in order to make the content meaningful while at the same time preventing previous knowledge of the material. The mythology story described a myth associated with celebrating the beginning of winter held by a fictitious group of people. The history story described the causes, course, and consequences of a war between two fictitious nations. The biology story described the flora of a fictitious island. The chemistry story described the accidental discovery and properties of a fictitious chemical element. The participants were then tested in either English or Spanish and answers were coded for accuracy of retrieved information and speed of retrieval (reaction time).

Spanish-English bilinguals showed a language-dependent memory pattern for both response accuracy and response speed when answering questions about the stories they heard. Bilinguals produced more correct answers, and responded faster, when the languages of encoding (story language) and retrieval (question language) matched than when they did not match. Subsequent analyses of response accuracy data revealed that the relative proficiency in the bilinguals' two languages mediated the language-dependent memory pattern, so that only *balanced* bilinguals, with similar levels of understanding in both English and Spanish, remembered information more accurately when the languages of encoding and retrieval matched than when they did not match. For *unbalanced* bilinguals (those who were better at understanding Spanish than English), accuracy in the match and mismatch conditions did not differ significantly. Both balanced and unbalanced bilinguals showed language-dependent memory patterns in speed of response data. Thus, accessibility of semantic memories in bilinguals appears to be influenced by proficiency in the two languages. This influence of proficiency on language-dependent memory may be easier to uncover in studies of semantic retrieval, because while autobiographical memories are subjective and cannot be scored for accuracy, semantic memories are based on factual information and can be judged as either accurate or inaccurate.

The Marian and Fausey findings corroborate the language-dependent memory hypothesis, and extend it to semantic memory. This study is consistent with monolingual research on the role of context in semantic memory for linguistic material. For instance, Tulving and colleagues found that semantic context played a critical role in remembering linguistic material such as word pairs (Thomson and Tulving, 1970; Tulving, 1972; Tulving and Thomson, 1973). Higham (2002) showed that cue-reinstatement facilitated retrieval of learned word pairs, and Thornton et al. (2002) found that retrieval of semantic memories in patients with Multiple Sclerosis who have memory deficits is facilitated by evoking the contextual environment in which semantic information was learned. Studies with monolingual speakers also suggest that using language with similar phonological features at encoding and retrieval improves some types of learning and memory (Bradlow et al., 1999; Nygaard et al., 2000; Singh et al., 2004). The experiment on context-dependent memory in academic learning extends laboratory-style research (using syllables and word lists) to more ecologically-valid research (using information students are likely to learn in science and humanities classes).

4.2 Semantic memory and language in real life knowledge

The Marian and Fausey study extended the hypothesis of language-dependent memory to semantic memory, specifically, to remembering academic information akin to the kind of information learned in educational contexts. The question remained whether language dependency influenced other types of semantic memory, and generalized to everyday, real-life knowledge. This question was the focus of Marian and Kaushanskaya (2007b) study.

Marian and Lu examined semantic memories of Mandarin-English bilingual speakers who were educated in both China and the United States. Bilingual participants were interviewed in both Mandarin and English, and were asked to recall common-knowledge information about the everyday world, such as geographical landmarks, famous personalities, and literary characters. At the end of the experiment, each participant was asked to indicate in which language the information was learned, Chinese or English. The question of interest was whether Mandarin-English bilinguals would retrieve more information, and be faster during retrieval in the match conditions than in the mismatch conditions. Findings corroborate those of Marian and Fausey, and indicate that language influences accessibility of semantic memories. Mandarin-English bilinguals retrieved significantly more information when the language of the interview matched the language in which that information was learned than when the two did not match.

In sum, both Marian and Fausey (2006) and Marian and Kaushanskaya (2007b) found evidence for language-dependent semantic memory. When considered together with earlier research on language-dependent memory in autobiographical narratives (Marian and Neisser, 2000), evidence for language-dependent memory appears reliable. In the next section, we consider the idea that language influences not only the accessibility of memories, but also their content. We mentioned the effect of language on emotional content earlier. Next, we focus on such content effects as representation of the self. Because language was found to influence autobiographical retrieval, and because autobiographical memories are linked with a person's identity, language-dependent memory effects on content, if they exist, are likely to be seen in self-construal. The influence of language on self representation is considered within the framework of linguistic relativity, according to which mental representations are language-specific.

5 Language and self-concept in bilinguals

Linguistic context at the time of memory encoding and retrieval may influence not only the accessibility of memories, but also their content. The idea that language influences thought has been conceptualized in terms of the linguistic relativity hypothesis, which is based on the differences between languages of the world on the one hand, and the subjective worldview on the other hand. In one of the most cited quotes on linguistic relativity, the linguistic anthropologist Edward Sapir wrote: "Human beings do not live in the objective world alone, nor alone in the world of social activity as ordinarily understood, but are very much at the mercy of the particular language which has become the medium of expression for their society." (1958, 209). Sapir's student, Benjamin Lee Whorf, further proposed that "we dissect nature along lines laid down by our native languages. The categories and types that we isolate from the world of phenomena we do not find there because they stare every observer in the face; on the contrary, the world is presented in a kaleidoscopic flux of impressions which has to be organized by our minds – and this means largely by the linguistic systems in our minds" (1940, 213).

The work of Sapir and Whorf laid the framework for what is now known as the Sapir-Whorf hypothesis. The stronger version of the hypothesis, *Linguistic Determinism*, proposes that if a language does not contain a linguistic label for a concept, the speakers of that language will not possess that concept. The weaker version of the hypothesis, *Linguistic Relativity*, states that language does not determine thought, but *influences* cognition by imposing certain constraints on the mental processes. Linguistic determinism has not found much support in empirical studies. For instance, even though the Dani language has only two words for color – *light* and *dark*, Dani people are able to differentiate other colors of the spectrum, i.e., red, blue, green, etc. (Rosch, 1972; Rosch and Olivier, 1972). While the effect of language on thought has not been found across the board (Malt et al., 2003; Li and Gleitman, 2002), evidence for a weaker version of linguistic relativity has been found in a number of domains. For instance, speakers of languages that grammaticize gender of inanimate objects tend to categorize objects based on gender similarities (Boroditsky et al., 2003), and speakers of a language that employ an absolute system of spatial reference (east/west) tend to have a better sense of direction than speakers of a language with a relative frame of reference (left/right) (Levinson, 1996). We propose that language influences not only how speakers of a language represent the external world, but, in a similar manner, how they represent their internal world, their self construal. As Kerby wrote, "The self is to be construed not as a prelinguistic given that merely employs language, much as we might employ a tool, but rather as a product of language" (1991, 4-5).

In this sense, when considered within the framework of linguistic relativity, the effect of language on memory and its content may consist of influencing the representation of the self – the way one chooses to describe oneself, one's behavior, feelings, etc.. As Gibson pointed out "Information about the self accompanies information about the environment, and the two are inseparable" (1979, 126). Multiple studies (see Wilson and Ross (2003) for a review) have shown that the way people talk about themselves and their personal experiences influences the way they remember events, with the past continuously rewritten to accommodate the ever-changing self-construal, and with self-construal frequently altered to accommodate memory. Since memory of past events influences a person's self and perception of oneself in relation to the social environment, we hypothesized that for a bilingual, speaking a particular language may influence his or her self-construal.

Marian and Kaushanskaya (2003, 2004) explored the influence of language on memory content by studying the effect of language on self-construal within the context of autobiographical memory in bicultural Russian-English bilinguals, focusing on the individualist/collectivist aspect of the self. The extent to which the self is defined in relation to society, and thus formulates the very basis of human behavior, is often seen as being located on the individualism-collectivism continuum (Triandis, 1995). In individualistic cultures, behaviors and attitudes are attributed to the individual's likes and dislikes, while in collectivist cultures, an individual is seen as part of the whole, and a person's behavior is seen as reflecting influences of society (Chiu, 1972; Heine and Lehman, 1995; Hong et al., 2000; Kitayama et al., 2002; Matsumoto et al., 2002; Ross et al., 2002). On the cultural dimension of individualism-collectivism, the former Soviet Union has been rated as more collectivist (Chirkov et al., 2003; Diener et al., 2000; Hofstede, 2001; Realo and Allik, 1999), while the United States has been rated as more individualistic (Hofstede, 1980;

Triandis, 1995). Marian and Kaushanskaya (2004) examined whether Russian-English bilinguals' self-construal is more collectivist in Russian narratives than in English narratives, and more individualistic in English narratives than in Russian narratives. Previously, differences in self-construal have been observed for bilinguals completing questionnaires in their two languages (Ross et al., 2002).

In Marian and Kaushanskaya (2004) study, frequency of personal pronoun usage was used as the linguistic measure of individualism-collectivism. When narratives were analyzed for personal pronoun usage, it was found that bilinguals tended to describe events using different pronouns depending on the language they were speaking at the time. It was found that Russian-English bilinguals tended to use more 1st person singular pronouns, such as *I, me, mine* when speaking English, but tended to use more 1st person plural pronouns, such *We, Us, Ours* when speaking Russian.

In addition to a linguistic measure of individualism-collectivism, a non-linguistic measure coding for the main actor in the story was also used. We predicted that when speaking English, bilinguals would produce more stories in which they themselves were the main actor, but when speaking Russian, bilinguals would produce more stories in which the role of main actor was shared with other people. Indeed, this is what was found: Russian-English bilinguals tended to tell stories in which they themselves were the main actors when telling stories in English, but when telling stories in Russian, Russian-English bilinguals tended to tell stories in which they shared the spotlight with someone else.

Both the linguistic measure (frequency of personal pronoun usage) and the non-linguistic measure (main actor) converged to suggest that Russian-English bilinguals expressed a more individualistic self-construal when speaking English, and a more collectivist self-construal when speaking Russian. In that sense, self-representations appear to be highly fluid, and shift in response to a language cue. When speaking Russian, a Russian-English bilingual will project a self-schema more in line with the Soviet, collectivist view, while when speaking English, the pattern will be reversed. This is akin to findings from the cognitive domain of SPACE, where a person can utilize multiple systems of spatial orientation, but tends to use the system imposed by the language he or she speaks (Levinson, 1996).

Given the experimental design of the study, it is difficult to attribute the effect of shifting self-representations to either language or culture. While it is possible that the bias in describing events using 1st person singular pronouns may influence the person's self-construal, it may also be that the bias of pronoun usage itself is due to the individualistic values of the American culture, which seep into language. In fact, the difficulty of teasing apart linguistic and cultural influences on cognitive processes is ubiquitous – language and culture are tightly connected, and cultural affiliations are often defined by shared language. It is difficult, if not impossible, to separate the two in a viable experimental manner, and often, the joint influence of both language and culture on thought has been demonstrated. For instance, Nisbett (2003) suggests that a tendency of Westerners to focus on object categories and a tendency of Easterners to focus on relationship between objects during a categorization task can be attributed to both the difference in the languages spoken in the two parts of the world (nouns, which are referential in nature, predominate in Western languages, like English and German, but verbs, which are relational in nature, predominate in Eastern languages, like Mandarin Chinese and Korean), and to the cultural differences between East and West, with the West encouraging individualism, and the East encouraging collectivism. It is clear that both language and culture contribute to the representations and processes involved in self-construal and now that language dependency effects on self representation have been observed, further studies can consider language dependency effects on memory content in domains that are not sensitive to cultural differences.

6 Language-dependent memory: Principles and mechanisms

Studying the interaction between language and memory in bilinguals provides a fertile ground for exploring theories of language-dependent recall, linguistic relativity, and self-concept. In a series of experiments on language-dependent memory with multiple groups of bilingual speakers, language was shown to act similarly to other types of context, and influence accessibility of memories. Memories were more accessible when retrieved in the same language in which they were originally encoded, and the retrieval process was more efficient when the language of retrieval matched the language of learning. As with many phenomena in the field of bilingual research, the effect of language-dependency was influenced by bilinguals' relative proficiency in the two languages. However, language-dependent memory appeared to be a robust enough phenomenon to play a role in both episodic and semantic remembering, as well as in representation of the self. Moreover, language dependent memory was found not only for memories that may have been verbally retrieved before, and thus rehearsed linguistically (like the autobiographical memories in the Marian and Neisser study), but also for memories that have never been retrieved before (like the semantic learning in the Marian and Fausey study). This suggests that while previous experience retrieving memories in a particular language may contribute to language dependent effects in some settings, other processes may offer better accounts of language-dependent memory and are therefore considered below.

The reliability of language-dependent memory may lie in the markedness of language. It is possible that for bilingual speakers, the linguistic cue is stronger than any other environmental contextual cue. For bilinguals, the language spoken at any time marks the events that take place around them, thus making language a highly salient part of encoding. In fact, it may be that in a bilingual's daily life, the language chosen to convey information serves to denote a change in meaning. On the other hand, we are inclined to predict that even in circumstances in which the choice of language is entirely arbitrary, language dependent memory will still be observed. Baddeley's (1982) suggestion – that when stimulus and context bear an arbitrary relationship to each other and are perceived as such, the addition of the appropriate context or its deletion or substitution by another will have no influence – may not hold for language dependent memory. That is, a bilingual may show language-dependent memory even in circumstances in which the relationship between content and language is arbitrary. One could empirically test the role of the relationship between stimulus and language context in an experiment in which bilinguals are presented with lists of words in either one or the other of their languages and memory is later tested in match or mismatch conditions. Our prediction is that memory for word lists would be better in the match than the mismatch conditions, in spite of the absence of a meaningful relationship between stimuli and language. We would also expect language-dependent memory effects to arise in situations in which language of encoding is not easily identifiable (e.g., when recalling a conversation with another fluent bilingual with whom one frequently uses both languages, making it difficult to recall in what language this particular conversation took place). These predictions are rooted in the observed generalizability of the language-dependent memory phenomenon and build on the hypothesis that language markedness is so strong that it persists in spite of absence of any meaningful relationship between input and language.

Language-dependent memory phenomena are situated within the field of context-dependent memory, and follow the same principles as other contexts subsumed by the encoding specificity principle. However, language-dependent memory may also be underlied by cognitive mechanisms that are specific to language. For instance, Slobin (2003, 177) noted that "it is quite likely that the language in which information is presented - both fictional and documentary - plays a role in the ways in which information is stored and evaluated." Slobin has also suggested that listeners and observers encode information so that it is easy to express linguistically. Encoding information in a way that will be consistent with subsequent retrieval can be formulated as a 'thinking for potential speaking' extension of Slobin's 'thinking for speaking' hypothesis. When applied to bilingual speakers, language-dependent retrieval may be related to bilinguals' expectations about the match and mismatch in the encoding and retrieval languages.

Bilinguals often have well-defined expectations for when they will have to speak each language. If bilinguals have expectations about when encoding and retrieval linguistic contexts will match, they might attend more heavily to those linguistic distinctions important to the encoding language rather than those of their other language. If bilinguals expect to face a linguistic context at the time of retrieval that is different from the linguistic context at the time of encoding, they may adjust their encoding strategies and encode different information than the kind of information they might encode if they expected the environments at encoding and retrieval to match. The outcome of this strategy may be the advantage experienced by bilinguals when retrieving information in the same language in which it was encoded, similar to the advantage that language-dependent memory predicts.

In addition to Slobin's 'thinking for potential speaking', another possible mechanism for language-dependent memory may be tied to mental representations underlying linguistic expression, and rely on principles of linguistic relativity. Within the framework of linguistic relativity, the content of memory may be affected by the language used to encode and retrieve memories. Language may be influencing how people remember events by imposing a specific worldview through the linguistic structure and cognitive dimensions it grammaticizes. Levinson writes, "...given the architecture of the [cognitive] system, once one puts serious semantic constraints on the output, the rest of the system will be forced to support, code, and operate on those features. And so the imprint of language-specific categories will run deep in cognitive processes" (2003, 301). For bilingual speakers, it may be the case that a match of encoding and retrieval linguistic contexts promotes recall of language-specific *representations.* These language-specific representations may act as an additional mechanism driving language-dependent memory. Most likely, a combination of mechanisms – language markedness, encoding strategy adjustments in 'thinking for potential speaking', language-specific representations, language as a mental frame and a cue – actively interact to yield language-dependent memory effects in bilingual learning. Further research is necessary to fully understand the complex relationship among the many interacting variables.

Research on interactions between language and memory in bilingual speakers carries multiple applied implications for the fields of psychotherapy, witness testimony, and education. For instance, the finding that, for Chilean Spanish-English bilinguals, information is more accessible when probed in the same language in which it was encoded, may provide at least a partial explanation for lower academic achievement levels reported for Hispanic students tested in US American schools (Coltrane, 2002; Llagas, 2003), who are likely to have encoded at least some semantic information in their first language and had to retrieve it in the academic context of the second language. Similarly, the finding that emotional expression is stronger when the languages of encoding and retrieval match than when they mismatch, as in Marian and Kaushanskaya (2004), may have direct consequences for psychotherapy, and be a more reliable tool for accessing memories than the traditionally used distinction of the native vs. second language (Bond and Lai, 1986; Gonzalez-Reigosa, 1976).

The generalizability of language dependency to different types of memory is thought-provoking, given that the ultimate goal of learning (especially in an educational setting) is to decontextualize knowledge. Future experiments on language-dependent memory could vary the length of time between learning and testing as well as the surface form of material and of questions probing learning, and could incorporate rehearsal components as well as cross-modal learning and testing (e.g., written language). It will also be useful to examine whether language is an important element of context for bilingual speakers only, or whether language-dependent memory would also reveal itself in bi-dialectal speakers (for instance speakers of Standard American English and African American English) and across different linguistic registers. These manipulations would enable us to test the ubiquity of language dependent memory and the different variables that influence its magnitude.

We'll close with the example of Mr. M. (Aragno and Schlachet, 1996), a bilingual client undergoing psychotherapy in English whose treatment breakthrough occurred when he translated a word from one of his dreams from English to Spanish (the language of his childhood). In a recurrent dream involving a bear, a cursive translation of the word *bear* to the Spanish *orso* jolted M.'s memory by cueing an association to someone whose nickname was Orso. The English translation equivalent did not provide access to the dream's meaning, the original Spanish label did. M.'s case falls somewhere at the extreme end of the continuum of language dependent memory effects, yet it is an example of language dependent memory as described and studied in this chapter. For those who speak two languages, language choice and use at encoding and retrieval may matter a great deal and may carry cognitive and emotional consequences.

Acknowledgements

The authors would like to thank Caitlin Fausey for her contributions to this work, Henrike Blumenfeld, Li Sheng, and Margarit Tadevosyan for their comments, and the National Institute of Health NICHD 1R03HD046952 grant for support.

References

Aragno, A. and P. Schlachet. 1996. Accessibility of early experience through the language of origin: A theoretical integration. *Psychoanalytic Psychology* 13: 23–34.

Baddeley, Alan D. and M. Woodhead. 1982. Depth of processing, context, and face recognition. *Canadian Journal of Psychology* 36: 148–164.

Bond, M. H. and T. M. Lai. 1986. Embarrassment and code-switching into a second language. *Journal of Social Psychology* 126: 179–186.

Boroditsky, L., L. Schmidt and W. Phillips. 2003. Sex, syntax, and semantics. In: D. Gentner and S. Goldin-Meadow (eds.), *Language in Mind: Advances in Study of Language and Cognition*. Boston: MIT Press, 61–79.

Bradlow, A. R., L. C. Nygaard and D. B. Pisoni. 1999. Effects of talker, rate and amplitude variation on recognition memory for spoken words. *Perception and Psychophysics* 61(2): 206–219.

Chirkov, V., R. M. Ryan, Y. Kim and U. Kaplan. 2003. Differentiating autonomy from individualism and independence: A self-determination theory perspective on internalization of cultural orientation and well-being. *Journal of Personality and Social Psychology* 84: 97–110.

Chiu, L. H. 1972. A cross-cultural comparison of cognitive styles in Chinese and American children. *International Journal of Psychology* 8: 232–242.

Coltrane, B. 2002. English language learners and high stakes tests: An overview of the issues. *ERIC Digest* Retrieved October 1, 2003, from htttp://www.cal.org.ericcll/ DIGEST.

Dalton, P. 1993. The role of stimulus familiarity in context-dependent recognition. *Memory & Cognition* 21: 223–234.

Davis, G. M. and D. M. Thomson. 1988. *Memory in Context: Context in Memory.* Chichester, UK: Wiley.

Diener, E., C. L. Gohm, E. Suh and S. Oishi. 2000. Summarity of the relations between marital status and subjective well-being across cultures. *Journal of Cross-Cultural Psychology* 31: 419–436.

Eich, E. 1980. The cue-dependent nature of state-dependent retrieval. *Memory and Cognition* 8: 157–173.

Emmerson, P. G. 1986. Effects of environmental context on recognition memory in an unusual environment. *Perceptual and Motor Skills* 63: 1047–1050.

Fernandez, A. and A. M. Glenberg. 1985. Changing environmental context does not reliably affect memory. *Memory & Cognition* 13: 333–345.

Gibson, J. J. 1979. *The Ecological Approach to Visual Perception.* Boston: Houghton Mifflin.

Gillund, G. and R. M. Shiffrin. 1984. A retrieval model for both recognition and recall. *Psychological Review* 91: 1–67.

Godden, D. and A. Baddeley. 1980. When does context influence recognition memory? *The British Journal of Psychology* 71: 99–104.

Godden, D. R. and A. D. Baddeley. 1975. Context-dependent memory in two natural environments: On land and underwater. *The British Journal of Psychology* 66: 325–331.

Gonzalez-Reigosa, F. 1976. The anxiety-arousing effect of taboo words in bilinguals. In: C. D. Spielberger and R. Diaz-Guerrero (eds.), *Cross-cultural Anxiety*. Washington, DC: Hemisphere, 89–105.

Heine, S. J. and D. R. Lehman. 1995. Cultural variation in unrealistic optimism: Does the west feel more invulnerable than the east? *Journal of Personality and Social Psychology* 68: 595–607.

Herz, R. S. 1997. The effects of cue distinctiveness on odor-based context-dependent memory. *Memory and Cognition* 25: 375–380.

Higham, P. A. 2002. Strong cues are not necessarily weak: Thomson and Tulving (1970) and the encoding specificity principle revisited. *Memory & Cognition* 30: 67–80.

Hofstede, G. 1980. *Culture's Consequences*. Beverly Hills: Sage.

Hofstede, G. 2001. *Culture's Consequences: Comparing Values, Behaviors, Institutions, and Organizations across Nations*. 2nd edition. Beverly Hills: Sage.

Hong, Y., M. W. Morris, C. Chiu and V. Benet-Martinez. 2000. Multicultural minds: A dynamic constructivist approach to culture and cognition. *American Psychologist* 55: 709–720.

Javier, R. A., F. Barroso and M. A. Muñoz. 1993. Autobiographical memory in bilinguals. *Journal of Psycholinguistic Research* 18: 449–472.

Kerby, A. 1991. *Narrative and the Self*. Bloomington, IN: Indiana University Press.

Kitayama, S., H. R. Markus and M. Kurokawa. 2002. Culturel, emotion, and well-being: Good feelings in Japan and the United States. *Cognition and Emotion* 14: 93–124.

Levinson, S. C. 1996. Frames of reference and molyneux's question: Cross-linguistic evidence. In: P. Bloom, M. Peterson, L. Nadel and M. Garret (eds.), *Language and Space*. Cambridge, UK: Cambridge University Press, 77–108.

Levinson, S. C. 2003. Language and mind: Let's get the issues straight! In: D. Gentner and S. Goldin-Meadow (eds.), *Language in Mind. Advances in the Study of Language and Cognition*. Boston: MIT Press, 25–46.

Li, P. and L. Gleitman. 2002. Turning the tables: Language and spatial reasoning. *Cognition* 83: 265–294.

Llagas, C. 2003. Status and trends in the education of hispanics. Retrieved October 1, 2003 from http://nces.ed.gov/pubs2003/hispanics.

Malt, B. C., S. A. Sloman and S. P. Gennari. 2003. Speaking versus thinking about objects and actions. In: D. Gentner and S. Goldin-Meadow (eds.), *Language in Mind: Advances in Study of Language and Cognition*. Boston, MA: MIT Press, 81–111.

Marian, Viorica and C. Fausey. 2006. Language-dependent memory in bilingual learning. *Applied Cognitive Psychology* 20(8): 1025–1047.

Marian, Viorica and Margarita Kaushanskaya. 2003. Autobiographical memory and language in bicultural bilinguals. In: J. Cohen, K. McAlister, K. Rolstad and J. MacSwan (eds.), *ISB4: Proceedings of the 4th International Symposium on Bilingualism*. Somerville, MA: Cascadilla Press, 1478–1486.

Marian, Viorica and Margarita Kaushanskaya. 2004. Self-construal and emotion in bicultural bilinguals. *Journal of Memory and Language* 51: 190–201.

Marian, Viorica and Margarita Kaushanskaya. 2007a. Cognitive constraints on cross-linguistic transfer and borrowing in bilinguals. *Applied Psycholinguistics* 28: 369–390.

Marian, Viorica and Margarita Kaushanskaya. 2007b. Language context guides memory content. *Psychonomic Bulletin and Review* 14(5): 925–933.

Marian, Viorica and Ulric Neisser. 2000. Language-dependent recall of autobiographical memories. *Journal of Experimental Psychology: General* 129: 361–368.

Matsumoto, D., T. Consolacion, H. Yamada, R. Suzuki, B. Franklin, S. Paul, R. Ray and H. Uchida. 2002. American-japanese cultural differences in judgements of emotional expression of different intensities. *Cognition and Emotion* 16: 721–747.

McDaniel, M. A., D. C. Anderson, G. O. Einstein and C. M. O'Halloran. 1989. Modulation of environmental reinstatement effects through encoding strategies. *American Journal of Psychology* 102: 523–548.

Murnane, K. and M. P. Phelps. 1993. A global activation approach to the effect of changes in environmental context on recognition. *Journal of Experimental Psychology: Learning, Memory and Cognition* 19: 882–894.

Murnane, K. and M. P. Phelps. 1995. Effects of changes in relative cue strength on context-dependent recognition. *Journal of Experimental Psychology: Learning, Memory, and Cognition* 21: 158–172.

Nabokov, V. 1954. *Drugie Berega*. New York: Izdatelstvo Imeni Chekhova, Chekhov House.

Nisbett, R. E. 2003. *The Geography of Thought: How Asians and Westerners Think Differently ... and why*. New York: Free Press.

Nygaard, L.C., S.A. Burt and J.S. Queen. 2000. Surface form typicality and asymmetric transfer in episodic memory for spoken words. *Journal of Experimental Psychology: Learning, Memory and Cognition* 26: 1228–1244.

Otoya, M. T. 1987. A study of personal memories of bilinguals: The role of culture and language in memory encoding and recall. Ph.D. thesis, Graduate School of Education of Harvard University.

Realo, A. and J. Allik. 1999. A cross-cultural study of collectivism: A comparison of american, estonian, and russian students. *The Journal of Social Psychology* 139: 133–142.

Rosch, E. 1972. Universals in color naming and memory. *Journal of Experimental Psychology* 93: 10–20.

Rosch, E. and D. C. Olivier. 1972. The structure of the color space in naming and memory for the two languages. *Cognitive Psychology* 3: 337–354.

Ross, M., W. Q. E. Xun and A. E. Wilson. 2002. Language and the bicultural self. *Personality and Social Psychology Bulletin* 28: 1040–1050.

Rovee-Collier, C. K. and H. Hayne. 1987. Reactivation of infant memory: Implications for cognitive development. In: H. W. Reese (ed.), *Advances in Child Development and Behavior*. New York: Academic Press, 185–238.

Rovee-Collier, C. K. and G. C. W. Shyi. 1992. A functional and cognitive analysis of infant long term retention. In: C. J. Brainerd, M. L. Howe and V. F. Reyna (eds.), *The Development of Long-term Retention*. Berlin & New York: Springer Verlag, 3–55.

Sapir, Edward. 1958. The status of linguistics as a science. *Language* 5: 207–214. (first printed in 1929).

Schrauf, R. W. and D. C. Rubin. 1998. Bilingual autobiographical memory in older adult immigrants: A test of cognitive explanations of the reminiscence bump and the linguistic encoding of memories. *Journal of Memory and Language* 39: 437–457.

Singh, L., J. L. Morgan and K. S. White. 2004. Preference and processing: The role of speech affect in early spoken word recognition. *Journal of Memory and Language* 51: 173–189.

Slobin, Dan Isaac. 2003. Language and thought online: Cognitive consequences of linguistic relativity. In: D. Gentner and S. Goldin-Meadow (eds.), *Language in Mind: Advances in the Study of Language and Thought*. Cambridge, MA: MIT Press, 157–191.

Smith, S. M. 1988. Environmental context-dependent memory. In: G. Davies & D. Thomson (ed.), *Memory in Context: Context in Memory*. London: John Wiley & Sons, 13–31.

Smith, S. M., A. Glenberg and R. A. Bjork. 1978. Environmental context and human memory. *Memory & Cognition* 6: 342–353.

Suedfeld, P. and E. Eich. 1995. Autobiographical memory and affect under conditions of reduced environmental stimulation. *Journal of Environmental Psychology* 15: 321–326.

Thomson, D. M. and E. Tulving. 1970. Associative encoding and retrieval: Weak and strong cues. *Journal of Experimental Psychology* 86: 255–262.

Thornton, A. E, N. Raz and K. A. Tucker. 2002. Memory in multiple sclerosis: Contextual encoding deficits. *Journal of the International Neuropsychological Society* 8: 395–409.

Triandis, H. C. 1995. *Individualism and Collectivism.* Boulder, CO: Westview Press.

Tulving, E. 1972. Episodic and semantic memory. In: E. Tulving and M. Roberts (eds.), *Organization of Memory*. New York: Academic Press, 381–403.

Tulving, E. 1985. How many memory systems are there? *American Psychologist* 40: 385–398.

Tulving, E. 1993. Varieties of consciousness and levels of awareness in memory. In: Alan Baddeley and L. Weiskrantz (eds.), *Attention: Selection, Awareness, and Control. A Tribute to Donald Broadbent*. London: Oxford University Press, 283–299.

Tulving, E. and D. Thomson. 1973. Encoding specificity and retrieval processes in episodic memory. *Psychological Review* 80: 352–373.

Wertheimer, M. 1938. Laws of organization in perceptual forms. In: W. D. Ellis (ed.), *Source Book of Gestalt Psychology*. New York: Harcourt, 71–88.

Whorf, B. L. 1940. *Science and Linguistics*. Cambridge, MA: MIT Press. Reprinted in: Language, Thought and Reality.

Wilson, A. E. and M. Ross. 2003. The identity function of autobiographical memory: Time is on our side. *Memory* 11: 137–149.

Concept formation, memory, and understanding

Renate Bartsch

1 Introduction

This article presents an alternative to the traditional notion of concepts and their assumed functions in descriptions and understanding. This new model of concepts and understanding, developed in Bartsch (1998) and Bartsch (2002), will function in developing an alternative to the traditional thinking about memory as a huge library or set of ready-made images or (propositional) representations of past events. The alternative is a model of the memory as a capacity of constructing remembrances. This alternative will be formulated on two different levels of description and theorizing, firstly on the philosophical level of phenomenological data and structures on these, and secondly on the level of neurological data and theorizing. To include this second, scientific level into our philosophical considerations makes it possible to uphold a nominalist position, in which there are no concepts as meanings of linguistic expressions, while at the same time we are able to explain how we can understand or conceptualize new situations on the basis of previously experienced situations, and how we can employ linguistic expressions to describe these new situations. And on the other hand, we can assign new situations to linguistic expressions as their satisfaction situations, that is true-making situations, on the basis of previous assignments of satisfaction situations to utterances.

What follows is a recapitulation of the Chapters 1 and 2 of Bartsch (2005)[1], which contain also discussions of psychological and neuroscientific research about memory, which has been omitted in this shorter version.

---

[1] With kind permission by John Benjamins Publishing Company, Amsterdam/Philadelphia. www.benjamins.com

2 Concept formation described on the experiential level

Concept formation is based on experiences and, at the same time, it is forming experiences as so and so aspectualized or, in other words, conceptualized. Our experiences get structured in understanding, as far as there are previous experiences with which they have similarities and contrasts, and/or with which they are associated by contiguity:

The phenomenological data that make us confident as semantically competent language users are that we are conscious of episodes and examples as falling under a concept, namely as being similar to other examples, or as being designated correctly by the respective term. We also understand situations as standing in certain contiguity relationships with other situations. We are conscious of stability and flexibility in conceptualizing (or aspectualizing) situations, and we are conscious of situations (more or less) fitting or not fitting into sequences of situations, which represent general concepts and contiguity relationships.

Generalizing and at the same time *associative concept formation* on the experiential level takes place as ordering of data, namely ordering of our experiences, according to contiguity and similarity under perspectives. Similarity is due to common properties in the data or relationships between data. Relational similarity is called analogy. We realize similarity between data without knowing to which property or relationship it is due. Taking into account contiguity of experiences is an ordering of data according to local, temporal, causal, action-participant, action-result, and other factual relationships, which leads to associations. Analogical ordering, that is ordering by relational similarity, presupposes recognizing contiguity.

Perspectives are induced by contexts generally, by linguistic and situational contexts, and especially by desires, interests, actions, activities, habits, and by questions asked in certain situations. Certain basic perspectives, as for example the perspective of form (which form does x have?), the perspective of color (of which color is x?), or the perspective of face (which face is it? What kind of face is it?) are innate as similarity spaces provided within our visual system.

Although concepts do not exist as mental entities, we can speak of concepts as constructs, primarily on the phenomenological level, and secondarily on the level of linguistic explication. On the phenomenological level, a concept can be defined as an equivalence-class of similarity sets or series of examples.

A *(quasi-)concept* expressed by an expression e under a certain perspective is an equivalence class of series of satisfaction-situations for utterances of e under this perspective. Two series (similarity sets) of situations are *equivalent* if and only if the internal similarity of their union is not diminished when they are united.

Each member of the equivalence class is an equally good representative of the (quasi-) concept. This means that different people, although they have different similarity sets or series of experienced satisfaction situations for a term used under a certain perspective, they still have the same (quasi-)concept associated with that term, if and only if their similarity sets of satisfaction situations for that term can be thrown together, united, without diminishing the internal similarity measure. This means that the respective representatives of the (quasi-)concept are equivalent, and hereby the (quasi-)concept is inter-subjective. These people thus accept of each other their respective examples or satisfaction situations.

A *concept* is a stabilized quasi-concept. It is equally well represented by each stabilized series of satisfaction-situations. Thus, for an individual, a concept is stabilized at a certain point of time, if the similarity set of examples or satisfaction situations at this time is equivalent with the grown similarity sets at later points in time.

Stabilization of concepts means that the internal similarity of the series of examples does not diminish by adding new satisfaction situations or examples. This stabilization we experience as the fact that by new examples we do not learn anything new, compared to what we already have learned. Our concept has become stable, at least for a time. Massive data to the contrary can destabilize the concept, i.e. diminish the internal similarity, if the new data are not kept separate as being judged as deviant, or as being due to metaphorical language use.

Metaphorical use can be assumed if a perspective change is involved, such that other aspects of similarity between the examples of use of the respective term are selected under the new, different, perspective. The new cases of use of the term are then understood as metaphorical and represent a different, new, concept, which together with the old concept forms a polysemic complex of concepts. *Polysemy* of a term thus occurs across different perspectives. This means that a term can be used differently in different contexts that establish different perspectives. Under a single perspective concepts stand in *opposition* or contrast to each other and have to be expressed by different terms.

Besides general concepts we form *historical concepts*, such as partial concepts of individuals (individual concepts), events, episodes, nations, epochs, and also evolutionary lineages, and natural kinds. Historical concepts are identified by local, temporal and causal contiguity relationships, and are characterized also by similarity relationships.

Experiential general concepts and the associations between them can be explicated by theories and herewith theoretical concepts, expressed by the same name as the corresponding experiential concepts, can be attached to the respective experiential concepts. Also new theoretical concepts can be created within a theory that have no direct experiential correspondence.

A *theoretical concept* expressed by a term e is the semantically characteristic syntagmatic distribution of the term within a theory, which is a coherent set of general sentences held true. The semantically characteristic distribution of a tern e are all the sentential contexts of the term e under universal quantification, i.e. all predicates that are true together with the term under universal quantification. A theoretical concept is thus implicitly defined by a theory. It is linguistically explicated within the theory. Theoretical concepts can be ordered in semantic networks and especially taxonomies. Placed within a taxonomy, a theoretical concept becomes a formal concept. It is defined by *genus proximum* and *differentia specifica* within the taxonomic order.

3 Concept formation described on the neurological level

On the other hand, distinguished from the data and terminology of phenomenology and semantics, there are the data and the terminology of neurology and neuro-physiology about what goes on in brain and body. We assume current models for the processing of nerve stimulations and neural activity within connectionist architectures, consisting of nets of neurons and growing or strengthening connections between neurons due to activity of neurons and activity along the connections between neurons. In learning processes, groups of neurons, neuronal patterns, stabilize because of the strengthening of connections between neurons. These patterns are more or less stable conceptual indicators, which, with a high probability, get activated from out certain input, and hereby they indicate this input. We call them *conceptual indicators.* They get associated in learning processes with neuronal indicators for linguistic expressions. By receiving input data in contiguity (related by space and time, cause-effect, action-instrument, action-result, actor-action etc.), conceptual indicators get associated to each other via strong connections and thus form relationships to each other, which mirror semantic networks. Our brain forms connectionist inter-relationships between the conceptual indicators by strengthening synapses used in proliferating activation between neurons during learning processes, which consist in experiencing the world and acquiring knowledge. The connections built up in this way are the connectionist neuronal basis of generalization or categorization of data to different degrees, and of association between the categories. The latter means that contiguity relationships are learned.

4 The correspondence of experiential facts and structures with models of neural connectionism

Phenomenological facts, experiences and actions, correspond with neuronal events and processes.

1. There is our experience of similarity and contrast of situations under certain perspectives on the phenomenological side, and there is the activation of certain groups of neurons, functioning as conceptual indicators, under pre-activation of certain global fields of conceptual indicators on the neural side. The pre-activation corresponds to perspectives taken, or attention spaces opened. Methodologically, the phenomenological data and structures are primary, because the corresponding conceptual indicators and structures between these can only be identified as that what they are in their function via their correspondence with the conscious phenomenological data, our experiences and actions, and the relationships between them.

2. The similarity between data, which we experience, corresponds to the activity of conceptual indicators due to causal effects of the input data on the perceptive organs. A perspective, on the neural side, is a pre-selection or pre-activation of a certain field of conceptual indicators due to contexts, circumstances, desires, and actions. The correspondence between kinds of objects and conceptual indicators is not necessarily 1-1. A category of objects that appear regularly in two very different types of contexts can have two separate conceptual indicators, due to the different contexts that have determined the input to a high degree. Hereby the objects are seen in two rather different ways. To speak with Frege (1892, 26), they have two "Weisen des Gegebenseins", two ways of representation. The same holds for an individual object and the corresponding partial individual concepts we have acquired of it. They can be rather different, such that they even might have, before one knows better, two different indices pointing to them on the map of individual concept indicators. When one knows their identity, they get linked via the identity linking between their respective terms, or they can be linked directly, if one encounters the identity regularly in experience. An individual concept indicator is a network of conceptual indicators connected with an index for the individual within the specific memory (see below). The

conceptual indicators serve to characterize the individual, when we refer to it. The individual concept indicators thus correspond to partial individual concepts, namely to (parts of) our knowledge we have about an individual. The context or situation of reference to the individual selects relevant parts of our knowledge about the individual, which corresponds to the selection of conceptual indicators in connection with the individual index.

3. We have experience of contiguity between data under perspectives: spatial, temporal, causal, and other relationships (short: contiguity-relationships) and contiguity between circumstances and the performance of actions on the phenomenological side. This contiguity corresponds with associations, connections between several conceptual indicators, including relationships between concept-indicators and habit/routine indicators (indicators for motor-activity, actions) on the neural side.

4. Linguistic conceptual analysis by general sentences held true and especially by those of definitional form (i.e. theoretical and formal concepts) on the phenomenological side corresponds on the neural side with activation of networks of conceptual indicators, and also with networks of linguistic term indicators.

5. Awareness of constituent structures of phrases, especially sentences, and of situations and images, which involves binding or synthesis of parts within wholes (see section 5) on the phenomenological side, corresponds with activation circuits between conceptual indicators and activated groups of neurons on sensorial fields/systems, on the neural side. Hereby, smaller circles are embedded within larger ones. This structure corresponds to constituent structure of situations and sentences (cf. the arguments for this connectionist architecture in Bartsch, 2002).

5 Understanding

We distinguish understanding a situation from understanding a linguistic expression, although both make use of the same principles and structures on the phenomenological level and, correspondingly, on the level of connectionist neural architecture.

1. *Understanding* a situation is conceptualizing the situation, by which aspects are distinguished within the situation. We therefore also speak of aspectualizing a situation. To understand a situation means to embed the situation into the conceptual system, established at this point in the development of concept formation in a person's history of learning. The embedding happens under preservation of stability of the conceptual system. What does that mean?

Above, an experiential general concept was defined as an equivalence-class of stabilizing series of examples that are similarity sets under a certain perspective, or under a group of perspectives. Two similarity sets were called equivalent if and only if they can be united (thrown together) without changing the internal similarity measure. That is, the two sets do not add anything to each other as far as the concept is concerned. They both represent the concept equally well. If the internal similarity measure of a set of examples, namely satisfaction situations for an expression *e*, does not change anymore by adding new examples or satisfaction-situations, then this growing set of examples completely represents the concept, which is the whole equivalence class, expressed by *e*. A situation can be understood, which means can be aspectualized or conceptualized under that concept, if and only if the situation can be added to, or fitted into, a similarity set representing the concept. This means that the situation can be added to a representative similarity set of previous experiences without diminishing its internal similarity measure. In this way, we understand a situation if and only if the situation is integrated into our concept representing set of examples 'salva stabilitate'. If we inter-subjectively entertain the same concept, that is if our concept representing similarity sets are equivalent, then the situation can be said to be embeddable into our inter-subjective concept *salva stabilitate*. Then we understand the situation in the same way, at least as far as this conceptualization goes.

Understanding a situation as one in which a certain individual is involved as a participant, for example as agent, means that the situation is embeddable into the partial individual concept (the representation we have of the individual) under preservation of coherence between the situations that define the partial life-history of the individual as we know it. To understand, for example, JOHN as an agent in a situation means that we find there within a smallest situation the individual concept of JOHN and the general concept of an AGENT bound together in a constituent, and bound together with some ACTION concept, for example the concept of EATING. This means that the situation contains a smallest situation,

1. which fits into the individual concept of JOHN, a coherent series of situations of John's life history as we know it, and

2. which fits into the general concept of an AGENT, namely into a similarity set of situations in which someone is an agent, and

3. which fits into the general concept of EATING, a similarity set of eat-situations.

Understanding a situation thus consists in adding it to, or integrating it into, the conceptual representations we have, namely into the series of previous examples of a general concept or into a series of experienced or known occurrences of an individual, under preservation of their stability and/or coherence.

Understanding a situation that in some respect does not fit into our conceptual system is possible by *metaphorical understanding*. This is also understanding by similarity, but now under a new perspective, which makes it possible to continue a series of examples of a term e in a new way, due to similarities that are selected under this new perspective. Hereby we form a new concept expressed by e

under another perspective, or another type of contexts, than the perspective that was relevant for the previous uses of the expression. A problematic situation, in which, for example, a man is called a snail, fits into the series of uses of *snail* under the new perspective and is now understood as, for example, a situation containing someone that can be called a snail under the perspective of behavior, especially with respect to his way of showing motor activity, rather than under the perspective of natural kind (cf. Bartsch, 1998). Under another perspective, for example of how the person feels or how he behaves socially, we might understand the metaphoric use of the word *snail* as creating a new concept that is a metaphor of the concept of sliminess or stickiness in the social sphere.

Even if we merely have similarity sets under certain perspectives without associated terms, namely representatives of concepts that are not linguistically expressed, a perspective change can create the possibility to integrate or understand data that do not fit into the available conceptual system. A new perspective may single out a new similarity set among the old data, or select data from an old similarity set such that the new unusual datum fits together with this newly selected similarity set, and thus gets integrated into it, and hereby is understood. In this creative way of understanding, in which a change to a new perspective takes place, a new concept is formed, which is a new way of understanding data.

A parallel story about understanding a situation can be told with reference to the neurological processes involved: Causal effects of the situation (received data) activate those groups of neurons that function as conceptual indicators and individual concept indices that have been established as such indicators and indices by confronting and experiencing earlier similar situations. Activation circuits are established that correspond to constituents of the situation. They are bound together in larger circuits of activation, which correspond to larger constituents, and to the whole situation.

Understanding a linguistic utterance first means that the utterance is understood as a linguistic episode. The linguistic understanding of a linguistic episode or utterance, as acoustic and phonetic, phonological, lexical and syntactic understanding of the utterance as an utterance of an expression (linguistic type, linguistic concept) has a similar built-up as the situational understanding. Hereby the utterance is conceptualized as a linguistic expression or utterance type.

Understanding the semantic value of an utterance, on the other hand, means understanding the expression within the utterance situation and the present context. Understanding here consists in construing satisfaction situations for the expression, and especially the sentence, by forming B-intersections, that is by forming binding-intersections as constituents: In a binding-intersection between two concepts the smallest situational concept is formed that is embeddable into both concepts under preservation of stability and/or coherence. This smallest situational concept is the type of all the satisfaction situations that satisfy not just both concepts separately (intersection), rather they satisfy both, the two concepts, and also the syntactic synthesis between them. For example, understanding the phrase *brown horse* does not only mean that the possible satisfaction situations for this expression have to fit into the concept BROWN and into the concept HORSE under preservation of stability. This would be the case already for a situation in which there is something brown, i.e. the situation fits (*salva stabilitate*) into a series of brown-examples, and in which something else is a horse, i.e. the situation fits (*salva stabilitate*) into a series of horse-examples. But this would not yet be a satisfaction situation for *brown horse*. Rather the expression moreover means that the satisfaction situation must be the smallest in which both conditions are fulfilled. This is an extra condition: according to the syntactic value of the construction each satisfaction situation of the expression must contain a single object that fits into the concept BROWN as well as into the concept HORSE, under preservation of stability. Understanding a phrase in this way 1. is a process of collecting the restrictions on possible satisfaction situations of the phrase by intersecting representations of the concepts involved (namely intersecting stabilizing sets of examples or satisfaction situations of the concepts involved), which is lexical understanding, and 2. is forming, according to the syntactic analysis, the smallest situational concepts that characterize within these intersections the satisfaction situations for the constituents of the phrase and finally for the whole phrase or sentence. Construing a smallest situation is illustrated by the following example.

Understanding the sentence *John beats Paul.* The possible alternative hierarchies of syntactic construction all lead to the same result, a representative set of the situational concept of John beating Paul. Such a set of situations in which John beats Paul can be represented by the smallest situation, or situation type, in which John beats Paul, here represented by E. It can be broken down into different constituent structures.

(1) E = **B**(**B**(**B**(John, Agent), Beat), **B**(Paul, Patient))

(2) E = **B**(**B**(**B**(Paul, Patient), Beat), **B**(John, Agent))

(3) E = **B**(**B**(Beat, **B**(John, Agent)), **B**(Paul, Patient))

(4) E = **B**(**B**(Beat, **B**(Paul, Patient)), **B**(John, Agent))

(5) E = **B**(**B**(**B**(John, Agent), **B**(Paul, Patient)), Beat)

(6) E = **B**(**B**(**B**(Paul, Patient), **B**(John, Agent)), Beat)

We see that the process of construing the complex situational concept consists in gathering constraints on the set of possible satisfaction situations for the sentence at issue; in understanding the sentence step by step, more and more constraints are placed on the set of possible satisfaction situations, by which the set becomes smaller. The process of understanding a sentence thus is a specification, which can be done in different orders, but which always involves certain fixed hierarchies, namely the combination of the role-concepts with the participant individual concepts, and the binding of these with the action concept. Otherwise, this conceptual semantic structure is flat, and can be broken down into different constituent structures, depending on pragmatic factors.

We have merely treated the conceptual understanding. Interpreting an utterance presupposes conceptual understanding, but it also needs interpreting determiners, anaphoric pronouns and deictic expressions, especially temporal and local deixis, which will not be treated here. It would require taking into account self-reference and awareness of ones own position in space and time, which is beyond the present topic.

There is a relationship between understanding a situation and understanding a sentence. We construe satisfaction-situations from sentences, and we construe sentences by understanding a situation and then describing it according to this conceptualization.

There is a parallel between B-intersections, binding between concepts according to constituent structures on the phenomenological side, and the embedding of smaller activation circuits into larger ones, on the neural side. The structure of activation circuits embedded into larger circuits emerges in consciousness as the structure of constituents embedded into larger constituents (cf. Bartsch, 2002, Chap. 3).

There is a further kind of understanding, namely understanding the other as performing speech acts and reporting propositional attitudes, and understanding the other by empathy and through trying to see something from the other's point of view. Inter-subjective and subjective aspects in conceptualization play a role in how far this understanding of the other goes. I shall not treat this topic here, but it is partly taken into account in Bartsch (1998), in the chapter on propositional attitudes.

6 Memory and remembering

Memory is at least divided into two kinds, mostly called semantic memory and fact-memory, or semantic memory and episodic memory. Since not all general concepts, including relationships, are linguistically, and especially lexically expressed, we more precisely could speak of the generalizing memory, or short *general memory*, and a part of it, which is the semantic memory, being directly associated with lexical items expressing general concepts. Besides the episodic memory we distinguish another individualizing memory, the individual concepts memory, which holds our concepts of individuals, including individual objects. The episodic memory and the individual concept memory together are referred to as the specific (*historic*) memory, distinct from the generalizing memory. Our memory is built up in learning processes and generally in experiencing situations, and also in understanding narratives. In a way, every experience is part of a learning process. It attributes to building up and to modifying general concepts, and it can give rise to a more or less lasting specific remembrance, in which an experienced situation or object is connected with emotional and motivational aspects and motor dispositions towards behavior and especially actions. Such aspects later on, when experienced again, can call up the previous situation in which they prominently figured, and thus can give rise to remember episodes related to the present situation, individuals, and places.

Remembering is a conscious state, but even if a remembrance of a previous episode similar to the current one is not achieved, the perception and understanding of the current situation can be modified or partly determined by the unconscious partial reconstruction process of the previous situation, and actions can be called up by the current situation via the unconscious links to the previous episode. Thus an action, or attitude, or emotional evaluation will be transplanted on, or associated with the current situation.

We have distinguished the general memory from the specific, or historical, memory, the latter being a memory of individual concepts (that are our concepts of individuals) and a memory of episodes and other courses of events.

The general memory comprises indicators of general concepts, and of routines and habits. The indicators of a general observational concept and of the corresponding routine concept of an action are linked by connections, which have been strengthened because both are mostly activated together. In learning an action we, at the same time, observe and imitate (on the level of motor and pre-motor activity) the action. Thus, what traditionally is called procedural memory, or routine memory, is taken to be part of the general memory, because routines are generalizations of self-performed concrete actions. The historical memory comprises indices of individual concepts, personal episodes, and facts.

We now describe the kind and structure of memory, as far as its main architecture and function is concerned. Historical memory is the capacity of (re-) constructing partial individual concepts of individuals one has known or has information about, and the capacity of (re-) constructing previous episodes. Remembrance is an act of remembering, i.e. is the result of this kind of (re-) construction. Memory, the collections of neurons functioning as indices by means of their connections to conceptual indicators and to sensorial and motor fields, is unconscious. It is a potentiality, a capacity or disposition to remember. Remembering, a result achieved by activating this capacity, is conscious.

The general memory is materialized as a brain area or field of groups of neurons functioning as conceptual indicators and as routine indicators, with their generalizing (hierarchical) and associative connections/relationships among each other. These indicators are established over time by convergence of the impacts of learning processes in which examples are organized under perspectives by similarity and contrast, as well as by contiguity, such that, for example, the indicator for chairs is connected with those for sitting and for tables. These groups of neurons only function as conceptual indicators by virtue of their connections to other indicators, that is their position within a structure of indicators, and by virtue of the connections of the indicators to fields which provide phenomenal qualities and are causally related to input from the surrounding world. These sensorial and motor, as well as the proprioceptual and the emotional and evaluative fields, provide the phenomenal material, which is the necessary medium in which conceptual structures can be couched, such that we can experience situations and objects.

The capacity we call the general memory is not located in one compound field of neuronal indicators for objects, situations, and especially actions and routines. These groups of neurons and their interconnections by themselves are of no interest. Rather they function as indicators, and are thus of interest to us, only by means of their connections to primary sensorial and motor fields, and to emotion and proprioceptual fields, and the causal connections of these primary fields to the body and its surroundings. Only in circuit interaction with these primary fields at the cutting edge between brain and world they are able to indicate anything, and are they suited to contribute to what we are conscious of, namely to our experiences. Our capacity of conceptualizing or understanding thus does not reside in a single (compounded) area; it is based on a global interaction involving conceptual fields, the sensorial-motor and other systems, and their bodily causal relations with our surroundings.

The historical, or specific, memory is materialized as a brain area or field of groups of neurons functioning as indices (for individuals or episodes) with their connections to conceptual and routine indicators of the general memory, and space-time ordering relationships, and with connections to emotion-indicators and evaluation-indicators on the respective fields. Other than an indicator, an index is not formed by processes taking place and converging over several, or even many different examples in learning across time. Rather an index is formed immediately with the experience of an episode, or with our acquaintance with an individual, or with the narrative creation of a historical entity. It will be consolidated by rehearsals of the episode in thinking about it, or during periods of sleep. The associative power of an index gets extended by associating sub-indices in the course of learning more about the individual or situation. An index for an individual may get connected with other indices of individuals and of episodes. Thus, an index can become more complex.

If we remember a past episode, the memory index of the past situation works just like an index for an individual. The constituent structure of activation circuits involving conceptual indicators is organized from out that index, which in itself is composed out of sub-indices. This constituent structure out of activation circuits corresponds to the constituent structure of binding-intersections between the respective concepts that characterize a situation. For a remembrance to occur, these activation circuits must include groups of neurons on sensorial and motor fields. Without phenomenal material emerging from these fields, the process of re-construction of a remembrance of an episode or of and individual would not have a remembrance as a conscious result. Rather it would stay on the conceptual fields and from there it could influence perception and action, but that would be unconscious for us. In such a case we cannot compare the new perception with the past episode, though the past episode has influence on our understanding of the new situation.

In a remembrance of an episode, the activation circuits form a whole of smaller and larger circuits that also include neurons on the sensorial, motor, emotional, and proprioceptual fields, whereby neurons dedicated to phenomenal expression provide phenomenal material (qualia) necessary for a conceptually structured episode emerging in consciousness.

The specific memory field, which contains episodic and individual indices, is closely connected with emotional, proprioceptional, sensorial and routine and motor fields, from where memories of episodes can be induced, besides from indicators of general concepts. In principle, memories are constructed by the connectivity that had been established by the similarities and associations between previous data. The similarities and contiguities leading to associations were selected under certain perspectives, which correspond to certain pre-activations, contextually and situationally induced. We see that the specific memory is not located in one single field, identified by neurologists as the hippocampus. Rather the capacity of memory is based on a global interaction between the field of memory indices, possibly the hippocampus, and the other fields presented in the architecture of Figure 1 below.

We have assumed that both kinds of memory, the general memory and the specific memory, have connections with the sensorial, motor, emotional, evaluative, and proprioceptional areas. By interaction circuits between indicators in these areas and indices in the historical memory we perceive and imagine episodes (linguistic as well as situational ones) and perceive, imagine, and recognize individuals.

7 The architecture of memory

In Figure 1 below, the proposed architecture of the working episodic memory is represented. All two-way directed arrows represent circuits consisting of a connection with one direction and a connection with a reciprocal direction. In the central field M of the episodic memory, an episode is registered by a group of indices. The indices are established in the process of understanding the original episode by selecting those neurons as indices which are strongest activated in M by activation traveling via connections from the sensorial and motor fields and the conceptual and routine maps and the emotional and evaluation maps and the proprioception maps. In the constituent circuits of activation established in understanding by the activity traveling along the forward connections and their reciprocal ones, the strongest connections will later on be the paths along which most likely the episode is recalled. The selected neurons are established as more or less stable indices for the respective, hereby memorized, episode by strengthening the connections between these neurons and the neurons activated at the same time in the other maps or fields in the repeated circuit activation in re-experiencing, re-understanding and emotionally reacting to the episode, as well as in subsequent imagining the episode in remembrance.

Considering semantic structures of episodes we can expect that the indices would work best in a process of binding general concepts together in ontologically relevant aspects, if the indices were to point or connect to indicators of individual concepts, of relationships of space-time order, and of general concepts and relations. And they have to connect to (currently employed) neurons on the sensorial fields, which hereby will be used in forming and imagining the remembered episode. If the currently experienced situation and the remembered situation are both distinctly conscious in perception and imagination, this must happen in alternation, and hereby they can be compared and even contrasted with respect to the details. But we can expect normally that the current situation and the previous situation get blended together within the currently perceived situation, and thus we see the current situation more or less in the light of the previously experienced situation, even when that situation is not or cannot be remembered distinctly. The memory indices of the previous episode get activated by the indicators involved in the activation circuits of the current episode on other fields, and also re-activate them. Thus a rhythmic state of activation of interconnected circuits builds up, which, when hitting the sensorial, motor, emotional and proprioceptual fields, brings about the consciously perceived current episode, which can be a merger of the old and the new, or which can alternate with the remembrance of the old episode.

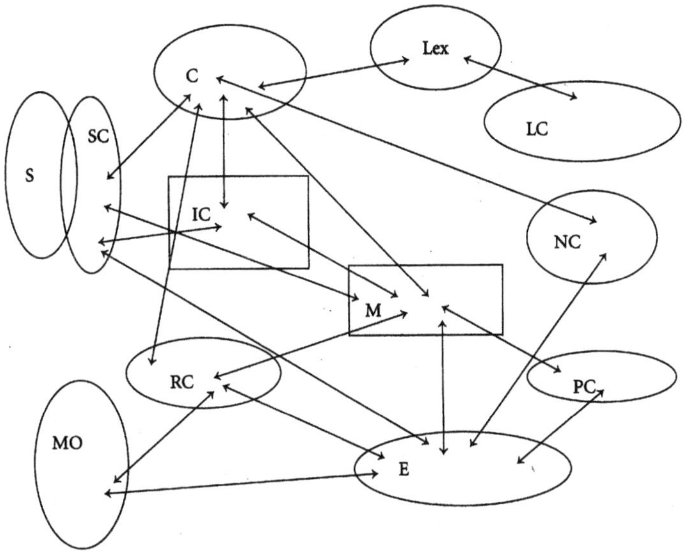

Figure 1. The architecture of episodic memory

Legenda:

M:	episodic memory center
MO:	(pre)-motor fields
RC:	routine maps (concepts/categories of routines)
E:	emotional fields and emotional concepts/categories maps
PC:	proprioceptual fields
NC:	maps for normative and evaluative concepts/rules
LC:	linguistic concepts: syntactic categories, syntactic patterns/rules
Lex:	lexical maps
C:	general concepts/ontological categories maps
IC:	individual concepts memory center
S:	sensorial fields
SC:	sensorial concepts/categories, including face map

In Figure 1, the boxes show the two central parts of the specific, historical, memory treated here, namely the individual concept memory and the episodic memory. The two-way directed arrows show connections to and from indicators and indices in the respective maps or fields that together can form compositions of activation circuits. In a remembrance of an episode the activation circuits form a whole of smaller and larger circuits that also include neurons on the sensorial, motor, emotional, and proprioceptual fields, whereby neurons dedicated to phenomenal expression provide phenomenal material (qualia) necessary for a conceptually structured episode emerging in consciousness.

The specific memory field, the centers that contains episodic and individual indices, is closely connected with emotional, proprioceptual, sensorial, and routine and motor fields, from where memories of episodes can be induced, besides from indicators of general concepts. In principle, memories are constructed by connectivity based on similarity and association.

Both kinds of memory, the general memory and the specific memory, have connections with the sensorial, motor, emotional, evaluative, and proprioceptual areas. By interaction circuits between indicators in these areas and indices in the historical memory center we perceive and imagine episodes (linguistic as well as situational ones).

The linguistic concept maps (LC) and the lexical maps (Lex) are connected in activation circuits with certain sensorial concepts maps for speech perception and with routine maps for articulation. This has not been represented in the figure.

The lexical maps (Lex) have per lexical item indicator associative relationships via connections to other indicators of linguistic items of its regular linguistic distribution, and also to the indicators of linguistic categories and sub-categories that characterize the linguistic distribution. Likewise, in parallel, the general concept maps have per concept indicator associative relationships via connections to other concept indicators for concepts that characterize the surrounding of the concept-realization in a situation. These indicators for associative relationships characterize contiguity relationships within and between situations. The regularly surrounding concepts functioning in these relationships are indicated by general ontological concept indicators such that in this way the conceptual frame of a concept and the corresponding syntactic-semantic frame of the concept-representing lexical item is represented in this structure of relationships between indicators. The frames give the basic conceptually motivated syntactic-semantic order in linguistic representations, which are expressed by conventional linguistic patterning and rules.

The individual concept center (IC) consists of indices for individuals. These indices, when activated, point via connections to 1. indicators of properties (general concepts) and indicators of relationships in connection with indices for other individuals, and 2. indices of episodes the individual is known to have been involved in. The central episodic memory field (M) and the IC-field together form a compound map of indices, to be called the specific memory (SPM), which consists of a field with indices for individual concepts, and a field of indices for episodes and, possibly, relations between them. This specific memory corresponds to having two kinds of basic entities in our ontology, namely individuals and situations/events.

We have distinguished indicators and indices, the indicators being assemblies of neurons that are activated with perceiving instances for a concept or relationship, including motor routines. In this way such an assembly functions as a conceptual indicator. The indicators with their connections to other indicators and to the sensorial, proprioceptual, emotional, and (pre-)motor areas form the generalizing memory, and especially a subsection of it, the semantic memory, in as far as the indicators are associated to linguistic expressions denoting the corresponding concepts. The indices, on the other hand, are assemblies of neurons in the episodic memory, those that refer to specific episodes, situations, events, and to individuals. An index for an individual, together with its connections to the concepts and relationships that are known to characterize and identify the individual, functions as an individual concept. Since not all episodes and objects which we encounter are remembered, we assume that there are many indices which loose their connections to the activated indicators of the index-establishing episode or object fast and are thus only binding together the respective concepts into the unity of the experienced episode or object for a short time. These memory indices then form a short-term memory, lasting for maybe 5 to 10 minutes or less, and when they have lost their connections they are available for shortly remembering new episodes or memories. In this way they still contribute to the generalizing and associating memory, this means to our concepts and routines, by binding these together into situations and situational concepts (types) of repeated situations. From research into the chemistry and physiology of the brain we know that it is a matter of the availability of certain chemicals, proteins and enzymes, that make connections function in the transmission of electric charge over the synapses, and that make the synapses grow broader and thicker, such that the connections get strong and serve for a long time for transmitting charges by means of neurotransmitters. The production and availability of the required chemicals varies for different brain areas and changes with the state of health and the states of being awake or asleep.

The indices get ordered at least partly by spatial and temporal relationships, which primarily must have been established by forming indicators for relationships of temporal and spatial order when experiencing basic bodily movements. Hereby, for example, positions of the hands, or the movements of the tongue in the mouth, can be felt in the proprioceptive areas as taking time, following each other, and as filling space and moving through space and hereby creating the experience of distances. From feeling space and time in bodily activity the relationships get enriched by finding such relationships also in outer space around the body, and then generally finding these relationships among objects and episodes in the outer world, which also get ordered in space and time. We have to assume such a development of temporal and spatial concepts because without a basis in our feeling of bodily activity we never could experience and thus be conscious of space-time order. We have assumed that the sensorial, proprioceptual, emotional, and (pre-) motor areas in our brain contain the neurons that are dedicated to produce feelings that are the phenomenal basis for being aware of something in a conscious manner. The indicators and indices themselves, by means of their connections, merely form a system of pointers that function via activation going along the established connections. We might sometimes indirectly be aware of brain activity in thinking, for example, when we try hard to remember a certain word, phrase or name, but for some time do not quite succeed and rather come up with unfit results that do not survive control. However, we cannot feel what is going on in our head in detail, or what processes of thinking are going on, except when the interaction circuits hit the areas that provide for the qualitative aspects, the qualia, of phenomenal effects. The whole system of pointers would not mean anything if it were not for the inclusion of the areas in the brain dedicated to phenomenal quality, namely the sensorial, motor, proprioceptual, and emotional fields. They make the connection to the world of bodies, objects, and episodes by being affected by this world in certain ways. These resulting affections get ordered in developing and re-activating, by circuit activation of these phenomenally dedicated areas with the general and the specific memory, i.e. the systems of indicators, indices, and their connections. These processes give rise to structured objects and episodes as the phenomenal results of the interaction circuits in a state of rhythmic activation between the phenomenally active areas, i.e. the conceptual, sensorial, motor, emotional, and proprioceptional areas, and the memory areas; and by connecting to linguistically specialized areas, they give rise to the appropriate linguistic representations.

8 Remembering, structured from out the episodic memory

In our brain the area we have called M is essential for having an episodic memory, i.e. for remembering past episodes, which we have encountered in our surroundings, or about which we have had linguistically coded information.

What this area really does is not quite clear. Neurologists have found out that if this area, the hippocampus, is damaged in patients, they cannot remember episodes they have experienced in the past and/or they cannot remember episodes they have experienced after the damage, depending on where exactly the lesion is, and on how extensive it is.

It is, by now, a passed-by stage to think of memory as a kind of huge library in which propositions and pictures are stored about previous experiences, and from where somehow such propositions and pictures can be drawn out into the open, i.e. into consciousness, when the memory is triggered in appropriate ways. This century-old picture for the storage of empirical knowledge in our minds we find already in Plato's dialogue Theaitetos, where he uses the metaphors of the waxen tablet and the pigeon house. In remembering we find an inscription on the waxen tablet, or we catch a pigeon from the many we have put into the house, each pigeon representing a stored episode or fact. Plato rejects these metaphors as inappropriate for how knowledge (episteme) is available to us, though he thinks they are partly correct for episodic knowledge (doxa). If this picture of storage is incorrect, as we now know, how then can we think about what memory is and how it functions?

It has been observed that remembering is more a reconstruction or reproduction of an episode, in which the same sensory areas in the brain are involved as have been involved when experiencing the original episode. Neuro-scientific experiments have shown that persons who have seen a certain picture, for example Mona Lisa, have for about 90% the same brain areas activated in the act of recollecting the picture, as they had when they previously perceived the picture. The 10% difference is easily explained, because in perceiving they had a slightly different, mainly more detailed, and circumstantial input to the brain's visual system than they had in the act of recollection; and in recollection aspects might have been added that had not originally been in the picture.

What then is the task of area M? We can think of it as a collection of indices, whereby a neuron or a small group of neurons serves as an index, or as a combination of indices. An index gets established as a neuron that is activated when the sensorial-cognitive-emotional- and motor, and proprioceptual systems form the perception and the whole personal uptake of an episode, which hereby is a perceived and therewith located, conceptualized, and emotionally evaluated episode, short: it is an understood episode. The activated parts of the brain, i.e. the activated conceptual indicators on the generalizing conceptual maps of ontological categories and of habits or routines, the individual concept indices and indicators, the neurons of the primary sensorial fields, the groups of neurons serving as conceptual indicators for basic forms, motions, colors, and faces on the maps of the visual system, and the conceptual indicators of other sensory modalities involved, as well as proprioception areas of motion and emotion, all take part in forming the experienced episode. All these get directly or indirectly connected by synaptic activity and accordingly growth, whereby connections are established and strengthened to one or more neurons in area M, which then function as episodic indices, possibly also activating each other (pointing to each other) and indicators for temporal and local ordering relationships, and activating back the indicators on the other areas from which they had been activated.

The activation happens along circuits: in assembly X of neurons: excited neuron (1) $\rightarrow$ outgoing activation of (1) $\rightarrow$ incoming activation for neuron (2) $\rightarrow$ excitement of neuron (2) in assembly Y $\rightarrow$ outgoing activation of (2) $\rightarrow$ incoming activation for (1) $\rightarrow$ re-excitement of neuron (1) or some others of assembly X. There have to be such circuits in order to strengthen and built up connections such that neurons in X can be activated from out area Y. If Y:= M, the episodic memory center, this means that what goes into M from out some origin X, must also be able to go out from M back to the original X. In this way an index in M can point to conceptual indicators that had been activated in the original perception of a situation or object to which the index in M is due, and thus can address the original contents that are remembered by inducing activation circuits between the respective conceptual indicators and the sensorial, motor, emotional and proprioceptional areas.

Note that we find no concepts on conceptual maps. We merely find groups of neurons that get activated with input of data from situations or objects of a certain kind. They are merely indicators of classification on the basis of similarities of incoming data. This amounts to the activation traveling along connections strengthened by previous similar input, and they have associative connections with indicators for other concepts which had been formed and stabilized by experiencing other situations or objects that regularly stand in contiguity relationships of various kinds with the first situations and objects. We can say that the groups of neurons are conceptual indicators, and as such have a referential semantic value, firstly by virtue of their connectedness with groups of neurons of the sensorial, motor, and emotional fields, activated by getting input from, and enacting on, the surroundings. Secondly, they have a structural semantic value by their connectedness to other conceptual indicators, following generalization or specification and following associations based on spatial, temporal, causal and other contiguity relationships.

The activation circuits for classificatory hierarchies and the ones for contiguity associations are typically of the following form:

(7) Classificatory hierarchy: X includes Y, for example "a rose is a flower": Y = FLOWER; X = ROSE.

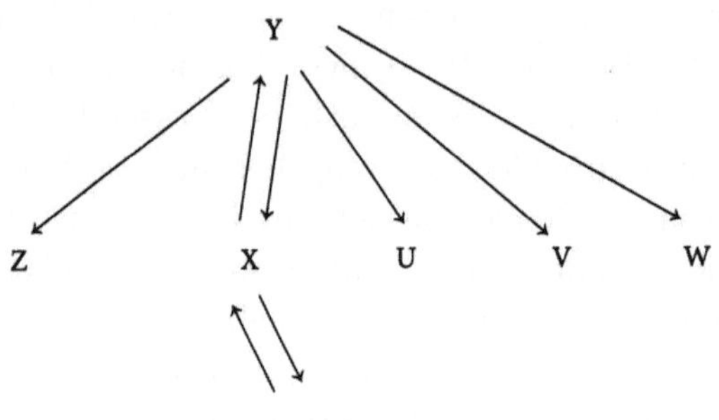

Figure 2. X includes Y

In seeing or imagining a rose the conceptual indicator for roses gets activated. The activation is spread further along an outgoing and incoming path to the indicator for flowers, which gets activated. It sends activation further to all the conceptual indicators for subsumed flower-concepts that had been learned. Since in this example only the ROSE-indicator is independently activated, only there the activation is strong enough to get an activation circuit going. The other indicators of different kinds of flowers get merely the fairly weak and broadly spread activation from the indicator of the hypernym, i.e. of the general flower-concept, and some more specific feature indicators by which certain flowers are similar to roses, and therefore activation circuits are not likely to be formed there. Here the activation simply dies out without establishing circuits, if no additional activation comes about by some perspective change, for example by turning the attention to the question of what other flowers are prone to similar kinds of mildew disease.

(8) Contiguity association: X has relationship R to Y

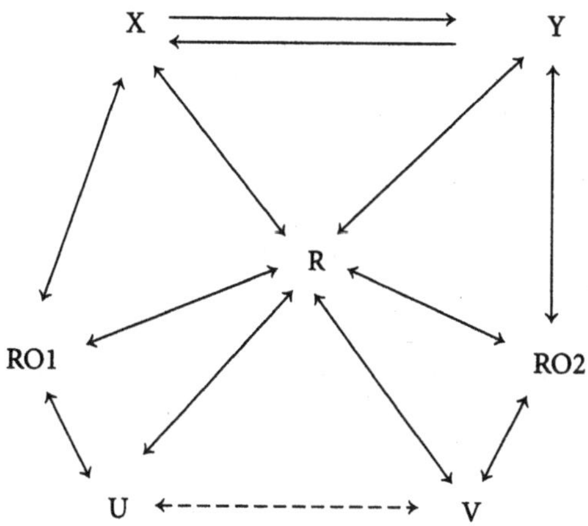

Figure 3. X has relationship R to Y

In order to avoid a drawing that gets too crowded by to many arrows, also here the doubly oriented arrow stands for an activation circuit. For a two-place relationship there must be two role-concept indicators which function to specify in which role X and in which role Y takes part in the relationship R. For example, if R is the causal relationship, ROLE 1 is Cause and ROLE 2 is Effect. The conceptual indicators involved are thus the ones for X, Y, R, RO1 and RO2. X and Y are activated in their causal relationship. Also for U and V the same relationship can be activated, if U and V receive independent activation.

That activation happens in circuits has been observed for the visual system and has a great explanatory power when assumed as an overall principle of brain architecture. The circuit structure generally provides a mode for representing constituent structure that can be found in experiencing situations, images, and linguistic expressions. This architecture implies that the indices can, when they receive some triggering activation from some brain part that had been involved in the experience of the original episode, send out activation along the previously established circuit-lines of sending back activity to those brain parts that had been the ones that originally have established the index in area M by activating the neuron or group of neurons that hereby had become indices. The indices in the area M must have been established with experiencing the original episode from out the neurons that express phenomenal quality, for example in the V1/V2 area of the visual system, where space-time contiguity ordering takes place in interaction with maps of form and motion, and self-perception, at least as far as one's own motor activity and directional orientation goes. In a parallel fashion, the respective maps of other sensorial modalities and proprioception can be involved. Likewise the indices in area M have to be associated via activated connections with the indicators of spatial and temporal concepts and of other concepts that had been activated by analyzing the original episode on the conceptual maps.

The circuits go along the connections that had been activated in the understanding of the original episode, and possibly other similar episodes, and episodes connected with the original one by space-time and other factual contiguity. The whole activation in circuits has to include the primary sensorial areas, the proprioception and motor areas, areas of bodily feelings, and emotional areas, in order to experience an episode, as perceived or imagined or remembered. The circuit structure of smaller embedded circuits and larger composed circuits provides the possible constituent structures for episodes, as well as for the sentences describing these. In Figure 3 we saw, for example, that the relationship R(X,Y) to two possible constituents, [XRO1]R and R[RO2Y] of the whole [XRO1RRO2Y], short XRY, which can be a constituent of a larger structure, here [XRY and URV].

In section 5 we saw that in understanding a situation, individual concepts have to be made use of, by integrating the situation under a role-concept into a partial individual concept available under preservation of coherence of the individual concept. Thus, a situation was understood as the one of John beating Paul by integrating or embedding it into the partial individual concept of JOHN as an AGENT and the partial individual concept of PAUL as a PATIENT and into the ACTION concept of BEATING while binding them together into the smallest situation, and thus representing the situational concept that characterizes all situations in which John beats Paul. On the other hand, a sentence like *John beats Paul* was understood by forming the B-intersection between the available partial individual concept of John and the role-concept AGENT, the B-intersection between the available individual concept of PAUL with the PATIENT-concept, and then the B-intersections of these concepts of JOHN as agent and PAUL as patient with the ACTION-concept of BEATING. This constituent structure of binding-intersections between concepts, now, corresponds to neuronal activation circuits along the connections between the groups of neurons serving as the respective concept indicators and indices. The smaller activation circuits are embedded into larger ones, and finally into the whole large circuit composed from all the constituent circuits. Now, also in remembering a past episode a same kind of constituent structure is necessary in the remembrance; syntactic systematicity, the right organization of contiguity as far as this basic conceptual built up is concerned, must be preserved in the remembered episode, such that the situation of John having beaten Paul is distinguished from the one of Paul having beaten John. This has to be steered from out the memory index.

In the example above, we have taken R (in Figure 3) as the BEAT-ACTION and RO1 as the role of AGENT, and RO2 as the role of PATIENT. When we understand a sentence that refers to a situation experienced in the past, the memory index of the past situation is activated from out the description given in the sentence via the conceptual indicators addressed by the lexical items in the sentence and the syntactic structure. (If we have no index of the situation established in the past, but get informed about it for the first time, such an index has to be created within the memory of reported facts, which is part of the specific memory.) The index then has additional access to other aspects of the past situation and we hereby can remember more about the past situation than is expressed in the sentence.

The memory index of the episode, a group of neurons, has to be composed out of sub-indices, smaller groups of neurons or singular neurons, which fix the respective constituents, such that the episode of Peter beating Paul is distinguished from the episode of Paul beating Peter. This requires that a sub-index connects strongly to the index of PETER and the indicator of the AGENT-concept, another sub-index to the index of PAUL and the indicator of the AGENT concept, and a third index to the indicator of the BEAT-concept. Hereby the general connections of the BEAT-indicator to the AGENT-indicator and to the PATIENT-indicator makes the overall activation circuit possible which combines the sub-circuits in one constituent structure, which must include the sensory-motor fields in order to result in a conscious remembrance.

Figure 4 shows the construction of the episode of Paul beating Peter. The upper index in M is the index referring to PETER, the middle index the one referring to the BEAT-situation and the lower one is the index referring to PAUL. The round-cornered rectangles represent previously established individual concepts indicators, consisting of individuating indices in connection with characterizing concept indicators. The rectangles represent concept indicators.

Instead of the general roles of an agent (RO1) and of a patient (RO2) we can think of special roles that are connected with each action concept. In this case this would be the beater-role (BR1) and the role of the beaten one (BR2).

In the compound memory index the middle index is the one for the basic situation, which is an event, action, state or process. It can be related to indices of other situations by temporal, and spatial relationships, and by other contiguity relationships. Thus the scene *Paul spits at Peter. Then Peter beats Paul.* can be re-constructed from out

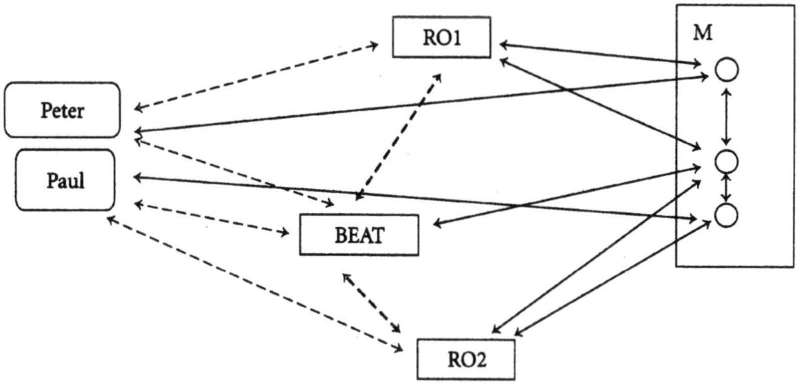

Figure 4. Memory activation of the episode "Paul beats Peter."

the memory indices in the way modeled in Figure 5. The same is true for achieving activation circuits for other constituents, namely those corresponding to modifier-noun and modifier-verb constructions.

The middle index, the one referring to the event or action, the situational index, can be connected to conceptual indicators characterizing the action, for example to the one for HARD. This would be the case if we remember a scene in which Peter beats Paul hard. By this we would construct the constituent BEATING HARD.

In remembering a situation in which there was a brown horse and a black blanket, the memory index for the situation must contain at least two sub-indices, which organize the binding of BROWN to HORSE and BLACK to BLANKET respectively, in order to distinguish this situation from one in which there is a black horse and a brown blanket. If the black blanket was on the brown horse, there has also to be a sub-index connecting to the indicator of the two-place relationship ON. The sub-index connecting to the indicator of HORSE must also have a connection to the indicator of the BOTTOM-ROLE-concept, relating to the indicator of the concept ON, and the sub-index connecting to the BLANKET indicator must also connect to the indicator of the TOP-ROLE, relating to the indicator of the concept ON.

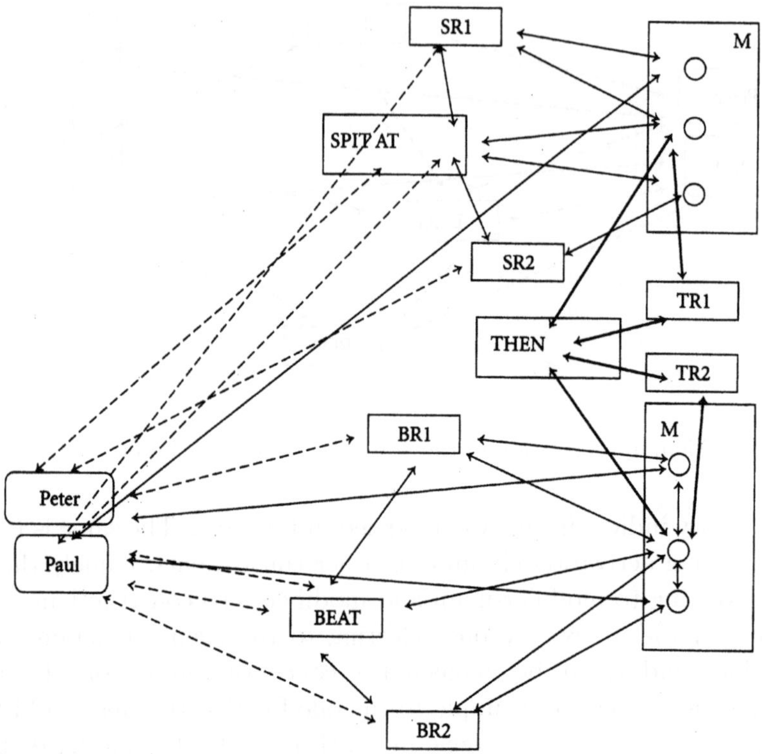

Figure 5. Circuit activation of "Paul spits at Peter. Then Peter beats Paul."

Figure 6 merely shows two sub-indices of the memory index of a situation in which there is a brown horse and a black blanket. The two sub-indices organize the two constituents, such that BROWN, HORSE, BLACK, BLANKET are not mixed up. The two constituents then activate the respective sensorial concepts and the phenomenally dedicated neurons in the visual system, such that a situation of a brown horse and a black blanket can be imagined. A remembrance of a situation with a brown horse and a black horse, and likewise the phrase *a black horse and a brown horse*, would be organized from out the memory indices as shown in Figure 7. We see that the indicator for the concept HORSE is connected with two different indices for

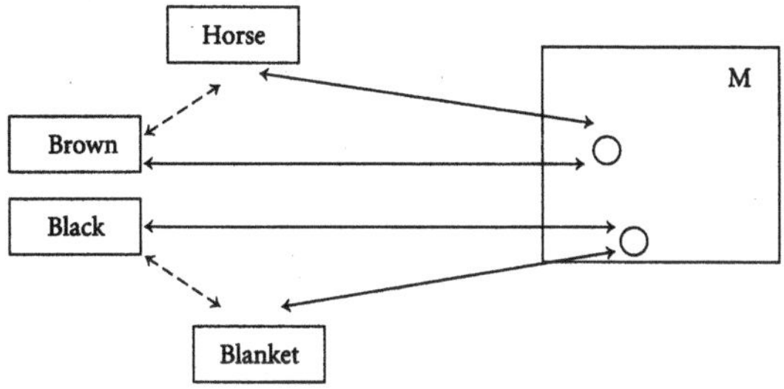

Figure 6. Memory activation of the episode "A brown horse and a black blanket"

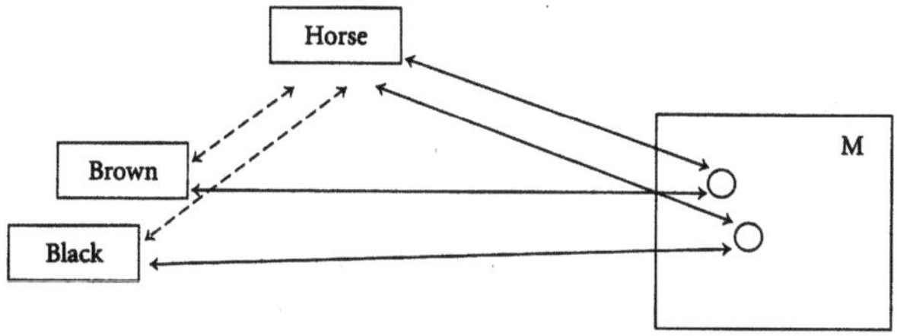

Figure 7. Memory activation of the episode "A black horse and a brown horse"

individuals in the specific memory, one is in circuit activation with the indicators for BLACK and HORSE, and the other with the indicators for BROWN and HORSE. On the other hand, a remembrance of a black and brown horse, and likewise the phrase *a black and brown horse*, would be organized from out the memory indices in a way that indicates that only one individual is involved (Figure 8).

The structuring of a remembered episode from out the memory indices follows, in the case of reliable remembrance, the way in which the original episode was structured as a perceived situation, or as the result of understanding a description and interpreting it in the world or some model. Remembering is a special act of imagination, namely one determined by indices in the episodic memory area M. In

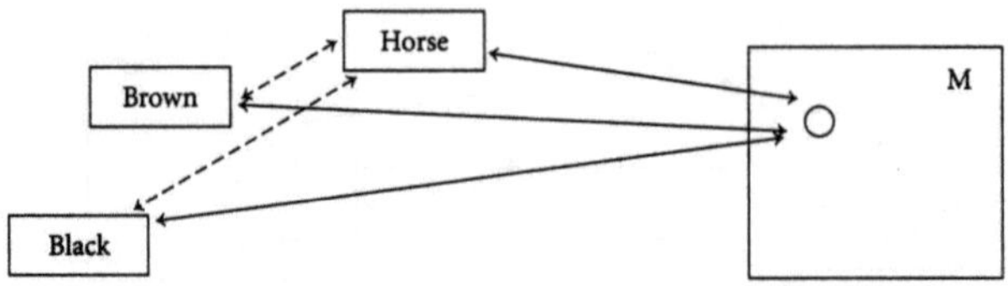

Figure 8. Memory activation of the episode “A black and brown horse”

our consciousness, this amounts to the imagination being embedded within one’s history, i.e. within the autobiographical memory, and hereby the image is understood as a remembered episode, and not just as a free fantasy. Remembering and imagining are often hard to distinguish, because remembering can include parts that were not present in the original episode, but come from other remembered episodes, or are added from cross-activation with and among conceptual indicators on the ontological conceptual maps and on the categorizing maps of the sensorial modalities and of the motor and emotional maps. Imagination for a large part can be understood as free combination of reconstructed parts of episodes indexed in area M. Thus memory plays an essential part as a basis for employing the power of imagination, also in our present experience of situations.

9 How memory works in understanding

In section 5 we have just answered this question for the general memory, and especially for the semantic memory. Also the historical, specific memory plays a role in understanding, of course as far as reference to individuals is concerned, which has been shown in the previous example. Also the episodic memory plays a role.

Above, it has been pointed out that the historical memory center consists of groups of neurons that serve as indices for individuals, places, and episodes. The memory-indices can function as such because they are connected to the general concept indicators that had characterized aspects of the previously experienced individual or episode. Likewise, the indices are connected to category indicators of the sensorial systems (indicators of sensorial concepts) and to neurons on the primary sensorial fields, which are dedicated to effecting certain sensational impressions, certain smells, sounds, faces, feelings of movements and other proprioceptional sensations, and emotions. A certain aspect, which is identical to one in the current situation, can call up the previous situation as a remembrance, via suitable connections. The remembered episode is constructed via the connections from the memory indices to conceptual indicators and neurons of the other fields, as modeled in section 6 and 7.

In understanding, the current situation is seen in the light of one or more previous similar situations: aspects from these situations can be unconsciously mixed up or partly be replaced for each other; and the current situation can be experienced with additional aspects from the old situations. The two situations or episodes can also be consciously compared or contrasted. Singular actions, but also routines that were connected with an old situation can be re-activated to become part of the current situation; they can be imagined, planned, or executed.

Above we saw that in understanding a situation, individual concepts have to be made use of, by integrating the situation under a role-concept into a partial individual concept available under preservation of coherence of the individual concept. Thus, a situation was understood as the one of John beating Paul by integrating or embedding it into the partial individual concept of JOHN as an AGENT and the partial individual concept of PAUL as a PATIENT and into the ACTION concept of BEATING, while binding them together into the smallest situation, and thus representing the situational concept that characterizes all situations in which John beats Paul. This constituent structure of binding-intersections between concepts corresponds to neuronal activation circuits along the connections between the groups of neurons serving as the respective concept indicators and indices. The smaller activation circuits are embedded into larger ones, and finally into the whole large circuit composed from all the constituent circuits. Also in remembering a past episode a same kind of constituent structure was necessary within the remembrance; the right contiguity relationships within the situation, as far as this basic conceptual built up is concerned, must be preserved in the remembered episode, such that the situation of Peter having beaten Paul is distinguished from the one of Paul having beaten Peter. This had been steered from out the complex memory index by the connections of its sub-indices to the indicators involved in the respective constituents.

The indices that constitute the episode must provide repeated activation for the circuit activation to hold for the time in which the remembrance occurs and in which we reflect on it. Furthermore, the indices can be connected to other episodes, which can be called up by activation of these connections. If, for example, if we experience often that Peter beats other boys, some of these previously experienced episodes of Peter beating others can be called up, since the connections are already strengthened by these repeated experiences. This also means that these episodes are typical within the individual concept we have of Peter. An individual concept thus is indicated by an index which is connected with indicators of typical properties of the individual, and which is connected with indices of episodes in which we have experienced the individual or about which we have been told. These properties and episodes contribute to understanding a new situation in which this individual is involved. The new situation is embedded into these old associative structures, and from there implications can be drawn unconsciously as associations coming up, or consciously by using these associated episodes or property assignments in controlled inferences we can make from the description of the new situation in conjunction with the descriptions of the old ones.

Both, the general memory of concepts and routines, especially the semantic memory, and the specific, historical memory, especially the individuating and the episodic memory, make up our understanding and even our perception of new situations and new sentences. And they provide the information on which our actions are based.

Understanding is subjective because it is based on our own history of experience. However, for a large part understanding is intersubjectively coordinated at the same time, through the workings of the historical memory that we partially share, and the partially common general memory, especially its linguistically guided semantic part. This inter-subjective part is, of course, the essential part for being able to get informed about the surroundings not merely by own experience, but by experience that is coordinated with others and by getting informed through others about all that what one does not or even cannot experience oneself, but what still is relevant for one's own orientation and possibility to act, and by getting informed of what is codified as public rules and norms. Concept formation is steered by the natural and social surroundings of the learning and experiencing individual, and about which it has to be informed, and on which it has to act; concept formation is subjective in part, depending on personal experiences; but concept formation is also inter-subjectively guided by the conventions and norms of the language communities, in which the subject lives. By means of language we can share our experiences in as far as they can be expressed by public means, and through the linguistic or pictorial expressions these experiences can become part of the memory of other persons, reconstructed in their partly subjective ways of understanding.

References

Bartsch, Renate. 1998. *Dynamic Conceptual Semantics: A Logico-philosophical Investigation into Concept Formation and Understanding.* Studies in Logic, Language, and Information. Stanford, Cal: CSLI and FoLLi Publications.

Bartsch, Renate. 2002. *Consciousness Emerging: The Dynamics of Perception, Imagination, Action, Memory, Thought, and Language.* Advances in Consciousness Research, Vol. 39. Amsterdam & Philadelphia: John Benjamins.

Bartsch, Renate. 2005. *Memory and Understanding: Proust's 'A la recherche du temps perdu' Seen in the Light of Dynamic Conceptual Semantics.* Amsterdam & Philadelphia: John Benjamins.

Frege, Gottlob. 1892. Über Sinn und Bedeutung. *Zeitschrift für Philosophie und philosophische Kritik* NF 100: 25–50.

Eternal objects, figuræ, and memory

Michael Fortescue

1 Eternal objects and figuræ

This article is concerned with the organization of linguistic memory. The perspective it takes combines a cognitive interpretation of Whitehead's philosophy of Process (as in Fortescue 2001) with Hjelmslev's more specifically linguistic framework. For Whitehead, memory - whether linguistic or otherwise - is a matter of enduring '*nexūs*' of sensory, kinaesthetic, and propositional forms that can be investigated from the point of view of two distinct but complementary perceptual modes, that of 'presentational immediacy' and that of 'causal efficacy'. The former concerns memory as a static 'system' of potential contrasts (Pattern), the latter the dynamic deployment of memory sequences in time (Process). Personal, episodic memory consists of an inextricable mesh of the two, with causal efficacy holding together complex clusters or sequences of (token) sensory images, and. language itself operates in the mixed mode of 'symbolic reference', whereby the use of words and whole utterances activates the semantic (and grammatical) contents of memory. Both aspects can be described in terms of Whiteheadian 'eternal objects', i.e. 'forms of definiteness', but it is especially the Pattern aspect of language that is in focus in the present context (for an elaboration of the Process aspect see Fortescue 2003). Corresponding to 'eternal objects' (of Pattern) Hjelmslev used the less problematical, more neutral term '*figura*'.

Whitehead was not very specific - let alone exhaustive - as to the number of sub-types of 'eternal objects' in his grand system. He was no Aristotelian taxonomist. The only distinction he discussed in any detail was that between eternal objects of the 'subjective' and of the 'objective' species (the latter correspond to the universal 'forms' of mathematics and will not concern us further here). The various types I propose on the list in section 2 below - in so far as they include sign types among them - correspond to the *figuræ* of a Hjelmslevian 'metasemiology' (though Hjelmslev came no nearer to a taxonomy of these than Whitehead did). It is important to note that they are just as concrete - relatable to the *sensa* of perception - as the categories of a 'lower level' semiotic analysis of a single language. In fact both eternal objects and *figuræ* are applicable to all possible levels of analysis, by virtue of being repeatable and communicable. They are relevant to substance as well as to form, and to both the content and expression planes of language. Hjelmslev equated his proposed metasemiology with an (in principle) exhaustive description of the ultimate components of 'substance' (Hjelmslev, 1963, 120ff).[1] Today we can bring to bear on that project advances in our knowledge of the content side of language, in prototype semantics, discourse pragmatics, modern metaphor theory, image schemas and force dynamics and other cognitively orientated forms of linguistics that were unavailable to Hjelmslev. What we might ask today is which *figuræ* analysable on a static descriptive meta-level are likely to have direct psychological implementation and which are not. They may equally well reflect discrete, binary contrasts or fuzzy 'prototypical' categories. Their degree of concreteness or abstractness is variable - all that matters is that the pattern concerned is repeatable and communicable.

By coming from 'outside language' the Whiteheadian approach may serve as a corrective to an over-indulgence in Peircean semiosis, from within which there is a risk that nothing can be seen beyond the impenetrable 'event horizon' of symbols and signs. Hjelmslev himself left open a way of escape from this predicament (which he

[1] Or rather what he called 'purport' (*mening*) as opposed to 'substance' (*substans*). The former term refers to the 'amorphous continuum' against which, he claimed, 'the net of linguistic form casts its shadow', thus creating 'substance', which for Hjelmslev presupposes the categories of language (op. cit.: 57). He was surely wrong (or at least purposely provocative) in this claim, if he really meant to suggest that pre-linguistic children do not recognize various types of salient 'natural kinds'. Elsewhere, note, he does talk of the possibility of an exhaustive description of linguistic content-purport as something requiring the collaboration of all the non-linguistic sciences, both physical and phenomenological (op. cit.: 78).

faced himself) in his suggestion of the possibility of a metasemiology. The Whiteheadian variant allows for the cognitive anchoring of semiotics and for 'meaning' to be approached from two complementary perspectives at once, the holistic and the analytic. Hjelmslev was temperamentally and intellectually disinclined to see that much of the content side of language is of a holistic and context-dependent nature (as opposed to its combinatorial aspects in isolation from non-linguistic context). The Whiteheadian approach that I espouse allows us to distinguish clearly the different 'societal' levels on which the same *figuræ* may be relevant, namely the level of the individual speaker/hearer, the level of the community of speakers of a specific language, and the purely descriptive metasemiological level embracing both of these. It also makes a clearer distinction between Pattern (which is what a metasemiology is concerned with) and Process (with which it is not, at least not directly). Hjelmslev himself, rather confusingly, used the term 'process' (*forløb*) to refer to texts as linguistic products, more specifically to their syntactic patterning (a matter of static 'content form' on the syntagmatic axis of language). Eternal objects cover a wider array of 'forms of definiteness' than Hjelmslev's *figuræ* - Hjelmslev was primarily thinking of types A and B illustrated in the following section. An essential step towards actually carrying through his metasemiological project lies, it seems to me, in seeing that types of linguistic intention, context-of-use, and process in general (but not individual processes themselves) may also be analysed in terms of *figuræ,* i.e. Whiteheadian eternal objects.[2]

[2] Hjelmslev did in fact suggest treating certain other kinds of *figuræ* (those corresponding especially to my types Cii and Eii below) under what he called a 'connotative semiotics' dealing with indexicality, style, emotional expression, etc., as an open-ended complement to an exhaustive, reductionist content 'metasemiotic'. A still broader 'metasemiology', by extracting the ultimate 'types' of elements behind all semiotic systems, can in principle be exhaustive. Note that a 'semiology' for Hjelmslev is a 'metasemiotic with a non-scientific (i.e. non-exhaustive) semiotic as an object semiotic' and is extendable beyond language systems as such, whereas a 'semiotic' is in principle exhaustive (reflecting the basic glossematic procedure of 'deduction'). Linguistics is thus a 'metasemiotic'.

In order to isolate *figuræ* of any kind, on both the expression and the content planes, Hjelmslev employed the notion of the 'commutation test' of paradigmatic alternation (Hjelmslev, 1963, 73f.). *Figuræ* are invariants, that is 'correlates with mutual commutation' (within a paradigm) - a change of an invariant on the expression plane results in a determinate change on the content plane, and *vice versa*. Those of the expression plane include the notion of the phoneme, for instance. As is well known, it was especially his search for the *figuræ* of the content plane - using the same methodology as for analysing the expression plane - that distinguished Hjelmslev from other structuralists. One major problem with that endeavour was that the 'paradigms' which the commutation test applied to content presuppose are ultimately anchored in cognitive categories independent of language (i.e. in 'substance'). Thus the content elements 'wood' and 'tree' (or their French and German equivalents rather) he saw as invariants within the same content 'paradigm', whereas Danish *træ*, which is more broadly polysemous, he saw as containing two variants (mutually substitutable) covering the same semantic area divided into two by the other languages. But that area itself, the substance divided up differently by the content paradigms of individual languages, is not wholly amorphous, it can be defined (at least in this case) in terms of prototypes of perception and/or 'natural kinds'. These are also invariants - invariants of substance. There is no reason to expect a particularly close or one-to-one relationship between the invariants of linguistic form and those of substance, but they both belong to the *figuræ* of a higher-order metasemiology. The search within the framework of a purely linguistic 'metasemiotics' for an exhaustive description of the minimal content *figuræ* (analogous to the expression plane glossemes) may well have been a wild goose chase, since the number of features required to distinguish all lexical meanings is enormous (if not infinite) and is moreover subject to the massive indeterminacy introduced by context. But is that also true of the search for content *figuræ* in a metasemiology? Is this also doomed to founder in the way that any reductionist componential analysis is bound to founder in the end?

To answer this one needs to ask how one would go about in practice applying the commutation test - via correlations between expression and content planes - to unearth the *figuræ*, the ultimate invariants, of a metasemiology, as Hjelmslev enjoins us to (op. cit.: 122f.). It would seem that this can only be done through applying an analysis of the correlations between the full range of content and expression distinctions actually made by the languages of the world ('purport' itself can not be divided into these two planes, note). This is part and parcel of the overall typology of the world's languages that Hjelmslev envisaged (op.cit.: 126). Linguistic form (*sprogform*), he suggested, is actually equivalent to purport form (*meningsform*), just seen from a different perspective (op. cit.: 123f.), though we can only get at the *figuræ* of the latter from the *figuræ* of the former. For Hjelmslev '*meningsform*' remained the way substance is modulated by pure form. This nevertheless represents an opening into the physical world of substance described by the natural and anthropological sciences - and also to the contents of individual memory. So the procedure, one might think, must be to unearth the minimal, irreducible semantic components behind all linguistic signs, across all languages, which, when changed, correlate with changes in expression in some part of some language. This is of course a still more open-ended task than when submitting the words of a single language to an exhaustive semantic analysis. However, it is surely still feasible if one limits the endeavour to a taxonomy of language-relevant *figuræ* **types** constrained by what is known of both the typology of human languages on the level of the community-of-speakers and of the cognitive processing of language on the level of the individual speaker.[3] What this procedure will not arrive at is an exhaustive listing of all specific

[3] This is easy enough to envisage for closed classes of elements - the grammaticalized categories with which linguistic typology is largely concerned - but it can also in principle be extended to content words in lexical areas which seem to be neatly characterizable in terms of a universal set of semantic primitives, such as domestic animals and kinship terms (from which Hjelmslev draws his few concrete examples). However, these are few and turn out to be either far less neat than envisaged or else to reflect a purely conventional, socially sanctioned taxonomy of social relations.

'atoms' of meaning of all kinds of words, a conceptual *smørgåsbord* from which individual words in individual languages put together their actual meanings. The trouble is, of course, that few words lack some degree of polysemy and, moreover, word meaning is largely organized along context-sensitive, prototypical lines. The only way out of this dilemma for Hjelmslev would have been to accept that, on the one hand, the 'substance' relevant to language is indeed structured to some significant degree independently of language itself, and, on the other, that the range of intentionality expressed through language use is itself structured, interacting with and affecting the overall pattern. These were steps Hjelmslev was unable to take himself.

Hjelmslev's most positive contribution to a viable metasemiology - the aspect of his work I am singling out in the present paper - was, to my mind, to see that the *figuræ* needed to analyse all levels of language structure (as semiotic or metasemiotic, as expression or content) are essentially of the same order, for the simple reason that *figuræ* are not signs themselves: his *figuræ* are non-signs ingredient in signs. His search for invariants (not just smaller and smaller variants) was at the heart of his method, whether on the expression or the content plane of language. Hjelmslev was well aware, however, that the *figuræ* of the content side are not the same as those of the expression side (there cannot possibly be any one-to-one mapping since the *nexus* that constitutes a symbolic sign is essentially arbitrary). He did not believe in a fixed, substantive set of universal semantic components in the manner of Leibniz' 'universal alphabet of meaning', but only in a weaker version of this, namely that there are universal formal principles by which sense components are combined to produce lexemes (cf. Lyons 1977, vol. 1: 331). But for some reason Hjelmslev drew back from his own proposal to investigate the *figuræ* of a universal metasemiology. In his later work (especially Hjelmslev 1954) he continued to search rather for *figuræ* of individual languages, seen now as organized into four 'vertical' strata.

In the Whiteheadian scheme of things the 'way things are' can be divided up into certain overall categories, the most important for present purposes being: (a) eternal objects (concepts, forms of definiteness); (b) *nexūs* ('societies' - including persons, enduring objects, and events as well as human societies); (c) propositions (relations between *nexūs* and eternal objects), and (d) prehensions (processes). A metasemiology must cover all types and sub-types of these - but not specific **tokens** of (b), (c), or (d), for example not the contents of individual memory (whether episodic or encyclopaedic) nor the individual words of a given language (these are 'weak *nexūs*'). It is essential to understand the societal level of which one is talking when applying these notions: on the level of the language community (the broader *nexus* validating the language behaviour in question) it is a matter of defining the complex eternal object that a socially transmitted language system represents (in all its inherited, repeatable aspects: grammar, norms of use, and vocabulary), whereas on the level of the personal *nexus* (or speaker/hearer) it is a matter of individual cognition and how the socially transmitted eternal object is 'represented' in the individual mind/brain. A metasemiology must link both these levels - what is common to them both (or rather all three) is the ingredient eternal objects themselves, since these must be the same for every speaker/hearer in order for effective communication using the language to take place at all, and (as regards the metasemiology) for translation to be possible between languages. It also covers (unlike the two subordinate, socially embedded levels) higher order typological generalizations only unearthed by comparing more than one particular language system.

2 Species of eternal object relevant to language as social inheritance

The present section concerns most immediately the first of the two levels defined above, namely that of the linguistic community as a whole; the question of the 'ingression' - or manifestation - of eternal objects in the individual speaker/hearer will be handled more specifically in the following section. The relationship between sign expressions and sign contents validated by the complex socially inherited eternal object has to be reestablished (i.e. learnt) by every single new speaker/hearer and, as it were, the content categories 'mapped' into experientially (subjectively) anchored meaning, so the language must in a sense be recreated from scratch each time with the help of input and context and certain inherent propensities of the mind/brain to look for systematic communicative intentions. On the individual cognitive level the signs of a language are *nexūs* (relations between clusters of *figuræ* of expression and of content in memory), whereas on the level of the community of its speakers they constitute part of the abstract overall pattern of the language which has no reality apart from in the mind/brains of individual speaker/hearers and their linguistic products. Moreover, the corresponding linguistic processes involved on the two levels are very different and must be treated separately: on the level of the individual speaker/hearer it is a matter of general cognitive prehensions (including acts of 'symbolic reference'), but on that of the language as an abstract entity at the level of the community, it is a matter of diachronic changes in the system itself (actually a reflection of changes in the society - the *nexus* - bearing it). The overarching metasemiology itself does not contain processes as such, only process types (just as it only contains word types, albeit defined in terms of a sub-set of the same *figuræ* as on the other levels). It is pure Pattern and has no independent ontological status at all.

Here, then, is a first pass at the minimal set of sub-types of eternal object (read '*figuræ*') that appear to be needed to discuss the phenomenon of language from a Whiteheadian perspective:

A. Concepts
   i. predicates (of activity, state, quality, etc.)
   ii. logical subject types

B. Relational/structural patterns
   i. morphosyntactic
   ii. phonological
   iii. (co)referential
   iv. logical-relational
   v. semantic

C. Types of subjective form
   i. discourse modulation functions
   ii. epistemic stance
   iii. validatory attitudes

D. Intentional types
   i. discourse acts
   ii. strategies (and patterns of inference)
   iii. behavioural norms
   iv. background communicative principles

E. Nexus types
   i. contexts of situation
   ii. social/historical and textual embedding
   iii. sign (e.g. word) types

F. Propositional types
   i. simple
   ii. complex

The types of 'prehensions' relevant to language (Process types, not actual token processes) could have been added here in so far as they too correspond to eternal objects.[4] I shall ignore this in the following, however, which focusses on language as Pattern.

Let us look at all of the types of eternal object listed above in more detail - I shall give a couple of examples of each category. Bear in mind that though all of them are relevant for language, they are not all linguistic as such, especially the first and last types, A and F, onto which linguistic items (themselves consisting of eternal objects) can be 'mapped'. The complex eternal object constituting the grammar of (say) English on the level of the community of its speakers can be said to be restricted to eternal objects of type B, but a language is more than its grammar: all linkages between its elements of expres-

4 Namely: a. Physical (including 'indicative'), b. Conceptual, c. Hybrid, d. Indicative, e. Propositional, f. Anticipatory, g. Intuitive judgments, h. Transmutation, i. Symbolic reference. See Fortescue (2001) for further elaboration.

sion and content, of structure and associated meaning, are passed on by the community to new speakers as a more or less unified 'package', as are the principles of how to use that package in society. In other words, the grammar of English (or any other language), inherited from generation to generation, is embedded in a broader social world - this is organized knowledge, it has to be learnt via a social *nexus* in which it is ingredient and cannot come straight from the eternal object itself.

This is not to deny the role of inherent constraints deriving from the internal structure and functioning of the mind/brain; these (including the propensity to communicate itself) are there in the internal organization of every potential speaker/hearer. They need not be reflected in the complex eternal object itself except indirectly, as the accreting product of history. Bear in mind at this point that the categories we are looking at from a metasemiological perspective as 'types' (in capital letters below) can be filled out at the community-of-speakers level with specific *nexūs* - in particular with specific signs (words, etc.) and associated contextual 'frames'. At the personal (cognitive) level these patterns will be instantiated within a broader, richer, more indeterminate and subjective *nexus* of associations, the product of individual experience and memory. In general, eternal objects of one type may make reference to (i.e. be ingredient in) those of any other type - thus structural configurations under type B may have their own functional 'meanings' with which they constitute a 'weak *nexus*' of type Eiii, and they may be further associated with certain Di and Ci intentions and Fi relations.

A. Concepts

i. predicates (examples: RUN, FLOAT, HIT, SQUARE, GREEN, RAPIDLY, REPEATEDLY)
ii. logical subject types (e.g. MAN, TREE, HOUSE, WATER)

These correspond roughly to the perceivable/imaginable activities, states, qualities, scalar values, etc., typically referred to by lexical content words (but may also be relevant to bound morphemes). They do not, however, presuppose lexical expression - no one language need have 'basic' words corresponding exactly to all or any of them. Concepts are from the Whiteheadian perspective 'unordered' (i.e. purely potential) themselves, but for the individual subject (speaker/hearer) they are manifest as associated clusters of sensory, kinaesthetic, or other more abstract 'affordances' such as children learn about during their pre-linguistic development.[5] Not only 1st order entities (things, persons, etc.) can be treated as logical subjects, note, but also (by 'transmutation') 2nd and higher order ones (states of affairs, propositions, etc.), but this is a matter of referential process. The eternal objects involved in defining Aii type eternal objects are simply bundles of Ai predicates reflecting stable, repeatable object (proto-)types. Both sub-types contain relatively complex concepts as well as simple ones - thus types of actions under (i) may involve associated subject types under (ii) (thus 'hitting' involves both an animate hitter and a thing - or person - hit, with or without the mediation of an instrument). On the personal (cognitive) level these associations (including those that bind words to concepts, forming symbolic 'bundles') are *nexūs*, on that of communities of speakers they are merely eternal objects of relation of a certain kind. One could well sub-divide (i) into actions vs. qualities, etc., and (ii) into stable countables vs. unstable

---

[5] I use this term much as MacWhinney (1999) does, following Gibson, to refer to sensory reactions to a word (e.g. images invoked), but I extend it here in the Whiteheadian vein to include action schemas and still more complex and/or abstract associations. These clusters of sensory associations are not relevant in their entirety to the descriptive meta-level, only on the cognitive level of individual speaker/hearers. Nevertheless, on the level of communities of speakers individual words obviously have determinate, socially transmitted 'values' - this is so because signs as relations between *nexūs* (types as well as tokens) are part of the complex eternal objects constituting individual languages. The *nexūs* involved can be very specific, namely binding individual words to an array of related meanings relevant to particular contexts, i.e. to specific event and entity *nexus* types (all themselves defined by other simpler types of eternal object). Concepts of greater specificity are generally accessed through association with words set in less tangible 'social' context/*nexus* types (as under E below). 'Abstract' concepts depend on such secondary *nexūs* which each individual learner has to reconstruct, often reorganizing existing, more concrete word-meaning *nexūs* in the process.

or unbounded masses, etc., but intermediate and overlapping types can generally be found.

B. Relational/structural patterns

i. morphosyntactic (e.g. CLAUSE, PHRASE, SUBJECT, MODIFIER, HEAD)
ii. phonological (e.g. PHONEME, LABIAL, PITCH ACCENT)
iii. logical-relational (e.g. ON-TOP-OF, AND, PREVIOUS-TO, BECAUSE-OF)
iv. (co-)referential (e.g. SAME-ENTITY-AS, SAME-NOUN-CLASS-AS)
v. semantic (e.g. INCLUDES, OPPOSITE-OF, ENTAILS, AGENT, TELIC, PERFECTIVE)

The first two sub-types correspond to the categories of structural contrasts relevant to the grammar of individual languages (expansions of words, phrases and clauses), independent of specific occasions of reference, predication, etc. Sub-type (iii) corresponds to the basic meanings of prepositions and conjunctions, etc., (iv) reflects rule-like patterns of agreement, cross-reference, etc. (associated with indicative prehensions), and type (v) covers 'semantic' patterns in the narrow sense - relations of entailment, hyponymy, antonymy, etc., holding between classes of lexical items (and forming the basis of taxonomies) and between entities and predicates (the basis of the argument structures associated with verbs) or within complex predicates (e.g. modality and aspect). The hierarchical organization of the various strata of language (phonemes, morphemes, sentences and texts) also belongs here, relating sub-types (i) and (ii). There are also higher-level metasemiological distributional/ implicational generalizations that can be made across languages. A fully specified functional grammar for a specific language contains a sub-set of all these elements (and their potential mappings to other categories).[6] Note

[6] This does not necessarily mean that there is any direct interpretation of such a grammar in process terms on the level of the individual speaker/hearer. The abstractions here correspond on that level largely to holistic 'feelings' of relatedness and structure in the Whiteheadian mode of 'causal efficacy'. On

that these eternal objects may all enter into complex linguistic signs under type Eiii below, but do not themselves constitute signs. Hjelmslev's treatment of morpho-syntax as static 'content-form' (combinatorial principles) makes perfect sense from this generalized 'Pattern' perspective; it is more problematic on the individual speaker's level (but this was not the level he was concerned with).

C. Subjective form types
   i. discourse modulation functions (e.g. FOCUS, TOPIC, FRAME)
   ii. epistemic stance (e.g. FACT, POSSIBILITY, NECESSITY)
   iii. validatory attitudes and emotions (e.g. AMAZEMENT, TENTATIVE, JOCULAR)

These sub-types cover all repeatable (i.e. communicatively recognizable) forms of meaning conveyed by aspects of communication that do not directly reflect propositional content, e.g. by prosodic patterns, interjections, discourse particles, attitudinal or rhetorical adverbials, etc., all of them expressive of emotional or other kinds of subjective perspective.[7] 'Epistemic stance' distinguishes propositions entertained or proposed as 'beliefs' from assumed 'facts' or hypothetical/ imaginary states of affairs, etc.

---

the meta-level there will always be a choice of different ways of analyzing the relevant patterns, i.e. by different theoretical treatments of the 'same' type of grammatical phenomena, since these have no ontological status. Different analyses may display varying degrees of descriptive economy and empirical generalizability.

7 The meanings of words expressing such elements are, of course, notoriously language-specific, and one may well ask whether such a discourse or rhetorical element such as '*well*' or '*in fact*', or exclamations like '*I say!*' or '*damn it all!*' in English can be broken down into a combination of universal *figuræ* at all. However, bear in mind that it is with types of discourse and expressive function we are dealing with here on the metasemiological level, not with individual words. The particular array of discourse functions a given particle in English performs can certainly be described in general terms, however complex and/or context-specific they may be. As with type Eiii *figuræ* below, individual words belong on the *nexus* level of the community of speakers.

D. Intentional types

i. discourse acts (e.g. REQUEST INFORMATION, ORDER, PROMPT, PROMISE)
ii. strategies (e.g. CALCULATE CONSEQUENCES, UNEARTH MOTIVATION)
iii. behavioural norms (e.g. TAKE-TURN, REPLY)
iv. background communicative principles (e.g. BE-RELEVANT, SUPPLY-JUST-ENOUGH-INFORMATION)

Illocutionary speech acts are only a special case of 'discourse act' here (one where there is a rather direct association between form of utterance and content); such acts are generally embedded in a higher order intentional ('perlocutionary') complex involving type (ii) factors. The sub-types here cover the repeatables that make up such complex aims, including conventional response types and turn-taking in conversation. 'Strategies' include patterns of inference, which allow logical progression from one proposition to another (including forms of 'practical' syllogism), and 'behavioural norms' include the basis of deontic modality, but also include the dimensions of variation that are covered by Coseriu's (Coseriu 1975) concept of 'norm' (non-systematic yet conventional - or at least statistically expected - aspects of usage).[8] The last sub-category (iv) covers the longer-term intentional stances corresponding to the heuristics, maxims and principles with which pragmatics is concerned (they form the basis for empathy).

Note that Whitehead's dynamic view of meaning, like Grice's 'meaning-nn' (speaker meaning - Grice 1957), covers both what is said and what is merely implicated, and corresponds to both Peirce's 'immediate' and 'dynamical' interpretant (respectively the feeling of

---

8 This is a layer of language mediating between *parole* and *langue* ('System'). It contains all the social variation out of which the individual speaker abstracts the essential system of 'functional oppositions', i.e. the complex eternal object defining the language concerned. One might say that System must be abstracted out of socially given Norm by every individual, and that abstraction is necessary precisely to allow stable internalization (and further transmission) of the language.

recognizing a sign and the resultant actions/reactions induced in the recipient - Peirce 1958/1931, vol. 8: 343.)

E. Nexus types

i. contexts of situation (e.g. TICKET-OFFICE, LECTURE, ENQUIRING-AFTER-STREET-DIRECTIONS)
ii. social/historical and textual embedding (e.g. HERE-AND-NOW, IN-THE-ERA-OF, IN-TEXT-OF)
iii. sign types (e.g. NOUNS, VERBS, FUNCTORS, INTERJECTIONS, PROPER-NAMES)

The first two of these sub-types cover all manner of 'frames', 'scripts', 'scenarios', 'routines', 'texts', etc., as well as types of spatiotemporal settings providing deictic anchoring (tense and spatial deixis), in fact anything in the contextual embedding of an utterance that has a socially shared bearing on its interpretation, from the immediate communicative situation through highlighted 'topics of discourse' to whole cultural settings.[9] The third sub-type, 'sign types', is of particular significance in relation to language, covering as it does the relation between morphemes, words, and larger units under B and their meanings (under A, etc.). What is reflected here in broad metasemiological terms is quite literally sign types, since signs themselves cannot be directly equated across language - only approximate overlaps in meaning (and shared lower level eternal ob-

9 Actually, '*nexus*' covers all varieties of 'association', but *nexūs* as such are not eternal objects - they cover 'societies' and 'enduring objects' constituted by virtue of their association to a common eternal object (and further interrelated by potential propositional relationships - for instance knowledge of specific 'facts'). This includes the particular 'mental models' of both 'episodic' and 'encyclopaedic' memory, which are therefore not included under this type of eternal object (though the *figuræ* of the latter enter into the contents of individual memory). Note that these *nexus* types are what is potentially recognized as pertaining to a given communicative situation by individual speaker/hearers - it is a matter of the match between a token situation and the corresponding type. The *figuræ* relevant to defining both the type and tokens will by and large be the same (though tokens will contain many irrelevant elements and may match the token only by a fairly rough relationship of analogy).

jects ingredient in them) can be so analysed. Signs can be of varying levels of complexity, from single morphemes to whole constructions involving a variety of both content and expressions *figuræ*. It is important to grasp that these patterns must be conventionalized to attain the status of eternal object here, and that there will always be a penumbra of semi-conventional patterns - in particular ones emergent from the 'natural' interplay of available linguistic means and ad hoc communicative means - that can only be regarded as 'potential signs'. 'New' eternal objects are continually arising like bubbles of froth emerging from - and often disappearing back into - the turbulent waters of actual language use, only some of them becoming 'captured' by the complex conventional object that is the language concerned ('new' here is not in conflict with 'eternal', by the way, when one understands the purely potential nature of eternal objects). On the community-of-speakers level, as mentioned earlier, the *nexūs* between specific words and their meanings (which for the individual speaker/hearer is a matter of associated eternal objects of any type and their potential combination in specific context types) themselves embody eternal objects of relationship since they are communicable and repeatable yet abstracted from any concrete occasion of usage. So on that level specific words of English like *fall* or *holiday* with their respective meanings can - as part of the 'eternal object' English - be said to exemplify the type. These meanings may range in degree of abstractness from perceptual types under A to socially defined 'forms of definiteness' that have no independent status apart from the words associating them to specific types of *nexūs* of type Eii (and, in turn, the types of eternal objects defining their typical perceptual affordances).[10]

[10] At the personal level these socially shared meanings may not be easily isolatable (except via dictionary definitions) from actual cognitive processes of use. This is not only because of complex additional associations in the mind/brains of individual speakers but also because of the degree of indeterminacy introduced by multiple layers of communicatively relevant background (type E eternal objects) in constraining or altering such 'basic' meanings in context (this may require inference as well as knowledge of grammar and vocabulary in order to be worked out).

F. Propositional types

i. simple (e.g. TRANSITIVE-ACTION, PURPOSEFUL-MOTION)
ii. complex (e.g. CAUSAL, TEMPORAL, REPORTATIVE)

These cover basic 'event structures' and relations of causality and temporal unfolding between successive propositions - they consist of associations between certain type Ai and Aii concepts and cover the 'underlying' propositional structures onto which linguistic sentences 'map' (by compression into fewer or expansion into a larger number of units, etc.), including basic 'force dynamic' schemas (Talmy, 1988), which can in turn be combined and extended. Token propositions, recall, are not themselves eternal objects but relate the latter to specific *nexūs* (or to Aii logical subject types).

3 The 'ingression' of figuræ of language Pattern in the individual mind/brain

All of the types of eternal objects listed above can in principle be related to particular structural sub-regions of the mind/brain, in particular of the cortex. They constitute the structure of linguistic memory. In themselves eternal objects are unordered: the associations pertaining between them depends on the particular processes in which they are involved. They emerge from different kinds of information impinging on different parts of the overall system.[11] The varying types of connection to other regions (whether this be a matter of long-distance neural links or of the diffusion and assimilation of 'copies' of more local patterns) constitute constraints on the kinds of processes passing through them. Note that the contents of individual/personal memory consists according to Whiteheadian doctrine of enduring objects (*nexūs* of an 'internal' sort), not of **eternal** objects (which nevertheless enter the constitution of the former); these are

[11] I assume that the cortex alone forms the basis for perception in the mode of presentational immediacy, whereas deeper regions of the mind/brain are probably involved in perception in the mode of causal efficacy. Some of the types of eternal objects listed above do presuppose access to deeper regions (notably those under type C referring to emotional tone).

only approximately repeatable for the individual subject (and change moreover with time) - they are only very indirectly 'communicable' between subjects. Circumventing the question of the perhaps largely indeterminate location of such enduring objects in individual memory, one could nevertheless envisage the following kind of distribution of the various eternal object types listed in section 2, based on what is generally known of the overall functioning of the brain today (although in detail the picture may well turn out to be wrong at various points).[12]

A. Concepts

i. Simple predicates of action, state and quality in proximity to the relevant sensorimotor association areas (including motor cortex for kinaesthetic action types); more complex ones are situated in higher level association areas ('tertiary' convergence zones) with links to logical subject types under (ii) - also to purely socially-determined E-type eternal objects. Such eternal objects determine what it feels like to perform or view, etc., the particular type of activity/action/state concerned, and are crucially involved in processes of propositional prehension.[13]

---

[12] I do not assume a sharp distinction between 'episodic' (autobiographical) memory and 'encyclopaedic' or 'semantic' memory. Damasio sees both of these as distributed widely in the convergence zones of the temporal and frontal cortices and not in principle separable. The associations and means of ingression of the second kind of memory traces are presumably more verbal (note that definitional meaning can in theory be 'read off' imagery in the form of verbalizable Whiteheadian propositions). Episodic memory is in principle constituted by the same *figuræ* as behind encyclopaedic knowledge, only containing as an essential anchor the individual's own 'self-image' (itself a *nexus* - the maximally distinct 'map' of the subject himself/herself, as projected perhaps to the right frontal lobe and at all events continually updated). All of this is, according to Damasio, one vast 'dispositional space' of potential affordances, distinct from 'image space', which is located closer to the primary sensory areas of the cortex. For Whitehead too such knowledge is only accessible through specific kinds of processes (prehensions) that evoke specific complexes of eternal objects (patterns or 'images').

[13] As MacWhinney points out, however, there is evidence that also right hemi-

ii. Simple or complex types of perceptual object in sensory association areas (convergence zones); all such concepts are associated with the processes of transmutation (categorization) and indicative prehension (reference). Like those under (i), these eternal objects are cross-associated with encyclopaedic knowledge structures under type E below.

B. Relational/structural patterns

i. Anchored in the classical 'speech centre' arc between the auditory and motor cortex of the left hemisphere around the Sylvian fissure - morphological patterns presumably closer to the temporal lobe, syntactic ones closer to the frontal lobe end (Broca's area); note that I assume the morpho-syntactic categories finding ingression here are those relevant to specific languages and are not necessary universal.

ii. Superior left hemisphere temporal lobe 'phonemic' representations (or kinaesthetic 'gestural' or visual 'orthographic' ones in adjacent areas), all associated both cortically and subcortically to Broca's area.

iii. Parietal lobe association areas (for 'quasi-spatial' mappings).

iv. Associated with - and possibly just a sub-part of - Bi syntactic patterning, but sensitive to higher level (textually organized) *nexūs* under E.

v. Left hemisphere temporal association areas - but also the prefrontal verb-mediation zone (as under Eiii) is presumably involved as regards Ai concepts of a dynamic kind.

---

sphere prefrontal areas are involved in activating 'action terms'. He sees frontal lobe activity in general working in concert with more posterior regions of the brain (e.g. via the dorsal visual 'where' stream) so as to access and interact with sensory affordances. He specifically discusses frontal lobe involvement in organizing the 'spatial' mappings of the parietal lobes in complex 'perspective shifting'. He suggests four different types of perspective, i.e. modes of interaction between the individual and events experienced or described by him: affordances (in the narrow sense); spatio-temporal reference frames; causal action chains; and social roles (MacWhinney, 1999, 246f.).

C. Types of subjective form

   i. Associated with right hemisphere frontal motor cortex (the locus of affective tuning of prosodic 'packages'?), but also with the attentional aspects of prefrontal areas.

   ii. Higher-level left hemisphere prefrontal association areas. iii. Sub-cortical linkage of the frontal cortex with deeper emotional centres.

D. Intentional types

   Higher level prefrontal association (convergence zone) areas.

E. Nexus types

   i. Parietal associative area 'mental maps' as well as higher level prefrontal 'social' frames.

   ii. Broadly distributed 'encyclopaedic' knowledge structures (mainly anchored in the temporal lobes?).

   iii. As regards lexical words at least, this presumably involves associations between the left temporal lobe region where phonemic word forms are anchored and the left-hemisphere regions where A-type concepts and E-type 'frames' are stored.[14]

F. Propositional types

   Presumably concentrated in pre-frontal regions.

It should be emphasized that the eternal objects relevant for the structural organization of the individual mind/brain at this cognitive level are not necessarily equivalent or even isomorphic to the maximal generalizations, universals, and/or 'primitives' discernible at a meta-level of linguistic description (or within the complex eternal objects that the grammars of specific languages represent at the community-of-speakers level). Yet if the 'same' eternal objects are relevant to all societal levels, as I have suggested, there must be mu-

[14] This appears to involve a specific left hemisphere 'mediating' region in the inferior frontal lobe for relating verb forms to their meanings (adjacent to Broca's area, crucial in sentence-generation), where also grammatical functors are associated to 'valency/argument frames'. The inferior temporal lobe contains an analogous region for the mediation of the meanings of nouns to their phonemic expression (Damasio and Damasio, 1992).

tual 'translatability' via a common sub-set of eternal objects. A case in point is Wierzbicka's semantic primitives like THING, DO or SAY (Wierzbicka, 1992), which may well be ingredient in clusters of affordances associated with individual words (especially via basic 'image schemas'), but which do not by any means correspond exactly to the irreducible, holistic meaning of certain 'basic' words in any given language, since the meanings of all words - however complex - can be holistically accessed in the mode of causal efficacy and, moreover, all content words are associated with further affordances (involving eternal objects beyond some primitive, 'underlying' set). The latter are accessible in the mode of presentational immediacy and are highly subject to contextual delimitation and highlighting.

I shall not attempt an account of the processes in which such meta-level eternal objects may find ingression on the individual cognitive level. Those eternal objects that can be reasonably related to cognitive processes for which there is independent evidence (and which display obvious intuitive relevance for the individual speaker/hearer) are, in theory, the best candidates for elevation to metasemiological status - in so far as one is guided by cognitive 'realism' at all. This applies *a fortiori* to Hjelmslev's content-form *figuræ* (not to mention Chomsky's 'innate' principles and parameters). Just considering linguistic patterning alone (individual or across languages) is not enough, for without taking psychological plausibility into account there can be no grounds for the preference for one alternative meta-description over another, apart from aesthetic ones based on economy and inclusiveness (which apparently sufficed for Hjelmslev, as it still does for Chomsky).

4 The representation of word meanings in the brain

What needs to be illustrated now is how a restricted sub-set of metasemiological eternal objects - or *figuræ* - can link language Pattern and language Process on the levels of both the community-of-speakers and the individual speaker. Bear in mind that a *figura* (on any level) can in principle be as specific or general as required, as long as its status remains that of a repeatable type. It should also be borne in mind that - to reformulate the keystone of structuralistic thinking - linguistic categories (whether lexical or morphosyntactic) are accessible to speakers of a given language by their contrasts with other categories, not by their (meta-)labels. The Whiteheadian angle on this is that the *figuræ* relevant to description at the meta-level are only experientially accessible to individual speakers through their recognition of contrasts (of expression or of content) and that clusters of such contrasts (again on either 'plane') may be prehended both analytically - through selectively highlighted sensory 'affordances' - or holistically, in the mode of causal efficacy. This combines the 'componential' and the 'prototypical' approaches to linguistic categories.

Let us consider what meta-level *figuræ* might be needed to describe the content of a single English word (as an element in the complex we call English at the community-of-speakers level), one that is neither too concrete nor too abstract, for example the word *holiday*. We will then ask how (and where) these might find ingression in the mind/brain of the individual speaker. The full array of affordances of this word can be said to contain the following types of eternal objects/ *figuræ* from the categories elaborated above:

Ai. Complexes of percepts in a full range of sensory modalities, i.e. associated images, including kinaesthetic ones of swimming, walking in hills, etc. - an indeterminate congeries of impressions from earlier holidays (e.g. from descriptions of and pictures from specific holidays, one's own or those of others).

Bv. The relationship to the meanings of other words in the same word class, the same lexical field or taxonomy, the relevant relations of hyponymy, meronymy, etc.; this minimally includes the contrast between periods of work and of holiday longer than one day's duration.

Cii. The emotional feeling tone associated with the word (generally - but not necessarily! - happy, combining relaxation and eager anticipation).

Eii. The social background which validates what counts as a *holiday*, notably contrasts with *work* within the frame of the *working year* (or that of the *working day*), or (for pupils and students) with *term time* in the yearly academic cycle.

The sub-parts of this overall array that are actually highlighted or foregrounded as relevant for a particular token utterance containing it will depend on numerous factors, but most crucial for present purposes is the immediate linguistic context - e.g. in a collocation like *take a holiday.*[15] Here certain of the Ai and Eii type *figuræ* above will be irrelevant (for example those to do with school terms), owing to the notion of 'taking' (what is one's by right) that is introduced by the head verb *take.* But this mutual inhibition/ highlighting goes both ways in such collocations - *holiday* in turn suppresses all but a pale trace of the full meaning of the verb. It has almost the status of a verbalizing dummy word here, but the inherent *figura* of 'willed/purposeful action' adhering to the verb is nevertheless still discernible - its choice is motivated, since it harmonizes nicely with the highlighted features of the *holiday* complex as described.

It is instructive to compare the situation in English with that in French, which has several more specific words corresponding to the single word in English. Thus *congé* is leave from work (or from military service), but enters collocations similar to those of the English word: *être en/ prendre un congé* ('be on/ take a holiday'), whereas *les vacances* refers today to the summer holidays (from work or school - i.e. *les grandes vacances*), and *un jour férié* (or, with a specific religious content, *fête*) is a day officially recognized as free from work. There is also - somewhat outdated today perhaps - *jour de sortie*, typically a day off, an excursion to the country, and (*être en*) *villégiature*

[15] Consider such common collocations as *bank holiday, holiday mood*, and *holiday traffic*, in which other elements of the complex associative affordances of *holiday* are highlighted. In the case of the first of these, association with shops being closed is central (an element absent or suppressed in collocations involving longer stretches of work-free vacation such as *on holiday*). In the expression *holiday traffic*, on the other hand, the aspect highlighted is quite a negative one: the relevant affordances of *traffic* here (that part of them to do with road traffic from the point of view of the driver, conversely highlighted by *holiday*) suppress the more positive aspects of the meaning of *holiday* by negative prehensions.

of a stay in the country or at a resort. The question is, what is common to all these meanings - what is it that despite the lack of precise overlap is common to both languages here, that permits translation between them? Can we speak of a common (even universal) lexical field? What is shared is the social framework allowing inferences from the use of these words, for example that 'being on holiday' - or *congé*, or *vacances*, etc. - precludes 'being at work'. There is both a degree of cultural commonality between England and France here but also important differences (e.g. as regards the official status of local saint's days and the ways specific 'holy days' are celebrated). Each language groups together different classes of affordances that cover larger or smaller areas of denotation, the only significant structural difference being that in English the overall congeries of affordances associated with 'holiday' are narrowed down solely by collocation and context, while French already has preselected labels for a number of such sub-parts. As for a common 'lexical field', this is probably a mirage - as is well known, a given word may belong to several cross-cutting 'lexical fields' (think of English *leave* or French *congé* - or even better *fête*). There is nothing to hold this 'field' together but the social frames themselves. These are largely shaped by language (through contrasts with other words in the respective languages such as *work* or *travail*) but are in essence independent of it. The role of underlying embodied 'image schemas' (which may provide common cognitive anchoring for verbs of movement and transfer, for example) is minimal with words like this, although complexes involving various such schemas may be evoked as part of their affordances.

One might ask at this point which core sub-part(s) of the overall cluster of affordances associated with the word *holiday* must be regarded as part of the inter-subjective social object 'English', i.e. essential common knowledge of its speakers as opposed to contingent and/or purely subjective associations the individual speaker may have formed with the word. The answer must surely be in terms of relationships within the system as a whole, just as structuralists have always insisted, i.e. a matter of contrasts (of inclusion or exclusion) between the form and the content of the word *holiday* and that of other English words associated with a common semantic 'substance'.

The *figuræ* defining such common regions of 'substance' include some of a socially defined nature (e.g. *work* or *term time* vs. *holiday*), which require extensive social learning for the word to be transmitted in a generally accepted array of meanings, but they in turn are built upon more basic spatio-temporal image schemas and the like. The essential thing is that the 'logic' of the word - the inferences that can be made from its normal usage and its potential unpacking into paraphrase equivalents, instances and definitions - is recognized, and for this its mode of anchoring in the relevant social frame(s) itself constitutes the 'core' meaning. Both the linguistic and the non-linguistic knowledge here is transmitted socially, whether by ostension or by tokens of use-in-context of the word (or - more likely - a combination of both). The precise denotational scope of the concept expressed by the word is open-ended and context-dependent, so an analysis of the word into precise content form *figuræ* is only possible on the individual language level (referring to specific cultural 'frames') and these need only have an approximate equivalence to those represented in the individual mind/brain of its speakers. The **types** of content *figuræ* of relation likely to be involved are of course common across all languages (antonymy, meronymy, etc.).

Here it is relevant to bring in Whitehead.'s fourth ontological category of 'contrast'. Contrasts are defined in "Process and Reality" as 'modes of synthesis of entities in one prehension' (Whitehead, 1978, 22–24). They relate further to holistic prehension in the mode of causal efficacy, for 'whatever is a datum for a feeling has a unity as felt... This unity is a contrast of entities'. At its most basic this is a matter of the recognition of foreground/background relations and the 'filling in' of partial *gestalts*. This supplements the analytic perception of clusters of specific *figuræ*. The structural relationships defining a given language are species of contrasts and of contrasts of contrasts, etc. - they may in principle be infinitely expanded by productive generation of new combinations of signs. Note that contrasts may be prehended between eternal objects; they lead to increased intensity of ingression of the eternal objects concerned. A proposition is a particular kind of (complex) contrast. Two or more contrasts may be incompatible for joint ingression relative to an on-going 'subjective aim' (or intention), or lead to prehension of a higher order contrast balancing them out - this is how the subjective aim 'orders' eternal objects by selection: it manifests the principle behind all cognitive processes that aims towards evoking the maximal number of relevant eternal objects subject to conditions of contrast. One can say that the structural contrasts between *figuræ* of both expression and content that constitute the language 'English' form a single complex eternal object, a coherent system that may be socially transmitted by the community to each new speaker.

Now, if it is agreed that the *figuræ* of the meta-level must include those that are relevant for the individual cognitive level, one must proceed to inquire where the (to some degree) indeterminate constellation of associations representing the meaning of the word *holiday*, for example, might be located/distributed in the individual mind/brain. How might the 'weak *nexus*' between the word's phonological representation and its meaning be distributed between different cortical regions? What, in Whiteheadian terms, are the different eternal objects impinging upon this locus, relating it to other, more sensory-specific cortical areas? First, it should be repeated that by 'eternal object' I mean simply a repeatable pattern of excitation experienced by a language-using subject when prehending such a pattern at any level of abstraction (from iconic isomorphism with the sensory input to a completely arbitrary relationship to input). Any eternal object, whether simple or complex, has a particular 'feel' to the prehending subject in the holistic mode of causal efficacy, but it can also generate specific kinds of imagery in the mode of presentational immediacy. These patterns contrast more or less systematically with other patterns. Since the Whiteheadian term has the wrong kinds of connotations for discussing the *nexus* level of the physical brain, I shall talk from this point on of *figuræ* rather than'eternal objects' - on the understanding that these terms are in fact equivalent.

We can envisage the 'input' to a neural aggregate or web corresponding to the meaning of the word *holiday* either as the excitation of a region of a 'convergence zone' by specific pathways from other regions or as the 'ignition' of a 'functional web' in the manner of

Pulvermüller.[16] The relevant associations to other cortical regions correspond to links to those areas mentioned in section 3 above as likely candidates for the principal loci of the different types of *figuræ*. As we have seen, for *holiday* there are potential links to most of the sub-types, i.e. to imagery of a number of sensory - including kinaesthetic - types and to prefrontal 'frame' scenarios and to sub-cortical regions involved in evoking emotional tone. Beyond the objective 'framework' of features and scenarios unique to this word and defining its meaning by contrast with that of all other words in the language, there are of course more contingent associations, e.g. in the case of *holiday* the 'feeling' of driving in a car (in a light-hearted mood) towards some familiar holiday destination, or perhaps the feel of reclining in a deck-chair in a garden in the summer, cold drink in hand - though these things are normally accessed holistically in the mode of causal efficacy, without necessarily generating precise imagery. There is, however, a great deal of indeterminacy here since episodic memory is involved, i.e. the accumulated tokens of 'being on holiday' in an individual's memory.

5 Conclusion

The principal moral I wish to draw from all this is that the holistic and the analytic approaches to meaning are complementary and both necessary. This applies to the morphosyntactic categories of grammar as well as to the lexicon, which comprises the building blocks of linguistic memory. The non-decomposable Hjelmslevian notion of the 'invariant' can surely be replaced by the 'invariant but nevertheless decomposable'. One can thus regard the semantic categories relevant to verb lexicalization patterns and satellite choices (as discussed by

[16] These distributed webs of Pulvermüller (2002), which may be activated - either partially or wholly - at different frequencies of resonance, are malleable Whiteheadian *nexūs* at the neural level and represent (rather than the individual neuron) the basis of all higher cognitive functions. As regards language, they link phonological and grammatical core regions around the Sylvian fissure with (in the case of content words) more peripheral and far-flung areas of sensory-specific affordances.

Talmy 1985) as universal *figuræ* that may combine into language-specific constellations associated with specific words and constructions. These may in turn act as holistic units with contextual affordances not part of any unique underlying 'image schema' in building up still more complex meanings (e.g. by derivation). In fact it is the addition of the holistic perspective that saves the Hjelmslevian project and allows it to be translated into a contemporary framework of cognitively orientated linguistics. Where Hjelmslev went wrong, as I have already suggested, was in regarding the nature of the relationship between linguistic form and non-linguistic substance (or 'purport') as one-way, insisting that the former always imposes itself on the latter and not *vice versa.* Today it is easier to see that the traffic is two-way, and that 'natural kinds' (including basic action schemas) do indeed impose themselves on natural language, albeit in idiosyncratic and culturally articulated ways. What is of interest is how language builds upon these cognitive building blocks, neutralizing and compounding them and metaphorically abstracting away from them in shaping the complex language-specific contents of linguistic signs.

We can now return to the question as to overall criteria for determining which *figuræ* of a typologically adequate metasemiology are likely to be relevant to psychological processes within individual speaker/hearers and which are not. Here we need to distinguish between those *figuræ* that refer to universal schemas (not necessarily expressed in language at all) and those that are language-specific and context-sensitive. Clusters involving both types of *figura* can, as I have argued, be experienced and deployed holistically. The systematic compositionality of morphosyntactic (including productive morphological) expression-content pairings only extends a certain distance into lexical organization (e.g. the area treated by Force Dynamics and the 'metaphorical' extension of physical level 'basic' verbs to possession and mental activity, etc.). The rest of the way surely *has* to be complemented by holistic processes of perception and production on the part of the individual speaker/hearer. At the metasemiological level any kind of empirically justified generalization across languages is potentially valid, but if one wishes to maintain psychological adequacy, this further requires limiting the analytical *figuræ* employed to more or less universal image schemas plus principles for combining and extending them with the help of other *figuræ* (both general or specific). Beyond that, all is determined by the lexicon and grammatical coding possibilities of individual languages, where lexical and grammatical meanings are only fully graspable holistically (and within specific contextual constraints). It is thanks to the universal pre-linguistic nature of the schemas (and of the processes of metaphorical/metonymic extension of signs in general) that these language-specific clusters can nevertheless be logically related and translated to and from one another apart from by vague and indirect association. The *figuræ* needed for describing both the affordances of specific words and the universal schemas relevant to their logically consistent usage constitute overlapping sub-sets of the same range of *figuræ* of 'content substance' that includes both the linguistic and the non-linguistic world. This was surely Hjelmslev's point - whether he was fully aware of it or not - when suggesting the possibility of a 'metasemiology'. What such a metasemiology amounts to is no more nor less than a descriptive framework for discussing the organization of linguistic memory, the basis of all higher forms of cognition.

References

Coseriu, Eugenio. 1975. System, Norm und Rede. *Sprachtheorie und allgemeine Sprachwissenschaft* : 11–101.

Damasio, Antonio and Hanna Damasio. 1992. Brain and language. *Scientific American* September 1992: 63–71.

Fortescue, Michael. 2001. *Pattern and Process: A Whiteheadian Perspective on Linguistics*. Amsterdam and Philadelphia: John Benjamins.

Fortescue, Michael. 2003. The pattern and process of language in use: A test case. In: J. Seibt (ed.), *Process Theories, Cross-Disciplinary Studies in Dynamic Categories*. Dordrecht: Kluwer Academic, 177–218. also online version in Axiomathes, International Journal in Ontology and Cognitive Systems, 14, 191–232.

Grice, H. P. 1957. Meaning. *Philosophical Review* 64: 377–388.

Hjelmslev, Louis. 1954. La stratification du langage. *Word* 10: 163–188.

Hjelmslev, Louis. 1963. *Prolegomena to a Theory of Language*. Madison: University of Wisconsin Press. (Original Danish version: Omkring sprogteoriens grundlæggelse 1943).

Lyons, John. 1977. *Semantics*. Cambridge: Cambridge University Press.

MacWhinney, Brian. 1999. The emergence of language from embodiment. In: Brian MacWhinney (ed.), *The Emergence of Language*. New Jersey: Lawrence Erlbaum, 213–256.

Peirce, Charles Sanders. 1958/1931. *Collected Papers*. Cambridge, Mass.: Harvard University Press.

Pulvermüller, Friedemann. 2002. *The Neuroscience of Language: On Brain Circuits of Words and Serial Order*. Cambridge: Cambridge University Press.

Talmy, Leonard. 1985. Lexicalization patterns: semantic structure in lexical forms. In: Timothy Shopen (ed.), *Language Typology and Syntactic Description*, volume 3. Cambridge: Cambridge University Press, 36–149.

Talmy, Leonard. 1988. Force dynamics in language and cognition. *Cognitive Science* 12: 49–100.

Whitehead, Alfred North. 1978. *Process and Reality*. New York: The Free Press. (corrected edition, original edition 1929, New York: Macmillan).

Wierzbicka, Anna. 1992. The search for semantic primitives. In: M. Pütz (ed.), *Thirty Years of Linguistic Evolution*. Amsterdam & Philadelphia: John Benjamins, 215–242.

Learning and relative frequency

Francisco Morales and John R. Taylor

1 Introduction: Frequency effects in language

A remarkable feature of natural languages is the unequal frequency of occurrence of their structural elements. With respect to the words of a language, it is a common place that these do not occur with equal frequency. Frequency effects, however, show up also in other domains, for example, in phonology, morphology, and syntax. Thus, the vowels of a language do not occur with equal frequency in running text (Figure 1)[1]; in a language with phonological tone, the tones are not distributed evenly over the morphemes of the language (Figure 2); while competing realizations of a morphosyntactic category do not share the field equally (Figure 3).

The phenomenon of relative frequency was first investigated systematically, in a variety of languages and for various structural elements, in the first half of the last century by George Zipf (1935/1965), who built on the pioneering work of F. W. Kaeding (1898) in the domain of word and syllable frequency. Subsequent studies by Greenberg (1966) confirmed and extended Zipf's observations. Whereas earlier researchers were forced to rely on manual analysis – it is reported that Kaeding employed over 5000 research assistants to sort and tally his millions of index cards (Leech et al., 2001, ix) – the availability of fast and inexpensive data processing by computer has seen a blossoming of the field of corpus linguistics, and the discovery of ever more subtle frequency effects in natural languages (Sinclair, 1991; Biber et al., 1989; Moon, 1998; Hunston, 2002).

[1] The data for this analysis was derived from the upwards of 150,000 words transcribed in the Spanish corpora of the CHILDES database, pertaining to interchanges with infants below the age of 3;0 (MacWhinney, 2000; Romero et al., 1992; Montes, 1987, 1992; López Ornat, 1994).

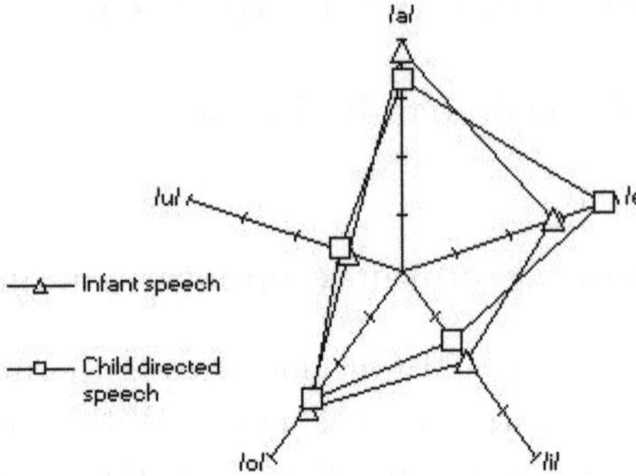

	/a/	/e/	/i/	/o/	/u/
Infant speech	30.6%	22.7%	15.5%	23.2%	8.0%
Child directed speech	26.4%	30.0%	11.7%	22.2%	9.7%

Figure 1. Relative frequencies of the five Spanish vowels in infant-produced speech and infant-directed speech

If the statistical properties of languages and their structural elements are now well documented, there is little consensus on the theoretical significance of this kind of data. A number of positions can be identified. As is well known, Chomsky (1957, 16–17) dismissed out of hand the very possibility that statistical data could be relevant to the goals of linguistic theory. So what, Chomsky quipped, if *I live in New York* might have a higher text frequency than *I live in Dayton Ohio*? (reported in Halliday 1991, 30). Greenberg, on the other hand, proposed to integrate frequency data into a theory of markedness, claiming that the unmarked term of an opposition will be more frequent than the marked term, simultaneously also proposing 'markedness' as a universal organizational principle of natural languages. Zipf (1935/1965) drew wider implications, seeing the statistical properties of languages in the context of regularities in other domains of behavior, whose causal principle was a 'law of equilibrium', which balanced tradition and innovation, uniformity and diversity (Pustet, 2004). Miller (1965), in contrast, interpreted Zipf's

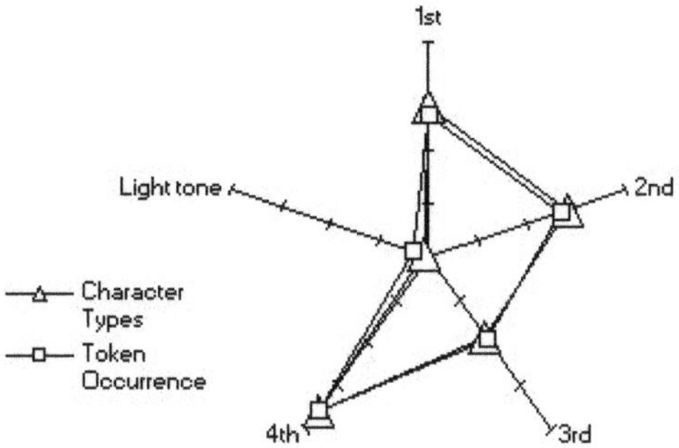

Tone	Characters (types)		Occurrences (tokens)	
	Characters	Percent	Tokens	Percent
1st	1959	25.19%	24690	23.71%
2nd	1972	25.35%	25130	24.13%
3rd	1300	16.71%	17853	17.15%
4th	2488	32.00%	33560	32.25%
Light tone	58	0.75%	2890	2.78%
Total	7778		104123	

Figure 2. Relative frequency of tones of Mandarin Chinese. Source: Liu & Ma (1986)

statistical data simply as the inevitable consequence of the stochastic nature of linguistic activity.

Recently, a number of researchers have attempted to establish links between the statistical properties of linguistic corpora and a speaker's mental representation of their language. For example, relative frequency has proved to be a crucial factor in explaining subtle phonological phenomena, such as the incidence of reductions, elisions, and assimilations (Bybee 2001; Bybee and Hopper 2001). Jurafsky et al. (2001, 229) draw the conclusion that 'probabilistic information about words, phrases, and other linguistic structure is represented in the minds of language users'. A person's knowledge of their language would therefore be determined, at least in part, by statistical

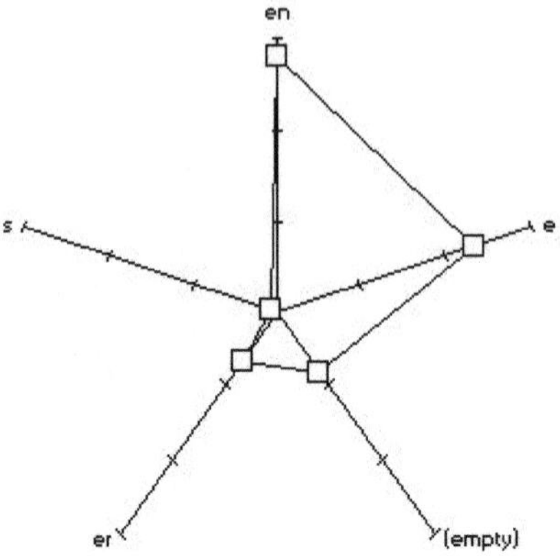

Plural Suffix	Percent
-en	42%
-e	35%
(empty)	12%
-er	10%
-s	1%

Figure 3. Token frequency of German plurals, based on the 200 most frequent nouns in 600,000 words of running text. Source: Janda (1991)

properties of the language samples to which they have been exposed (Ellis, 2002). Conversely, statistical properties of a text would be the consequence of speakers producing text in accordance with their mental representation of their language, including their knowledge of relative frequency. Language knowledge would therefore model the properties (including the statistical properties) of input data (Taylor, 2007).

In this paper we take a new look at the relation between a language and its users. We take it as axiomatic that a language is exquisitely adapted to the learning capabilities of its users. It is common cause that a language has to be acquired anew by each generation of its speakers. Properties of a language which enhance learnability will be easily acquired, while properties which hinder acquisition will not. Aspects of a language which are not attuned to its speakers' learning capabilities will simply not survive transmission to subsequent generations of speakers. Our hypothesis is that the different frequencies of occurrence of a language's structural elements are a feature of a natural language which promotes its learnability. A language will be easier to acquire to the extent that its words, morphemes, phonemes, tones, inflectional classes, syntactic structures, etc. do not occur with equal frequency.

We test this hypothesis on category learning in artificial neutral networks. Networks are trained on a number of types, each represented by one or more tokens. The networks are then tested on new tokens of the respective types. The experimental variable is the number of training tokens for each of the types. Put simply, we compare two conditions. On one condition, each type is trained on an equal number of tokens per type. On the other condition, the types are trained on variable numbers of tokens. The crucial question is whether networks trained on condition 2 perform better than networks trained on condition 1, even though, collectively, the total number of training tokens on condition 2 is less than the number of training tokens on condition 1.

2 Experiments

The objective of the series of experiments reported here is to explore whether, and in what ways, modifications to the relative number of tokens per type during training will affect the performance of a network while testing. In particular, we look for evidence of superior performance vis-à-vis networks trained with a uniform distribution of token per type while using a smaller overall number of training tokens.

2.1 Methodology

The artificial neural network employed to conduct these experiments is a knowledge-based Evolving Connectionist System, called ECOS (Kasabov, 1998, 2000, 2001, 2002; Kasabov and Song, 2002). This system can be broadly characterized as a multi-modular architecture evolving in a problem space of not necessarily fixed dimensions and exhibiting fast, incremental, constructive, pattern-based learning as a function of, among other things, one-pass data propagation. There exist a number of ECOS models suitable for different kinds of knowledge acquisition in function of the implementation of Zadeh-Mamdani fuzzy rules or Takagi-Sugeno fuzzy rules, among others.

In essence, the behavior of ECOS systems revolves around the creation and modification of localized prototype clusters representing the training data in an n-dimensional problem space. The training procedure utilizes distance measures to calculate the location of input signatures against the receptive fields of existing clusters. Input signatures that fall within the receptive field of a given cluster modify its location as well as its receptive and activation fields. Input signatures that fall outside of the receptive fields of all existing clusters give birth to new clusters. The ECOS learning process thus populates and partitions the solution space. During the testing process, the distance between test signatures and prototype clusters is measured against the latter's activation fields and classification of the former ensues.

The network model chosen for these experiments was a stripped-down version of the simplest ECOS system as presented in Kasabov (2002) and employed Euclidean distance measures for training and testing.

The data used in these experiments derived from a subset of the English-language corpora assembled in the CHILDES database (MacWhinney, 2000). This subset of the database comprised all those transcriptions that captured the speech of infants under 3 years of age together with that of their caretakers[2].

The 1850 transcribed verbal exchanges involved 216 children that collectively totaled 5,272,392 tokens (words). Frequency counts of lexicon reoccurrence identified 33,976 unique types in the infant-

---

[2] specifically, Bates et al. 1988; Bernstein 1982; Bloom 1970; Brown 1973; Clark 1978; Demetras 1989b,a; Haggerty 1929; Higginson 1985; Howe 1981; MacWhinney 2000; Theakston et al. 2001; Nelson 1989; Ninio et al. 1994; Demetras et al. 1986; Sachs 1983; Suppes 1974; Valian 1991; Van Houten 1986; Wells 1981

directed speech and 19,951 unique types in the infant-produced speech. Despite the fact that the various transcription styles of the different researchers rather likely resulted in an inflated number of unique types, the large sample size makes it safe to assume that the most frequent types on each list correspond to the most frequent words that infants immersed in English-speaking environments hear, learn, and consequently replicate. The following are the 30 most frequent content words directed at infants: *that, what, yes, there, no, go, this, get, one, want, here, put, where, right, ok, look, not, see, like, now, up, all, out, well, think, down, come, then, little*, and *just*. These words, or subsets of these words, constituted the training and testing sets for all experiments described in this paper (unless otherwise explicitly specified).

In order to conduct the experiments, the 30-word set was digitally recorded (22,050 Hz, 16 bit, mono) by two adults, a male and a female speaker with markedly dissimilar accents. To maximize contrast between words while reducing the induction of excessive and unnatural similarities, the entire word set was recorded 28 times (*that, what, yes*, etc., as opposed to *that, that, ..., what, what, ...*, etc.). Recordings were then sliced and 22 instances (tokens) of each type were manually selected as samples to be used for training and testing the networks. Finally, the order of token recordings was randomly shuffled within each type to eliminate possible prosodic effects.

For the following experiments, these digital recordings were preprocessed as follows. Each token recording was divided into non-overlapping 20 millisecond windows where each window received a coefficient based on a 10 mel-scale cepstrum table. A discrete cosine transform (DCT) was then applied to standardize different word lengths to the input requirements of the network (100 input nodes, in this case). Simply put, each token recording was transmuted into a 100-digit signature.

2.2 Experiment I

Experiment I provides a simple illustration of the effects of relative frequency of token distribution on the classificatory capabilities of a network. The data set for this experiment employed only the first 10 types (*that, what, yes, there, no, go, this, get, one, want*) from the male speaker. The training set consisted of 4 randomly selected tokens of each type (from the 22 available) and the testing set consisted of 4 randomly selected tokens of each type (from the 18 still available). Two identical networks with identical default (and immutable) learning parameters were trained as indicated in Table 1.

Table 1. Training configurations for Experiment I.

Network A					Network B				
1:	*				1:	*			
2:	*				2:	*			
3:	*	*	*		3:	*	*	*	
4:	*	*	*		4:	*	*	*	
5:	*				5:	*			
6:	*				6:	*			
7:	*	*	*		7:	*	*	*	
8:	*				8:	*			
9:	*			<—	9:	*	*		<—
10:	*	*			10:	*	*		

Table 1 shows that network A was trained with the following variable configuration of tokens per type: [1 1 3 3 1 1 3 1 1 2] while network B was trained with the variable configuration [1 1 3 3 1 1 3 1 2 2]. That is, networks A and B were trained with exactly the same tokens (not only the same number, but the very same token signatures) with the exception of type 9 in network B, where an additional token signature was used for training (see the leftward arrows in Table 1). This small difference in training – and this difference alone, since both networks were identical *and* had the same default immutable learning parameters[3] – gave rise to a disparity in perfor-

[3] Training was conducted serially over a fixed sequence for all experiments in this paper. Networks were trained first on token(s) of type 1, then on those of type 2, and so on. Also, within each type, networks were first trained on token 1, then token 2, and so on. The only experimental variable was the number of tokens per type. Therefore, any discrepancies in behavior between two networks differing in, for example, one token of type 9 is due exclusively

mance when both networks were presented with the same testing set of 4 tokens per type (Table 2). The dash ('-') in Table 2 indicates that a test token was correctly classified. A number replacing the dash indicates the type to which the corresponding test token was incorrectly assigned. For instance, all tokens of type 7 were correctly classified by both networks, while the first token of type 3 was classified incorrectly as type 10 by both networks.

Table 2. Test results on Networks A and B

Network A					Network B					
1:	-	-	-	-	1	-	-	-	-	
2:	-	-	-	-	2:	-	-	-	-	
3:	10	-	-	-	3:	10	-	-	-	
4:	-	-	7	7	4:	-	-	7	-	<—
5:	4	-	-	-	5:	4	-	-	-	
6:	7	9	-	-	6:	-	10	-	-	<—
7:	-	-	-	-	7:	-	-	-	-	
8:	-	-	-	-	8:	-	-	-	-	
9:	10	-	-	6	9:	10	-	-	-	<—
10:	-	-	-	-	10:	-	-	-	-	

These similarities in performance are to be expected as both networks were trained with the very same tokens except for the additional token of type 9 for network B. This additional training token aided network B in the classification of test token 4 for type 9. The interesting and unexpected finding concerns the effect that this additional training token in type 9 had on other types (marked by the left-pointing arrows).

Unlike network A, network B shows correct classification for test token 4 for type 4 and test token 1 for type 6, as well as a novel misclassification of token 2 for type 6. In short, a tiny modification in the relative frequency of tokens per type during training influenced the performance of the network during testing that extends beyond the type affected by the modification.

to the presence or absence of that token.

Even more striking is a comparison between the performance of networks A and B with that of a third network, network C, which was trained with all four available tokens:

Network A: $^{17/40}[\ 1\ 1\ 3\ 3\ 1\ 1\ 3\ 1\ 1\ 2\ ]_{32/40}$
Network B: $^{18/40}[\ 1\ 1\ 3\ 3\ 1\ 1\ 3\ 1\ 2\ 2\ ]_{35/40}$
Network C: $^{40/40}[\ 4\ 4\ 4\ 4\ 4\ 4\ 4\ 4\ 4\ 4\ ]_{38/40}$

Networks A and B employed a total 17 and 18 training tokens, respectively, of the 40 available tokens, while network C employed all 40 available training tokens. When tested against the same set of test tokens, the accuracy of networks A, B, and C was 80% (32 out of 40 test tokens were correctly classified), 87.5% (35 out of 40), and 95% (38 out of 40), respectively. While network C, not unexpectedly, performed better than networks A and B, the relatively small increase in performance was obtained at the cost of having to more than double the number of training tokens. It would seem, then, that networks A and B were making better use of the training tokens than network C, the ratio of total training tokens to accurately classified testing tokens being 1:1.88, 1:1.94, and 1:0.95 respectively. Observe, also, that networks A and B performed at 100% accuracy on the identification of types 1, 2, and 8, *even though only one token of these types had been used for training.* Given these findings, there would seem to be merit in investigating more systematically the contribution to a system's performance of the relative frequency of token distribution over types.

2.3 Experiment II

The results on Experiment I might have been a chance outcome resulting from the specific selection of tokens and types used for training. Experiment II was designed to investigate this possibility by eliciting all possible combinations of between 1 and 4 tokens over the 10 types, then training one network per combination, and finally, testing all networks against the same testing set. The training and testing data sets employed in Experiment I were used again, namely, the first 10 types (and corresponding tokens) of the data set obtained

Table 3. Performance of 4^10 networks over 4 test tokens per type

	25	26	27	28	29	30	31	32	33	34	35	36	37	38	39	40	Total
10									1								1
11								2	6	2							10
12			1			4	5	9	18	14	4						55
13		1	2	3	5	19	19	31	61	51	26	2					220
14		2	8	21	20	51	69	93	169	162	83	26	1				705
15		3	27	49	81	127	197	265	365	421	254	100	13				1902
16		8	53	111	189	283	437	665	791	930	620	296	68	4			4455
17	1	14	96	200	346	578	966	1365	1635	1766	1260	795	198	18	2		9240
18		22	146	312	611	1018	1826	2523	2982	3095	2449	1630	505	79	7		17205
19		22	201	464	919	1644	2862	4192	5099	5302	4126	2933	1072	190	24		29050
20		15	235	583	1301	2253	4145	6372	7989	8275	6557	4759	1843	422	52	2	44803
21		17	236	666	1580	2829	5337	8854	11349	12100	9836	6954	2804	794	101	3	63460
22		12	222	690	1655	3230	6263	11175	14797	16396	13651	9440	4037	1132	174	11	82885
23		13	172	623	1605	3290	6721	12938	17573	20638	17457	11975	5258	1582	248	17	100110
24		6	122	479	1386	3011	6824	13575	18985	23801	20904	14235	6355	2004	318	30	112035
25		1	78	332	1025	2586	6298	12910	18711	25156	23424	15868	7184	2356	338	37	116304
26			37	181	703	2015	5271	11217	16822	24370	24165	16624	7768	2475	359	28	112035
27			14	83	408	1401	4004	8814	13844	21381	23051	16430	7811	2513	332	24	100110
28			3	40	187	849	2744	6203	10363	16960	20258	15042	7540	2401	279	16	82885
29				12	78	445	1658	3906	6927	12388	16038	12816	6762	2194	225	11	63460
30				1	22	201	873	2163	4146	8127	11432	10108	5625	1901	197	7	44803
31					3	63	395	1038	2181	4755	7311	7254	4353	1525	169	3	29050
32						14	135	444	1004	2408	4116	4711	3065	1192	116		17205
33						2	33	145	386	1069	2001	2722	1953	853	76		9240
34							4	39	112	398	824	1359	1125	551	43		4455
35								8	20	112	279	576	549	341	17		1902
36								1	1	22	72	199	238	167	5		705
37										2	11	55	85	66	1		220
38											1	9	25	20			55
39												1	4	5			10
40														1			1
Total =	1	136	1653	4850	12124	25913	57086	108947	156337	210101	210210	156919	76241	24786	3083	189	1048576

from the male speaker. There being 4 to the 10th power combinations with repetition of 4 elements over 10 places, a total of 1,048,576 identical networks (with identical and immutable learning parameters) were trained each with a different configuration of tokens per type. All networks were subsequently tested against the same set of test tokens, yielding the results shown in Table 3. Column labels indicate the number of testing tokens correctly classified, rows are preceded by the total number of training tokens that were employed, while the intersect tallies the number of configurations (networks) that satisfied both parameters. Zero values are not shown and no network recognized less than 25 testing tokens (columns omitted). Only one configuration amounted to a total of 10 training tokens, namely ${}^{10/40}[\ 1\ 1\ 1\ 1\ 1\ 1\ 1\ 1\ 1\ 1\ ]_{33/40}$, and only one configuration amounted to a total of 40 training tokens ${}^{40/40}[\ 4\ 4\ 4\ 4\ 4\ 4\ 4\ 4\ 4\ 4\ ]_{38/40}$. These uniform configurations recognized 33 and 38 test tokens (of the 40 possible) respectively.

A quick read through the table reveals that there were 24,785 configurations whose overall accuracy was equal to that of the maximum training configuration ${}^{40/40}[\ 4\ 4\ 4\ 4\ 4\ 4\ 4\ 4\ 4\ 4\ ]_{38/40}$, and which necessarily employed fewer tokens for training. In fact, there were four configurations which achieved this level of accuracy with a total number of only 16 training types:

${}^{40/40}[\ 4\ 4\ 4\ 4\ 4\ 4\ 4\ 4\ 4\ 4\ ]_{38/40}$
${}^{16/40}[\ 1\ 1\ 2\ 2\ 1\ 2\ 4\ 1\ 1\ 1\ ]_{38/40}$
${}^{16/40}[\ 1\ 1\ 2\ 3\ 2\ 2\ 2\ 1\ 1\ 1\ ]_{38/40}$
${}^{16/40}[\ 1\ 1\ 2\ 4\ 1\ 1\ 3\ 1\ 1\ 1\ ]_{38/40}$
${}^{16/40}[\ 1\ 1\ 3\ 2\ 1\ 1\ 4\ 1\ 1\ 1\ ]_{38/40}$

Note also that there were 3,272 configurations that performed better than the maximum uniform configuration ${}^{40/40}[\ 4\ 4\ 4\ 4\ 4\ 4\ 4\ 4\ 4\ 4\ ]_{38/40}$, 189 of which performed with 100% accuracy. The most accurate and economical of these variable configurations were the following:

${}^{20/40}[\ 1\ 1\ 2\ 4\ 2\ 1\ 4\ 3\ 1\ 1\ ]_{40/40}$
${}^{20/40}[\ 1\ 2\ 2\ 4\ 2\ 1\ 3\ 3\ 1\ 1\ ]_{40/40}$

Table 4. Performance of 4^10 networks over 6 test tokens per type

	34	35	36	37	38	39	40	41	42	43	44	45	46	47	48	49	50	51	52	53	54	55	56	57	Total
10											1														1
11										2	3	4		1											10
12					1		1	2	1	12	13	9	11	4	1										55
13					2	4	12	8	17	33	37	40	35	16	10	6									220
14				2	3	12	37	33	75	87	108	101	102	68	51	17	8	1							705
15			3	3	15	30	70	112	174	218	288	273	273	193	136	75	33	6							1902
16		1	7	10	22	66	144	238	342	515	592	672	620	522	360	208	104	24	8						4455
17		5	6	24	44	102	220	393	633	930	1171	1412	1347	1151	856	558	275	88	21	4					9240
18	1	3	15	27	74	134	313	551	948	1527	2040	2403	2649	2363	1843	1330	607	288	74	14	1				17205
19	1	8	9	32	86	177	378	694	1303	2055	3048	3875	4463	4204	3592	2649	1484	708	214	58	11	1			29050
20		7	7	31	77	184	433	777	1542	2593	3977	5347	6517	6861	6066	4824	3129	1592	630	170	32	7			44803
21		4	5	11	69	189	395	777	1628	2876	4669	6565	8404	9683	9338	7777	5728	3291	1468	466	102	14	1		63460
22		2		8	43	135	305	700	1530	2774	4891	7166	9904	11932	12646	11289	9157	5902	2989	1162	297	50	3		82885
23				2	23	79	201	522	1236	2462	4577	6986	10115	13407	15034	14856	12713	9185	5360	2413	781	150	8		100110
24				1	8	37	100	360	822	1864	3795	6192	9347	13250	16114	17035	15978	12608	8178	4277	1622	407	39	1	112035
25					3	11	49	172	479	1225	2735	4801	7803	11699	15409	17635	17628	15413	10846	6519	2896	859	118	4	116304
26						4	13	66	236	648	1641	3261	5694	9315	13284	16198	17588	16460	12894	8447	4515	1486	275	10	112035
27						1	3	12	87	280	821	1935	3644	6342	10039	13529	15567	15960	13627	9655	5829	2256	493	30	100110
28								3	20	76	337	940	1935	3858	6659	9836	12405	13704	12819	9906	6581	2969	763	74	82885
29									2	17	94	378	857	1959	3795	6329	8547	10610	10754	9033	6592	3351	1023	119	63460
30										2	17	103	323	786	1867	3446	5185	7138	8057	7361	5821	3372	1164	161	44803
31											1	23	70	258	743	1575	2686	4125	5318	5339	4544	3014	1185	169	29050
32												2	8	55	224	596	1152	2074	2989	3322	3163	2419	1046	155	17205
33														7	50	171	402	845	1438	1799	1897	1679	841	111	9240
34															7	28	104	295	568	788	982	1031	594	58	4455
35																3	18	75	178	295	413	524	368	28	1902
36																	1	13	39	85	143	231	189	4	705
37																			6	18	33	77	84	2	220
38																				2	6	18	29		55
39																						3	7		10
40																							1		1
Total =	2	30	52	151	470	1165	2674	5420	11075	20196	34856	52488	74121	97934	118124	129970	130499	120405	98475	71133	46261	23918	8231	926	1048576

In other words, there were training configurations, characterized by a variable number of tokens per type, which outperformed the maximum uniform configuration possible – $^{40/40}$[4 4 4 4 4 4 4 4 4 4]$_{38/40}$ – and which used *only half* the total number of training tokens.

For Experiment IIb, a second testing set was assembled by randomly selecting 6 tokens out of the 14 tokens still unused for each type (from the male speaker). Testing each *already trained* network with this 60-token testing set yielded the results shown in Table 4. No configuration (network) performed below 34 correctly identified testing tokens, nor above 57 (of 60 possible), and appropriate columns have been omitted. Again, the maximum uniform configuration $^{40/40}$[4 4 4 4 4 4 4 4 4 4]$_{38/40\ 56/60}$ was not the most accurate. Rather, the variable configuration $^{21/40}$[1 2 3 3 3 2 3 1 2 1]$_{37/40\ 56/60}$ performed equally (overall) for this second testing set (as did 8,229 others) using almost half the total number of training tokens that the maximum uniform configuration used. Furthermore, 926 networks (configurations) performed better, the most economical being $^{24/40}$[2 1 3 3 3 3 3 2 2 2]$_{35/40\ 57/60}$.

Observe that each column (equal performance) in both tables shows a similar pattern of increase in the number of configurations, which then falls after peaking roughly in the middle. A plot of Table 4 is shown in Figure 4.

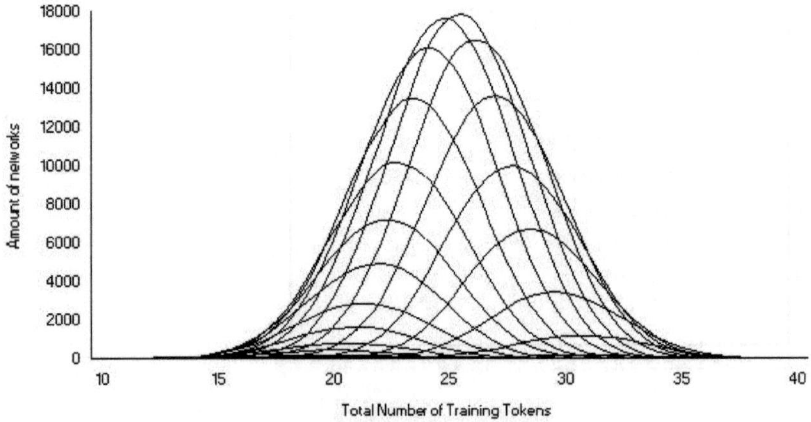

Figure 4. Performance of 4^10 networks over 6 test tokens per type

Each line draws from a column of data in Table 4 and evolves left to right distributing configurations by total number of training tokens (the x-axis stands for total number of training tokens and the y-axis for the number of networks). The bell shapes can be partly justified by taking into consideration that, when tallying up the contents of each configuration, combinations with repetition of 4 elements over 10 places results in a symmetrical bell distribution peaking over 25 tokens (Figure 5). For a visual illustration, observe the y-axis values (number of configurations) in both plots; all bells in the former (Figure 4) must fit under the bell in the latter (Figure 5).

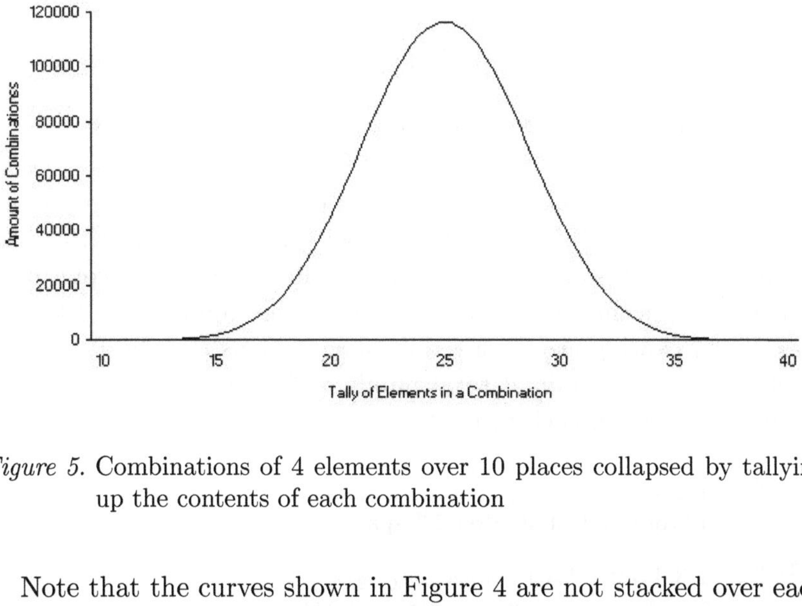

Figure 5. Combinations of 4 elements over 10 places collapsed by tallying up the contents of each combination

Note that the curves shown in Figure 4 are not stacked over each other in random fashion. The attentive reader may have noticed (Tables 3 and 4) that the peaks, the maximum values for each column, line up in cross section. Experiment IIc employed the 8 tokens (per type) left available to test each of the 4ˆ10 *already trained* networks, yielding the three-dimensional surface shown in Figure 6 (table omitted).

Recapitulating: 4ˆ10 networks were trained with no more than 4 training tokens per type and then were tested serially on testing

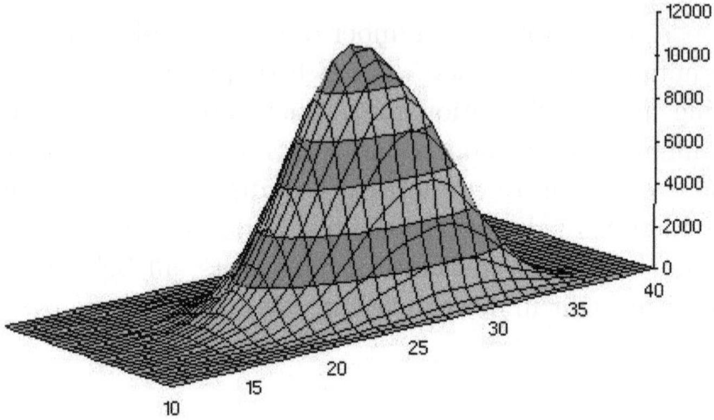

Figure 6. Performance of 4^10 networks over 8 test tokens per type

sets consisting of 4-tokens per type (Experiment IIa), 6- tokens per type (Experiment IIb), and 8- tokens per type (Experiment IIc). Cumulatively, the first test set consisted of 40 tokens, the second of 60 tokens, and the third of 80 tokens, all together adding up to 180 samples. The following are among the configurations with best accuracy combined with a minimal total number of training tokens, as they progressed through each test set:

$^{20/40}$[1 1 2 4 2 1 4 3 1 1] $_{40/40\ \ 47/60\ \ 71/80}$
40 total out of 40 after 1st space

$^{26/40}$[1 1 3 4 3 2 4 4 3 1] $_{40/40\ \ 56/60\ \ 72/80}$
96 total out of 100 after 1st and 2nd spaces

$^{28/40}$[1 4 3 4 3 2 4 4 2 1] $_{40/40\ \ 56/60\ \ 74/80}$
170 total out of 180 after 1st, 2nd, and 3rd spaces

Briefly, and as an example, only two tokens of type 9 were employed in the last configuration listed to train a network to correctly classify 17 (out of 18) test tokens of the same type. Collectively, these results provide evidence that relative frequency of token distribution affects performance systematically and that some variable configurations can achieve better performance than more 'expensive' uniform configurations.

In order to dispel worries about the results being a function of the data used, all the above experiments were repeated with words 11 through 20 (*here, put, where, right, ok, look, not, see, like, now*) and then again with words 21 through 30 (*up, all, out, well, think, down, come, then, little, just*) from the data set obtained from the male speaker. In order to extend the results beyond a single speaker, all the experiments were repeated once more with the data set obtained from the female speaker. Collectively, these experiments involved training and testing 6,291,456 networks with 1,320 different tokens belonging to 30 types and two speakers. Results for all experiments yielded outcomes comparable to those presented so far in as much as relative frequency of token distribution systematically affected performance while identifying in the process a number of variable configurations that outperformed more 'expensive' uniform configurations.

In order to dispel concerns that the results might have been a function of preprocessing or of the recording quality, all experiments where repeated again with recordings made at 11,025 Hz and 8 bit, and then replicated once more employing 13 ms windowing. Finally, the architecture of the network was altered from 100 input nodes to 80, thus requiring modifications to the preprocessing that transmuted recordings into 80-dimensional signatures. For safe measure, all experiments were replicated one last time by altering the input layer to 140 nodes and consequently adjusting the preprocessing to produce 140-dimensional signatures. Again, results from all experiments showed that relative frequency of token distribution affected performance in the manner described above.

There also was the question of whether the behavior observed was a privilege of high frequency words or whether it could be extended to other sets of words. To answer this question, both the male and female speakers recorded the numbers 1 to 10 in English, Spanish, and Japanese. Each of these sets was then employed to replicate the experiments outlined above and results were akin to those reported so far.

Although tens of millions of networks were trained and tested with thousands of different tokens, the number of types per experiment was restricted to 10 and the range of tokens per type available during training was limited to between 1 and 4. This constraint was based on the physical computer resources required and the exponential nature of the problem, as a single experiment involving 4^10 (1,048,576) networks required around 2 weeks of dedicated uninterrupted processing. An experiment involving all 30 types and a range of 1 to 4 training tokens per type would require training and testing 4^30 (1,152,921,504,606,846,976) networks. Even maintaining the number of types at 10 but increasing the maximum number of tokes to 6 would require 60,466,176 networks.

2.4 Experiment III

Rather than focussing on eliciting all possible configurations and testing each with a fresh network, alternative search algorithms were designed to look for specific kinds of variable configurations. To this purpose, Experiment III was designed to employ all 30 types (from the CHILDES analyses data) and to contrast uniform learning against frequency-based learning from a different point of view. The data set from the male speaker was used for this series of experiments. The 22 tokens per type were randomly divided into a training set of 10 tokens per type and a testing set of 12 tokens per type.

In Experiment IIIa, a network was trained with 1 token per class and the accuracy of recognition was measured against the 12 tokens per type of the testing set. A second network then was trained with 2 tokens per class and the accuracy of recognition was measured against the same testing set. The process continued until a network was trained with all available tokens from the training set (10 tokens per type). The results are shown in Table 5.

As expected, accuracy of classification increases as more tokens per type are provided. This uniformity of token presentation would be abnormal (indeed, impossible) in natural language learning, where types occur with varying frequencies. It is worth observing, however, that more tokens per type do not imply correspondingly better learn-

Table 5. Uniform learning while increasing the number of training tokens per type

Tokens per Class	Total Training Tokens	Accuracy
1	30	48.06%
2	60	62.78%
3	90	55.56%
4	120	63.33%
5	150	61.67%
6	180	59.44%
7	210	72.50%
8	240	69.44%
9	270	66.11%
10	300	73.89%

ing, although an overall improvement is apparent, and the maximum uniform case (10 tokens per type) outperforms all others.
There being 30 types, the second network employed a total of 60 training tokens to attempt to correctly identify 360 test tokens and was successful in 62.78% of these cases (226 tokens). The last network – the maximum case – employed a total of 300 tokens to attempt to identify the same 360 novel tokens and was successful in 73.89% of these cases (266 tokens).

Figure 7 shows that, despite gradual increases in classification accuracy, uniform learning becomes increasingly more costly in terms of the ratio of training to testing tokens. The second network (2 training tokens per type) demonstrated a success ratio of 1:3.76 while the last network (10 training tokens per type) had a success ratio of 1:0.86. In other words, it could be said that the last network was hindered by some form of 'collision' between its training tokens.

Experiment IIIb employed the same training and testing sets as well as identical networks. A search algorithm was allowed to systematically vary (left-to-right, winner only, advance) the relative frequency of tokens, producing training sets with varying numbers of tokens per type. Each resulting training configuration was fed to a (fresh) network and several configurations were found that performed

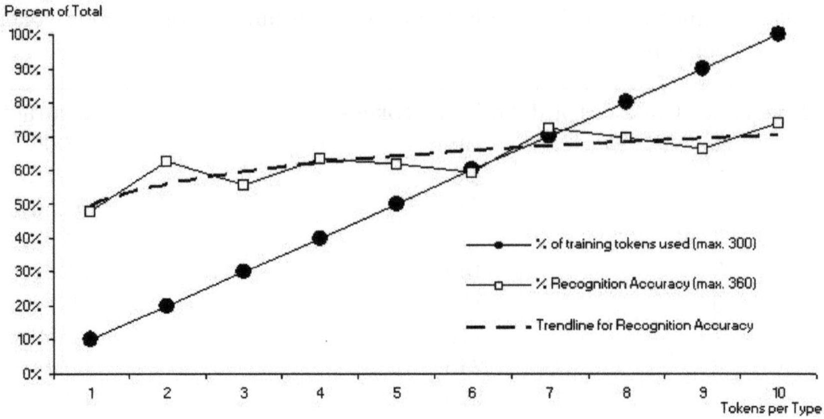

Figure 7. Graphic representation of Table 5

with better accuracy than the maximum uniform case (10 tokens per type) of Experiment IIIa. The results are shown in Table 6.

All variable configurations shown in Table 6 outperformed the maximum uniform configuration from Experiment IIIa and did so with as few as 92 tokens in all, less than a third of those employed by the maximum case (Table 5). It can be safely assumed that these are not the absolute best variable configurations and that, were additional time and resources available, more adequate (perhaps optimal) configurations could be found. The point, however, is made. Types interact with each other as the region of space that each occupies is modified not only by its own tokens but by those of its neighbors.

Table 6. Sample of frequency-based learning from Experiment IIIb

#	Configuration	Accuracy	Total Tokens
1	[10 1 1 10 1 1 1 1 10 10 1 9 1 1 1 1 10 1 1 1 1 1 1 10 1 1 1 1 1 1]	74.44%	92
2	[10 1 1 10 1 1 1 1 10 10 1 9 1 1 1 1 10 1 1 1 1 1 5 10 1 1 1 1 1 1]	75.83%	96
3	[10 1 1 10 8 1 1 1 10 10 1 9 1 1 1 1 10 1 1 1 1 1 5 10 1 1 1 1 1 1]	77.78%	103
4	[10 1 2 10 8 1 1 1 10 10 1 9 1 1 1 1 10 1 1 1 1 1 5 10 1 1 1 1 1 1]	78.06%	104
5	[10 1 2 10 8 1 1 4 10 10 1 9 1 1 1 1 10 1 1 1 1 1 5 10 1 1 1 1 1 1]	79.44%	107
6	[10 1 2 10 8 1 1 4 8 10 1 9 1 1 1 1 10 1 1 1 1 1 5 10 1 1 1 1 1 1]	79.72%	105
7	[10 1 1 10 10 1 1 4 8 10 3 9 1 1 3 2 10 3 9 1 1 2 5 10 1 1 1 1 1 1]	84.72%	122
8	[4 9 7 2 5 10 10 7 10 5 4 9 2 1 5 2 4 1 1 1 1 1 1 1 1 1 1 1 1 1]	79.72%	109

Table 7. Sample of frequency-based learning from Experiment IIIc (left-to-right search)

Pass #	Configuration	Accuracy	Total Tokens
1	[6 1 1 1 1 1 1 1 1 1 1 1 1 1 1 1 1 1 1 1 1 1 1 1 1 1 1 1 1 1]	43.61%	35
2	[6 9 1 1 1 1 1 1 1 1 1 1 1 1 1 1 1 1 1 1 1 1 1 1 1 1 1 1 1 1]	55.00%	43
3	[6 9 1 2 1 1 1 1 1 1 1 1 1 1 1 1 1 1 1 1 1 1 1 1 1 1 1 1 1 1]	56.11%	44
4	[6 9 1 2 5 1 1 1 1 1 1 1 1 1 1 1 1 1 1 1 1 1 1 1 1 1 1 1 1 1]	57.77%	48
5	[6 10 1 2 5 1 1 1 1 1 1 1 1 1 1 1 1 1 1 1 1 1 1 1 1 1 1 1 1 1]	58.88%	49
6	[6 10 10 2 5 1 1 1 1 1 1 1 1 1 1 1 1 1 1 1 1 1 1 1 1 1 1 1 1 1]	59.44%	58
7	[6 10 10 2 7 1 1 1 1 1 1 1 1 1 1 1 1 1 1 1 1 1 1 1 1 1 1 1 1 1]	60.55%	60
8	[6 10 10 2 7 10 1 1 1 1 1 1 1 1 1 1 1 1 1 1 1 1 1 1 1 1 1 1 1 1]	63.88%	69
9	[6 10 10 10 7 10 1 1 1 1 1 1 1 1 1 1 1 1 1 1 1 1 1 1 1 1 1 1 1 1]	65.00%	77
10	[4 10 10 10 7 10 1 1 1 1 1 1 1 1 1 1 1 1 1 1 1 1 1 1 1 1 1 1 1 1]	65.83%	75
11	[4 10 10 10 8 10 1 1 1 1 1 1 1 1 1 1 1 1 1 1 1 1 1 1 1 1 1 1 1 1]	67.22%	76
12	[4 10 10 10 8 10 9 1 1 1 1 1 1 1 1 1 1 1 1 1 1 1 1 1 1 1 1 1 1 1]	70.27%	84
13	**[4 10 10 10 8 10 9 6 1 1 1 1 1 1 1 1 1 1 1 1 1 1 1 1 1 1 1 1 1 1]**	**74.16%**	**89**
14	[4 10 10 10 8 10 9 6 1 4 1 1 1 1 1 1 1 1 1 1 1 1 1 1 1 1 1 1 1 1]	75.27%	92
15	[4 10 10 10 8 10 10 6 1 4 1 1 1 1 1 1 1 1 1 1 1 1 1 1 1 1 1 1 1 1]	75.55%	93
16	[4 10 10 10 8 10 10 6 1 4 6 1 1 1 1 1 1 1 1 1 1 1 1 1 1 1 1 1 1 1]	76.11%	98
17	[4 10 10 10 8 10 10 6 2 4 6 1 1 1 1 1 1 1 1 1 1 1 1 1 1 1 1 1 1 1]	76.38%	99
18	[4 10 10 10 8 10 10 6 2 4 6 1 1 1 2 1 1 1 1 1 1 1 1 1 1 1 1 1 1 1]	76.94%	100
19	[4 10 10 10 8 10 10 6 2 4 6 1 1 1 2 1 8 1 1 1 1 1 1 1 1 1 1 1 1 1]	77.22%	107
20	[2 10 10 10 8 10 10 6 2 4 6 1 1 1 2 1 8 1 1 1 1 1 1 1 1 1 1 1 1 1]	77.50%	105
21	[2 10 10 10 8 10 10 10 2 4 6 1 1 1 2 1 8 1 1 1 1 1 1 1 1 1 1 1 1 1]	78.05%	109
22	[2 10 10 10 8 10 10 10 5 4 6 1 1 1 2 1 8 1 1 1 1 1 1 1 1 1 1 1 1 1]	78.88%	112
23	[2 10 10 10 8 10 10 5 5 4 6 1 1 1 2 1 8 1 1 1 1 1 1 1 1 1 1 1 1 1]	79.44%	107
24	[2 10 10 10 8 10 10 5 8 4 6 1 1 1 2 1 8 1 1 1 1 1 1 1 1 1 1 1 1 1]	79.72%	110
25	[2 9 10 10 8 10 10 5 8 4 6 1 1 1 2 1 8 1 1 1 1 1 1 1 1 1 1 1 1 1]	79.72%	109
26	[2 9 10 10 8 10 10 5 8 4 4 1 1 1 2 1 8 1 1 1 1 1 1 1 1 1 1 1 1 1]	80.55%	107
27	[2 9 10 10 8 9 10 5 8 4 4 1 1 1 2 1 8 1 1 1 1 1 1 1 1 1 1 1 1 1]	81.38%	106
28	[2 9 10 10 8 9 10 5 8 4 4 1 1 6 2 1 8 1 1 1 1 1 1 1 1 1 1 1 1 1]	82.50%	111
29	[1 9 10 10 8 9 10 5 8 4 4 1 1 6 2 1 8 1 1 1 1 1 1 1 1 1 1 1 1 1]	82.77%	110
30	[1 9 10 10 8 9 10 5 8 4 4 1 1 6 4 1 8 1 1 1 1 1 1 1 1 1 1 1 1 1]	83.05%	112
31	[1 9 10 10 8 9 10 5 8 4 4 1 1 6 4 1 8 6 1 1 1 1 1 1 1 1 1 1 1 1]	83.61%	117
32	[1 9 10 10 8 9 10 4 8 4 4 1 1 6 4 1 8 6 1 1 1 1 1 1 1 1 1 1 1 1]	83.88%	116
33	[1 9 10 10 8 9 10 4 8 4 4 1 1 6 4 2 8 6 1 1 1 1 1 1 1 1 1 1 1 1]	84.16%	117
34	[1 9 10 10 8 9 10 4 8 4 4 1 1 6 4 2 8 6 1 1 2 1 1 1 1 1 1 1 1 1]	84.44%	118

Configurations 1 through 7 were obtained from a start configuration different to the one used to obtain configuration 8. The objective was to show that the shape of variable configurations is rather flexible and that the internal structure of a type changes with that of surrounding types (compare types 1 and 2 in configurations 7 and 8). Note also, that configuration 8 is 'top-heavy', that is, the first 17 types carry the job of configuring an optimal space for all 30 types. Experiment IIIc was designed to test a modified search algorithm that would show favoritism towards a subset of types and that would attempt to produce 'top-heavy' configurations akin to configuration 8 in Table 6. Results are shown in Table 7.

Table 7 shows that pass #13 (bold frame) employed a total of 89 training tokens to achieve a level of accuracy comparable (slightly better in fact, 74.16% versus 73.89%) to that of the maximum uniform configuration in Experiment IIIa. This version of the algorithm (left-to-right, winner only, restart) was unable to find a configuration with accuracy over 84.44% having modified up to type #21 in the process. Of relevance, however, is that the configuration in pass #13 modifies the relative frequency of tokens for types 1 through 8 to affect the performance accuracy of the network over all 30 types.

In Table 8, the previous algorithm is reversed to search right-to-left, that is, choosing a different subset of types to vary, and again shows how persistent and flexible the effects of frequency variation are on overall performance. As can be seen, the 8 right-most types (pass #13, bold frame) achieved a level of accuracy just as good (slightly better in fact) as the maximum case in Table 5 with only 82 training tokens (versus 300, a ratio of 1:3.65). This version of the search algorithm was unable to find a configuration with an accuracy over 81.94% having in the process run over 22 types and modified up to type #9 in the process.

Summing up, results from Experiment III collectively show that it is possible to obtain variable configurations that crudely simulate a slope of frequency distributions where a subset of all types carry the task of setting up a problem space beneficial for less frequent types, even if these are minimally represented.

3 Contextualization of the experiments

The effects of frequency on a network's performance have been shown to be independent of speaker (male and female), data set (within and across languages), data gathering and preprocessing (sample rate, windowing, and signature size), and modification of the ECOS architecture (input and output layers). A further issue is whether these results can be replicated with other computational models.

Table 8. Sample of frequency-based learning from Experiment IIIc (right -to-left search)

Pass #	Configuration	Accuracy	Total Tokens
1	[1 1 1 1 1 1 1 1 1 1 1 1 1 1 1 1 1 1 1 1 1 1 1 1 1 1 1 1 1 5]	44.44%	34
2	[1 1 1 1 1 1 1 1 1 1 1 1 1 1 1 1 1 1 1 1 1 1 1 1 1 1 1 7 1 5]	49.16%	40
3	[1 1 1 1 1 1 1 1 1 1 1 1 1 1 1 1 1 1 1 1 1 1 1 1 1 1 1 7 1 7]	50.83%	42
4	[1 1 1 1 1 1 1 1 1 1 1 1 1 1 1 1 1 1 1 1 1 1 1 1 1 1 3 7 1 7]	51.66%	44
5	[1 1 1 1 1 1 1 1 1 1 1 1 1 1 1 1 1 1 1 1 1 1 1 1 1 1 3 8 1 7]	53.05%	45
6	[1 1 1 1 1 1 1 1 1 1 1 1 1 1 1 1 1 1 1 1 1 1 1 1 1 10 3 8 1 7]	54.72%	54
7	[1 1 1 1 1 1 1 1 1 1 1 1 1 1 1 1 1 1 1 1 1 1 1 1 1 10 3 8 1 8]	61.38%	55
8	[1 1 1 1 1 1 1 1 1 1 1 1 1 1 1 1 1 1 1 1 1 1 1 1 1 10 3 8 2 8]	62.22%	56
9	[1 1 1 1 1 1 1 1 1 1 1 1 1 1 1 1 1 1 1 1 1 1 1 1 1 10 9 8 2 8]	65.55%	62
10	[1 1 1 1 1 1 1 1 1 1 1 1 1 1 1 1 1 1 1 1 1 1 1 1 1 10 9 8 4 8]	66.11%	64
11	[1 1 1 1 1 1 1 1 1 1 1 1 1 1 1 1 1 1 1 1 1 1 1 1 10 10 9 8 4 8]	72.22%	73
12	[1 1 1 1 1 1 1 1 1 1 1 1 1 1 1 1 1 1 1 1 1 1 1 2 10 10 9 8 4 8]	72.77%	74
13	**[1 1 1 1 1 1 1 1 1 1 1 1 1 1 1 1 1 1 1 1 1 1 9 2 10 10 9 8 4 8]**	**74.72%**	**82**
14	[1 1 1 1 1 1 1 1 1 1 1 1 1 1 1 1 1 1 1 1 1 1 9 1 10 10 9 8 4 8]	74.72%	81
15	[1 1 1 1 1 1 1 1 1 1 1 1 1 1 1 1 1 1 1 1 1 1 9 1 10 10 9 8 2 8]	75.55%	79
16	[1 1 1 1 1 1 1 1 1 1 1 1 1 1 1 1 1 1 1 1 4 1 9 1 10 10 9 8 2 8]	75.55%	82
17	[1 1 1 1 1 1 1 1 1 1 1 1 1 1 1 1 1 1 1 1 4 1 9 1 10 10 9 8 1 8]	75.83%	81
18	[1 1 1 1 1 1 1 1 1 1 1 1 1 1 1 1 1 1 1 1 4 1 9 2 10 10 9 8 1 8]	76.11%	82
19	[1 1 1 1 1 1 1 1 1 1 1 1 1 1 1 1 1 1 1 1 4 1 9 2 10 10 9 8 2 8]	76.66%	83
20	[1 1 1 1 1 1 1 1 1 1 1 1 1 1 1 1 1 1 1 1 4 1 10 2 10 10 9 8 2 8]	76.94%	84
21	[1 1 1 1 1 1 1 1 1 1 1 1 1 1 1 1 1 2 1 1 4 1 10 2 10 10 9 8 2 8]	77.22%	85
22	[1 1 1 1 1 1 1 1 1 1 1 1 1 1 1 1 5 2 1 1 4 1 10 2 10 10 9 8 2 8]	77.50%	89
23	[1 1 1 1 1 1 1 1 1 1 1 1 1 1 1 1 5 6 1 1 4 1 10 2 10 10 9 8 2 8]	77.77%	93
24	[1 1 1 1 1 1 1 1 1 1 1 1 1 1 1 1 5 6 2 1 4 1 10 2 10 10 9 8 2 8]	78.61%	94
25	[1 1 1 1 1 1 1 1 1 1 1 1 3 1 1 1 5 6 2 1 4 1 10 2 10 10 9 8 2 8]	78.88%	96
26	[1 1 1 1 1 1 1 1 1 3 1 1 3 1 1 1 5 6 2 1 4 1 10 2 10 10 9 8 2 8]	79.16%	98
27	[1 1 1 1 1 1 1 1 1 3 1 1 3 1 1 1 7 6 2 1 4 1 10 2 10 10 9 8 2 8]	79.44%	100
28	[1 1 1 1 1 1 1 1 4 3 1 1 3 1 1 1 7 6 2 1 4 1 10 2 10 10 9 8 2 8]	81.38%	103
29	[1 1 1 1 1 1 1 1 4 3 1 1 3 1 1 1 7 6 2 5 4 1 10 2 10 10 9 8 2 8]	81.66%	107
30	[1 1 1 1 1 1 1 1 4 3 1 1 3 1 1 1 7 6 1 5 4 1 10 2 10 10 9 8 2 8]	81.94%	106

In order to address this question it is important to discuss what constitutes 'learning' for the ECOS system. First, and as with other connectionist models, learning can be taken to be the classification accuracy of a network when faced with novel tokens belonging to those types it has been trained with. A high percentage of accuracy implies that learning has taken place while a low percentage of accuracy implies that learning has been deficient. Although this is an overly simplistic definition of learning, both for the sentient and the mechanical, the experiments presented so far provide evidence that this kind of learning can be promoted by employing training frequency as the sole experimental variable.

Second, and particular to the ECOS system, learning is a function of the number of clusters a network creates during training. If each training token has created its own cluster, learning has been minimal. If, however, individual clusters have come to represent several training tokens, learning has taken place. In other words, the ratio (training token):(cluster) is an indication of whether the system has been able to abstract relevant 'knowledge' from the training set.

Recalling the training procedure described in Section 2.1, when a training token falls outside of all existing clusters, the token creates a new cluster. This new cluster is a point in the problem space, namely, the position of the token. Note that in the case where each and every token creates a new cluster (rather than accrete), the behavior of ECOS is similar to a nearest-neighbor algorithm (Fix and Hodges Jr, 1951; Aha, 1997; Aha et al., 1991). In this situation, the problem space simply ends up being populated with the training set and, therefore, novel tokens are classified according to what amounts to a nearest-neighbor decision rule. This observation is of relevance because in Experiments I and II, networks tended to create as many clusters as there were training tokens. In other words, these ECOS networks behaved like k-nn systems. On account of this, Experiment II was replicated using nearest-neighbor decision rules (rather than ECOS) and it was found that, indeed, the effects of relative frequency of token distribution over types in k-nn models reproduced the results reported in this paper. It is safe to assume, therefore, that the results can be extended to at least some of the many exemplar and prototype models in the literature (for a comprehensive review, see Devroye et al. 1996). It should be noted that although research on exemplar-based artificial and natural learning have evolved largely independently of each other, there abounds AI and psychological literature attesting to common ground (Heit, 1994, 1997; Murphy and Medin, 1985; Nosofsky, 1986, 1992; Kruschke, 1992; Langley, 1999). Nonetheless, it is debatable whether, and in what way, it is ultimately feasible or legitimate to correlate artificial and natural learning, let alone extrapolate this specific simulation of the effects of frequency in computer models to language acquisition in humans.

One limitation of the simulations reported here concerns the small number of types that were used. The problem, namely, is that of designing experiments which employ a data set which realistically reflects natural language frequencies, that is, a data set which combines highly frequent words (HFW), represented by very many tokens, and highly infrequent words, represented by comparatively few tokens. It is estimated that in English, for example, 90% of spoken language is constructed out of about 1,000 word families, and that if these word families are expanded to account for all their constituent types, there are upwards of 4,000 words, approximately half of which are HFW (Nation, 1990, 2001). If one were to hypothesize that the phonological shapes of these 4,000 types somehow configure a problem space that lays the ground for ease of acquisition and accurate subsequent processing of low frequency words (LFW) – such that a lesser number of tokens of LFW is sufficient for this task – the complexity of the dynamics involved are beyond the capacity of the token signatures (number, quality, and relation between of features) employed in these experiments and far beyond available computational resources. The complexity is not diminished by the recognition that a person with average knowledge of English is said to be familiar with some 5,000 word families, while a person with expert knowledge is said to be familiar with some 20,000 word families (Goulden et al., 1990; Zechmeister et al., 1995). The problem is non-trivial (even for the human brain) and is reflected in the process of first language acquisition, where children spend their first years mastering only a small subset of the aforementioned types. Since there are many 'optimal' variable configurations (as demonstrated here), it is within the bounds of the feasible to consider that such massive experiments would yield desirable results. In any case, the experiments presented here cannot prove that there is a direct relation between frequency of occurrence in language and optimal learnability. What these experiments can show, however, is that there exist certain distributions of token signatures that configure a problem space in such a way as to enhance learning through frequency variation.

Nonetheless, a point of contact can be found between frequency and learning in light of these experiments. As explained, the exponential nature of the problem forces experimentation to be conducted on reduced sets of types. This constraint is also found in natural languages, where a comparatively small subset of the lexicon is dramatically more abundant in use. As mentioned, HFW, in the form of about 4,000 types, account for approximately 90% of spoken and more than 80% of written English (Nation, 2001). Consequently, some types are staggeringly more frequent than others, the range going from 60,000 per million down to 1 per million and below (Ellis, 2002, 167). An inevitable outcome of this seemingly poor exploitation of the lexicon is the high degree of polysemy that characterizes HFW versus LFW (Zipf, 1945; Polikarpov, 1999). We can make sense of these facts in view of the experiments reported in this paper. If the frequency of occurrence of HFW is to command the optimal distribution of the problem space for all types in the lexicon, then this subset of types must be kept at a level of proliferation that the brain can handle.

Finally, the relevance of the collection of features employed to represent the data should not be underestimated (Langley, 1999). The number, quality, and relationships between features constituting token signatures are cardinal factors in determining the viability of any learning system. In Experiments I and II, the size and quality of token signatures were appropriate for 10 types and these populated the problem space sparsely. In Experiment III, however, clusters were made to evolve in order to adequately represent 30 types. Had the number of types continued to increase, additional features would have been required as the dimensionality of the problem space – a function of the number of features used – is bound to increase along with the size of the data set. In other words, while 100 features may be sufficient to distinguish a few hundred tokens belonging to a couple of dozen phonological types, a data set with thousands of types and hundreds of thousands of tokens would require untold numbers of features. Otherwise, as the density of the data increases, so does the chance of type collisions. At the same time it should be noted that in any language there are going to be more meanings than there are words, and that the expression of the former will be to a large extent restricted to a set of HFW. Since mental spaces can be conceived as topological systems on account of the existence of chromotopic and tonotopic neurological areas in the cortex (Elman et al., 1998; Pulvermüller, 2002), it also appears reasonable to question whether the number of features available to describe percepts is less abundant than the number of features available to describe concepts. However, as some authors propose (Barsalou, 1992, 1999b,a; Pulvermüller, 2002), if the meaning of a word resides in the cumulative collection of sensorial experiences, then the depth and complexity of features required to account for the relative wealth of semantic entities can be found in the exponential composition of token signatures from different mental spaces corresponding to different perceptual modalities or domains of perceptual experience. In short, it may boil down to dividing and conquering the problem space into autonomous subspaces whether across or within linguistic/cognitive domains.

4 Conclusions

Let us imagine a language as a maximally efficient system, whose structural resources are exploited to the full. Suppose, to take a simple example, that a language has six stop consonants distinguished by three places of articulation and by a binary voicing contrast. In such a hypothetical language, each of the six stops would occur with equal frequency, corresponding to the optimal exploitation of the place and voicing features. Or suppose that the verbs of a language can be assigned to three inflectional paradigms. In the imaginary language, each inflection class would be represented by an equal number of verb types, while the three inflection classes would occur with equal frequency in running speech.

It is well established that such an 'ideal' language does not exist. Wherever we look in a natural language, we find variations in the frequency of occurrence of its structural elements. In some cases, admittedly, the variation might be attributed to 'external' non-linguistic factors. The supposedly higher text frequency of *I live in New York* vs. *I live in Dayton Ohio* would be a consequence of the circumstantial fact that more people happen to live in New York than live in Dayton Ohio. External circumstantial factors, though, are hardly able to explain the fact that the first conjugation of French verbs (the *chanter*-class) contains many more tokens than the *finir*- and *vendre*-classes, even less the fact that in discourse tokens of the third conjugation *vendre*-class outnumber those of the other classes (Bybee, 1995). Frequency effects permeate natural languages at all levels of description, to such an extent that one might suppose that variation in frequency is a 'design feature' (Hockett, 1987) of natural languages.

We suggest that this property of natural languages reflects the adaptation of languages to the learning capabilities of their speakers. The structural elements of a language have to be learned by each generation of speakers, and learning can only take place on the basis of input data. One might suppose that learning will be a simple linear function of frequency of input – the more frequent a particular element, the better it will be learned. (A slightly more sophisticated hypothesis would be that learning will be a power function of input frequency, cf. Ellis 2002). The facts of natural languages, however, are difficult to square with this 'common sense' view. For example, the hypothesis predicts that relatively infrequent elements of a language will be correspondingly difficult to acquire. Over time, and over generations of learners, such elements will become even less frequent, until they eventually vanish from the language completely. The hypothesis that learning is a linear (or power) function of input frequency predicts that natural languages will sooner or later converge on the maximally efficient language system mentioned above, in which all structural elements have an equal frequency of occurrence. There is no evidence, however, that languages do tend towards this maximally efficient state. On the contrary, frequency variation is a robust and endemic property of natural languages.

Our experiments offer a clue as to why this should be so. Our hypothesis is that variation in input frequency promotes acquisition, not only of the more frequently occurring elements of the system, but also of the less frequently occurring elements. Indeed, frequency variation of the input data is itself liable to promote learning of the full system, including the elements which have been encountered on very few, or even on only a single occasion.

References

Aha, David. 1997. *Lazy Learning*. Norwell, MA.: Kluwer.

Aha, David, Dennis Kibler and Marc Albert. 1991. Instance-based learning algorithms. *Machine Learning* 6: 37–66.

Barsalou, Lawrence. 1992. *Cognitive Psychology: An Overview for Cognitive Scientists*. Hillsdale, N.J.: Erlbaum.

Barsalou, Lawrence W. 1999a. Perceptions of perceptual symbols: Author's response to commentary. *Behavioral and Brain Sciences* 22(4): 637–660.

Barsalou, Lawrence W. 1999b. Perceptual symbol systems. *Behavioral and Brain Sciences* 22(4): 577–609.

Bates, Elizabeth, I. Bretherton and L. Synder. 1988. *From First Words to Grammar: Individual Differences and Dissociable Mechanisms*. Cambridge, MA: Cambridge University Press.

Bernstein, N. 1982. Acoustic study of mothers speech to language-learning children: An analysis of vowel articulatory characteristics. Ph.D. thesis, Boston University, Boston.

Biber, Douglas, Susan Conrad and Randi Reppen. 1989. *Corpus Linguistics: Investigating Language Structure and Use*. Cambridge: Cambridge University Press.

Bloom, Lois. 1970. *Language Development: Form and Function in Emerging Grammars*. Cambridge, Mass.: MIT Press.

Brown, Roger. 1973. *A First Language: The Early Stages*. Cambridge, Mass.: Harvard University Press.

Bybee, Joan. 1995. Regular morphology and the lexicon. *Language and Cognitive Processes* 10: 425–455.

Bybee, Joan. 2001. *Phonology and Language Use*. Cambridge: Cambridge University Press.

Bybee, Joan and Paul Hopper (eds.). 2001. *Frequency and the Emergence of Linguistic Structure*. Amsterdam: Benjamins.

Chomsky, Noam. 1957. *Syntactic Structures*. The Hague: Mouton.

Clark, Eve V. 1978. Awareness of language: Some evidence from what children say and do. In: Anne Sinclair, Robert J. Jarvella and Willem J. Levelt (eds.), *The Child's Conception of Language*. Berlin: Springer Verlag, 17–43.

Demetras, M. 1989a. Changes in parents' conversational responses: A function of gramatical development. Paper presented at ASHA, St. Louis, MO.

Demetras, M. 1989b. Working parents conversational responses to their two-year-old sons. Working paper, University of Arizona.

Demetras, M., K. Post and C. Snow. 1986. Feedback to first-language. *Journal of Child Language* 13: 275–292.

Devroye, Luc, Laszlo Györfi and Gabor Lugosi. 1996. *A Probabilistic Theory of Pattern Recognition*. New York: Springer.

Ellis, Nick. 2002. Frequency effects in language processing. *Studies in Second Language Acquisition* 24: 143–188.

Elman, Jeffrey, Elizabeth Bates, Mark Johnson, Annette Karmiloff-Smith, Domenico Parisi and Kim Plunket. 1998. *Rethinking Innateness: A Connectionist Perspective on Development*. Cambridge, MA: MIT Press.

Fix, Evelyn and Joseph L. Hodges Jr. 1951. Discriminatory analysis. Nonparametric discrimination: Consistency properties. Technical Report 4, USAF School of Aviation Medicine, Randolph Field.

Goulden, Robin, Paul Nation and John Read. 1990. How large can a receptive vocabulary be? *Applied Linguistics* 11: 314–363.

Greenberg, Joseph. 1966. *Language Universals*. The Hague: Mouton.

Haggerty, L. 1929. What a two-and-one-half-year-old said in one day. *Journal of Genetic Psychology* 38: 75–100.

Halliday, Michael A. K. 1991. Corpus studies and probabilistic grammar. In: K. Aijmer and B. Altenberg (eds.), *English Corpus Linguistics*. London: Longman, 30–43.

Heit, Evan. 1994. Models of the effect of prior knowledge on category learning. *Journal of Experimental Psychology: Learning, Memory, and Cognition* 20: 1264–1282.

Heit, Evan. 1997. Knowledge and concept learning. In: Koen Lamberts and David Shanks (eds.), *Knowledge, Concepts, and Categories*. Hove, East Sussex: Psychology Press., 7–41.

Higginson, R. P. 1985. Fixing-assimilation in language acquisition. Ph.D. thesis, Washington State University.

Hockett, Charles. 1987. *Refurbishing our Foundations: Elementary Linguistics from an Advanced Point of View*. Amsterdam: Benjamins.

Howe, C. 1981. *Acquiring Language in a Conversational Context*. New York: Academic Press.

Hunston, Susan. 2002. *Corpora in Applied Linguistics*. Cambridge: Cambridge University Press.

Janda, Richard. 1991. Frequency, markedness, and morphological change: On predicting the spread of noun-plural -s in Modern High German and West Germanic. In: *ESCOL'90 (Eastern States Conference on Linguistics)*. 136–153.

Jurafsky, Daniel, Alan Bell, Michelle Gregory and William Raymond. 2001. Probabilistic relations between words: Evidence from reduction in lexical production. In: Joan Bybee and Paul Hopper (eds.), *Frequency and the Emergence of Linguistic Structure*. Amsterdam: Benjamins, 229–254.

Kaeding, Friedrich Wilhelm. 1898. *Häufigkeitswörterbuch der deutschen Sprache*. Steglitz bei Berlin: Selbstverlag des Herausgebers. [Frequency dictionary of the German language].

Kasabov, Nikola. 1998. ECOS - a framework for evolving connectionist systems and the 'ECO' training paradigm. In: S. Usui and T. Omori (eds.), *Proceedings of ICONIP '98 - The Fifth International Conference on Neutral Information Processing*. Kitakyushu, Japan: IOS Press, 1232–1235.

Kasabov, Nikola. 2000. ECOS - Evolving Connectionist Systems - a new /old paradigm for on-time learning and knowledge engineering. In: N. Kasabov (ed.), *Future Directions for Intelligent Systems and Information Sciences*. New York: Physica–Verlag, 3–12.

Kasabov, Nikola. 2001. Evolving fuzzy neural networks for on-line supervised/unsupervised, knowledge-based learning. *IEEE Trans. SMC - part B: Cybernetics* 31(6): 902–918.

Kasabov, Nikola. 2002. *Evolving Connectionist Systems: Methods and Applications in Bioinformatics, Brain Study and Intelligent Machines*. London, New York & Heidelberg: Springer.

Kasabov, Nikola and Q. Song. 2002. DENFIS: Dynamic, evolving neural-fuzzy inference systems and its application for time-series prediction. *IEEE Trans. On Fuzzy Systems* 10(2): 144–154.

Kruschke, John K. 1992. ALCOVE: An exemplar-based connectionist model of category learning. *Psychological Review* 99: 22–44.

Langley, Pat. 1999. Concrete and abstract models of category learning. In: *Proceedings of the Twenty-First Annual Conference of the Cognitive Science Society*. Vancouver: Lawrence Erlbaum, 288–293.

Leech, Geoffrey, Paul Rayson and Andrew Wilson. 2001. *Word Frequencies in Written and Spoken English: Based on the British National Corpus*. London: Longman.

Liu, Lianyuan and Yifan Ma. 1986. Mandarin tonal distribution and tonal frequency. *Yuwen Jianshe* 3: xx.

López Ornat, Susan. 1994. *La Adquisición de la Lengua Española*. Madrid: Siglo XXI.

MacWhinney, Brian. 2000. *The CHILDES Database: Tools for Analyzing Talk*, volume 2. 3rd edition. Mahwah, NJ: Lawrence Associates.

Miller, George. 1965. Introduction. In: George Zipf (ed.), *The Psychobiology of Language. An Introduction to Dynamic Philology*. Cambridge, Mass.: MIT Press, v–x.

Montes, R. 1987. Secuencias de clarificación en conversaciones con niños (morphe 3-4). Ph.D. thesis, Universidad Autónoma de Puebla.

Montes, Rosa G. 1992. Achieving understanding: Repair mechanisms in mother-child conversations. Ph.D. thesis, Georgetown University.

Moon, Rosamund. 1998. *Fixed Expressons and Idioms in English: A Corpus-based Approach*. Oxford: Oxford University Press.

Murphy, Gregory L. and Douglas L. Medin. 1985. The role of theories in concept coherence. *Psychological Review* 92: 289–316.

Nation, I. S. Paul. 1990. *Teaching and Learning Vocabulary*. Massachusetts: Newbury House.

Nation, I. S. Paul. 2001. *Learning Vocabulary in Another Language*. Cambridge: Cambridge University Press.

Nelson, Katherine. 1989. *Narratives from the Crib*. Cambridge, MA: Harvad University Press.

Ninio, Anat, Catherine Snow, Barbara Pan and Pamela Rollins. 1994. Classifying communicative acts in children's interactions. *Journal of Communication Disorders* 27: 157–188.

Nosofsky, Robert M. 1986. Attention, similarity, and identification-categorization relationship. *Journal of Experimental Psychology* 115(1): 39–57.

Nosofsky, Robert M. 1992. Exemplars, prototypes, and similarity rules. In: A. F. Healy, S. M. Kosslyn and R. M. Shiffrin (eds.), *From Learning Theory to Connectionist Theory: Essays in Honor of William K. Estes*. Hillsdale, NJ: Erlbaum, 149–167.

Polikarpov, Anatoliy A. 1999. Cognitive model of lexical system evolutions and its verification. *Human Language Electronic Bulletin, www.humlang.newmail.ru* .

Pulvermüller, Friedemann. 2002. *The Neuroscience of Language: On Brain Circuits of Words and Serial Order*. Cambridge: Cambridge University Press.

Pustet, Regina. 2004. Zipf and his heirs. *Language Sciences* 26: 1–25.

Romero, Silvia, Aida Santos and Dora Pellicer. 1992. *The Construction of Communicative Competence in Mexican Spanish Speaking Children (6 Months to 7 Years)*. Mexico City: University of the Americas.

Sachs, Jacqueline. 1983. Talking about the there and then: The emergence of displaced reference in parent-child discourse. In: K. E. Nelson (ed.), *Children's Language*, volume 4. Hillside, NJ: Lawrence Erlbaum Associates, 1–28.

Sinclair, John. 1991. *Corpus, Concordance, Collocation*. Oxford: Oxford University Press.

Suppes, P. 1974. The semantics of children's language. *American Psychologist* 29: 103–114.

Taylor, John R. 2007. Metaphors of linguistic knowledge: The generative metaphor vs. the mental corpus metaphor. In: Iraide Ibarretxe-Antuñano, Carlos Inchaurralde and Jesús-M. Sánchez-García (eds.), *Language, Mind, and the Lexicon*. Frankfurt: Peter Lang, 69–104.

Theakston, Ana L., Elena V.M. Lieven, Julian M. Pine and Caroline F. Rowland. 2001. The role of performance limitations in the acquisition of verb-argument structure. *Journal of Child Language* 4: 127–152.

Valian, Virginia. 1991. Syntactic subjects in the early speech of American and Italian children. *Cognition* 40: 21–81.

Van Houten, L. 1986. Role of maternal input in the acquisition process: The communication strategies of adolescent and older mothers with their language learning children. Paper presented at the Boston University Conference on Language Development.

Wells, C. G. 1981. *Learning through Interaction: The Study of Language Development*. Cambridge: Cambridge University Press.

Zechmeister, Eugene B., Andrea M. Chronis, William L. Cull, C. A. D'Anna and N. A. Healy. 1995. Growth of a functionally important lexicon. *Journal of Reading Behavior* 27: 201–212.

Zipf, George. 1945. The meaning-frequency relationship of words. *The Journal of General Psychology* 33: 251–256.

Zipf, George. 1965 (1935). *The Psychobiology of Language. An Introduction to Dynamic Philology*. Cambridge, Mass.: MIT Press.

Nouns and verbs in the mental lexicon

Barbra Novak and Sydney Lamb

1 Introduction

From the connectionist perspective of the mental lexicon, information corresponding to a 'lexical entry' of a conventional lexicon is widely distributed. According to the relational network model (Lamb, 1999), the whole lexeme (its entire network representation) is widely distributed; however, the lemma, the central node of the lexeme, is localized in a specific area of the brain. The lemma itself carries no information; rather, the information is in the connections between the lemma and other nodes. These other nodes include the phonological representations of the lexeme, the semantic representations of the lexeme, and so forth. These nodes are located in widely distributed areas of the brain – the phonological production node in the frontal lobe, the phonological recognition node in the posterior temporal lobe, the semantic node in the temporal lobe, etc. All of these nodes combine to form the whole lexeme, under the relational network model.

A prevailing issue is that of rationalizing the observation that Wernicke's aphasics have greater difficulty with nouns than verbs, while Broca's aphasics have the opposite problem. If the lexicon is indeed a widely distributed network, as proponents of the connectionist view posit, how does an anterior/posterior differentiation between nouns and verbs exist? Explanation of this question in light of recent work concerning the connectionist theory in addition to evidence from aphasiology leads to a surprising but reasonable conclusion.

This paper will discuss prior research on nouns and verbs in the mental lexicon so as to evaluate the proposition that nouns and verbs are discretely represented in the mental lexicon, or, in other words, that lemmas of nouns and verbs are separated and represented in different areas of the brain: nouns in the left temporal lobe and verbs in the left frontal lobe. However, it is first necessary to establish some background on Broca's and Wernicke's aphasia because of the abundance of research concerning aphasiology discussed throughout this paper.

Broca's aphasia results from trauma to the area in the inferior frontal gyrus known as Broca's area. Whereas the comprehension of a Broca's aphasic is largely intact, his/her speech is typically non-fluent and agrammatic; the output is commonly referred to as 'telegraphic' because it consists of an abundance of content words (e.g. nouns) coupled with a lack of function words (e.g. prepositions). Conversely, trauma to the posterior superior temporal gyrus (Wernicke's area) results in Wernicke's aphasia, which is characterized by impaired comprehension and fluent, grammatical, neologistic speech. Additionally, individuals with frontal lesions, such as Broca's aphasics, often demonstrate impaired verb processing (Bates et al., 1991; Damasio and Tranel, 1993; Daniele et al., 1994; Lamb and Zhang, 2002; Shapiro and Caramazza, 2003), whereas individuals with posterior lesions, such as those with Wernicke's aphasia, frequently demonstrate impaired noun processing (Bates et al., 1991; Damasio and Tranel, 1993; Daniele et al., 1994; Lamb and Zhang, 2002); therefore, aphasics provide an excellent source of information regarding how and where nouns and verbs are represented in the mental lexicon.

As will be apparent by the conclusion of this paper, research supporting the hypothesis of discrete representations of nouns and verbs in the mental lexicon far exceeds the contrary proposition of a widely distributed lexicon without distinct local representations.

2 A brief overview

Research conducted over the past twenty years has provided great insight into the organization of the mental lexicon. Noteworthy is the fact that the research varies in subject selection (aphasics, subjects with other neurological deficits, and neurologically intact subjects) and methodology (positron emission tomography (PET), event-related potentials (ERPs), repetitive transcranial magnetic stimulation (rTMS), and neuropsychological tests). Some of the research discussed in this paper does not support the notion of discrete nominal and verbal representations in the mental lexicon, failing to provide sufficient evidence of anatomically distinct representations of nouns and verbs in the brain.

Research supporting the hypothesis of distinct nominal and verbal representations provides different explanations regarding the representation of nouns and verbs in the mental lexicon, including syntactic/morphological accounts, semantic-conceptual accounts, and lexical accounts.

Syntactic accounts rely on the assumption that verbs are more closely associated with syntax than nouns. It is postulated that verbs are more difficult to process because they are inextricably associated with syntax. Furthermore, verbs do not stand independently as nouns can, because verbs cannot be dissociated from their arguments. It has also been suggested that the selective verb deficit of an agrammatic may be the cause of his/her agrammatism (McCarthy and Warrington, 1985). Once again, this hypothesis relies on the notion that verbs are more intimately associated with syntax than nouns. However, there is some contrary evidence that demonstrates subjects with frontal lobe lesions who have a selective verb deficit in the absence of agrammatism (Daniele et al., 1994).

Additionally, morphological accounts rely on the assumption that verbs carry more inflectional morphology than nouns (Bates et al., 1991). As will be discussed later, there is strong evidence in opposition to syntactic/morphological accounts of the double dissociation between nouns and verbs (Bates et al., 1991; Daniele et al., 1994).

Semantic-conceptual accounts of the noun-verb dissociation rely on the fact that prototypical nouns represent objects and prototypical verbs represent actions. Proponents of this hypothesis suggest that lexical representations for actions are located close to the motor cortex (frontal lobe), because this is where motor planning occurs. Conversely, lexical representations for objects are located close to the sensory cortices (temporal lobe), presumably because objects are known primarily through perception. However, this does not explain abstract nouns and non-action verbs. The proximity principle, which posits that adjacent areas of the brain control related functions, provides a valid explanation for the semantic-conceptual account of the noun-verb dissociation. Nevertheless, the results gained from some of the research discussed below cannot be explained via a semantic-conceptual account of the noun-verb dissociation (Miceli et al., 1984; McCarthy and Warrington, 1985; Lamb and Zhang, 2002).

Finally, lexical accounts of the noun-verb double dissociation have been suggested; however, skeptics of this hypothesis remain (Bates et al., 1991). Proponents of the lexical account suggest that lemmas of nouns and verbs are discretely represented in the mental lexicon, independent of syntax, morphology and semantics.

The following section will begin an extensive review of available research covering discrete representations versus common representations of nouns and verbs in the mental lexicon. To reiterate, proponents of hypotheses supporting discrete representations of nouns and verbs posit that lemmas of nouns and verbs are represented in different anatomical areas of the brain. Conversely, proponents of hypotheses supporting common representations of nouns and verbs suggest that no anatomical differences exist in the representations of nouns and verbs.

3 Claims of discrete representations for nouns and verbs

This section will analyze existing research supporting the hypothesis that nouns and verbs are differently represented in the mental lexicon. Many researchers have found evidence that nouns and verbs are represented in separate and distinct anatomical areas in the brain – specifically, nouns in the temporal lobe and verbs in the frontal lobe.

Much of the research performed on this topic utilizes the language abilities of neurologically impaired subjects as evidence for discrete representations of nouns and verbs. For example, McCarthy and Warrington (1985) described the selective verb deficit of ROX, whose agrammatism was a result of cortical atrophy. ROX demonstrated impaired retrieval and comprehension of verbs, but intact retrieval and comprehension of nouns. ROX's verb impairment, demonstrating relative sparing of nouns, indicates that nouns and verbs are discretely represented in the lexicon. Zingeser and Berndt (1990) explored the noun-verb deficit differences exemplified by agrammatics and anomics. The subjects, five agrammatics, five anomics and five normal controls, performed single word elicitation and connected speech tasks consisting of unambiguous nouns and verbs for which frequency and length were controlled. The results indicate that agrammatics have a relative verb deficit, whereas anomics have a relative noun deficit. Additionally, Caramazza and Hillis (1991) investigated the impairments of two subjects, H.W. and S.J.D., to determine if grammatical class is represented separately within each modality-specific lexicon. H.W. presented with a left parietal lesion adversely affecting verbs in oral production only; conversely, S.J.D. presented with a left frontotemporal lesion coupled with a verb deficit in written production only. Caramazza and Hillis (1991) concluded that the specific deficits of these patients do not stem from damage to a specific grammatical category in a modality-independent lexicon, but rather, grammatical category knowledge may be redundantly represented in each output modality lexicon. Damasio and Tranel (1993) studied three subjects, AN-1033, Boswell, and KJ-1360. AN-1033 and Boswell demonstrated impaired noun retrieval and presented with lesions in the left fronto-parietal operculum, posterior temporal region, inferior parietal lobule, and left anterior and middle temporal lobe. Conversely, KJ-1360 had impaired verb retrieval resulting from a lesion in the left premotor cortex. Damasio and Tranel (1993) concluded that there are relatively separate lexical systems for nouns and verbs – specifically, the left anterior and middle temporal cortices for nouns and the left frontal cortices for verbs. Yet another case study involved EBA, an anomic aphasic with left frontal and temporal lesions, who demonstrated greater impairment of nouns relative to verbs in spoken output (Hillis and Caramazza, 1995). Although EBA's auditory comprehension of both nouns and verbs was intact, her orthographic comprehension of verbs and phonological production of nouns were impaired. This indicates not only that lexical knowledge of different grammatical categories, specifically nouns and verbs, are processed by different neural mechanisms, but also that separate neural structures are dedicated to orthographic and phonological representations for each grammatical category. Furthermore, Rapp and Caramazza (1997) found additional evidence of the modality-specific representation of grammatical categories as demonstrated by P.B.S., a left-handed subject presenting with a lesion in the left parietal, posterior frontal and temporal regions, which include both Broca's and Wernicke's areas. P.B.S. produced a greater number of written nouns than spoken nouns. Though verb use was not normal in either modality, the extent of the spoken verbal deficit was not easily determined because of the large number of neologisms produced in the place of verbs. P.B.S.'s deficits provide further evidence of the modality-specific organization of grammatical classes. Recently, Shapiro and Caramazza (2003) described the selective verb impairment of subject RC, who had damage to the left inferior frontal cortex. They postulated that the noun-verb dissociation in RC's speech could have been due to semantic differences between nouns and verbs, but RC's incorrect production of pseudo-words used as verbs could not be attributed to a semantic deficit. This led them to the conclusion that RC exhibited a morphological impairment affecting verbs more than nouns. Additionally, they speculated that damage to part of the left midfrontal gyrus superior to Broca's area (Brodmann area 9) may have been the cause of RC's verb deficit. Shapiro and Caramazza (2003) concluded that left prefrontal damage results in an impairment of grammatical knowledge about verbs, sparing the semantic knowledge of verbs and other action words.

Additional insight about the representations of nouns and verbs in the mental lexicon has been provided by experiments on neurologically intact individuals. Shapiro et al. (2001) suppressed the excitability of a portion of the left prefrontal cortex in normal subjects through the use of repetitive transcranial magnetic stimulation (rTMS). In rTMS, a coil positioned against the subject's head sends magnetic pulses to the brain, resulting in the temporary suppression of excitability of the targeted area (Shapiro et al., 2001). First, subjects were asked to produce singular and plural forms of nouns or third-person singular and plural forms of verbs; they then performed the same task with pseudo-words. A delay in the subjects' productions of verbs indicated that verbs are processed in the left prefrontal cortex, and consequently, nouns are not. A semantic explanation for the noun-verb dissociation does not fully account for the difference because both action and non-action verbs were utilized for this task. Furthermore, the conclusion of Shapiro et al. (2001) is consistent with that of Shapiro and Caramazza (2003) that the left prefrontal cortex controls retrieval of grammatical information about verbs, as evidenced by the delay in production of pseudo-words used as verbs.

An abundance of cross-linguistic evidence is available supporting the hypothesis of discrete representations of nouns and verbs in the left temporal and left frontal lobes, respectively. Pulvermüller et al. (1996) and Pulvermüller et al. (1999) investigated the noun-verb dissociation in German through EEG recordings of normal subjects performing a lexical decision task. The 30 Hz responses were stronger at recording sites close to the motor cortices in response to verbs. Additionally, the 30 Hz responses were stronger at posterior occipital sites over visual cortices in response to nouns, indicating that nouns and verbs are discretely represented in the brain. Miceli et al. (1984) examined the noun-verb double dissociation in Italian. They administered object and action naming tests to 20 subjects: 5 agrammatics, 5 anomics and 10 normal controls. The agrammatics demonstrated a marked deficit in action naming; therefore, they were selectively impaired in processing verbs. Miceli et al. (1984) concluded that nouns and verbs are distinct word class categories which are organized separately within the lexicon. In another study, Miceli et al. (1988) investigated the noun-verb dissociation of seven subjects with lesions in various loci. They concluded not only that the lexicon is organized into grammatical classes of words, but also that grammatical class information is redundantly represented in both input and output lexicons. Additional evidence of the noun-verb dissociation in Italian is provided by Daniele et al. (1994). They described the deficits of three subjects: R.A., who had atrophy of the posterior frontal lobes, including the posterior portion of the left inferior frontal gyrus, G.G., who had atrophy of the posterior left frontal lobe, and G.P., who had atrophy of the left temporal lobe. The results were as expected given the locations of the subjects' lesions: R.A. and G.G. demonstrated a verb deficit, whereas G.P. demonstrated a noun deficit. Daniele et al. concluded from this evidence that neural systems in the posterior frontal lobe may play an important role in the production and comprehension of verbs. Additionally, they asserted that neural systems in the temporal lobe may play an important role in the production and comprehension of nouns. Laudanna et al. (2002) presented a visual lexical decision task to 54 normal subjects, all native speakers of Italian. The results support the view forwarded by Caramazza and Hillis (1991); Hillis and Caramazza (1995) and Rapp and Caramazza (1997) – specifically, that grammatical category is represented within lexical representations of different modalities. Furthermore, Laudanna et al. (2002) argue that verbs and nouns are represented differently in the input lexicon.

Additional cross-linguistic evidence comes from analyses of Chinese (Bates et al., 1991). Chinese provides strong support for the hypothesis of distinct nominal and verbal representations. Chinese has virtually no inflectional morphology for nouns or verbs. It would therefore appear likely that if the noun-verb dissociation occurs in the speech of Chinese Broca's and Wernicke's aphasics, the dissociation cannot be due to a difference in nominal and verbal morphology. Indeed, after the administration of naming tasks to 6 Broca's aphasics, 7 Wernicke's aphasics and 11 normal controls, the results indicated that Broca's aphasics have a selective verb deficit, and conversely, Wernicke's aphasics have a selective noun deficit. Based on these results, Bates et al. dismissed the morphological account of the noun-verb dissociation and determined that further investigation of the lexical account was appropriate. The strength of the lexical account was tested via Chinese compound words. Many Chinese words are compound, being comprised of a verbal and a nominal component. Thus, if a noun-verb dissociation within these compound lexical items presents, it would signify a sublexical representation of nouns and verbs in the lexicon. The results indicated that Broca's aphasics demonstrate a selective advantage in the production of the nominal segment of the compound word, whereas Wernicke's aphasics have a selective advantage in the production of the verbal segment. Bates et al. (1991) suggested that the lexical account must therefore be altered in order to explain the fact that a Chinese compound word is not represented as a whole in the lexicon, but rather separately as two lexical components (noun and verb). They proposed that the noun-verb dissociation must be due to differences in representation at the sublexical level.

Lamb and Zhang (2002), utilizing data from Bates et al. (1991), also investigated Chinese compound words: both verbal and nominal compounds. They determined that Broca's aphasics have greater difficulty with the verbal component, as it pertains to both verbal and nominal compounds; conversely, Wernicke's aphasics have greater difficulty with the nominal component of verbal compounds, while demonstrating more diverse difficulties with nominal compounds. Additionally, their research provides evidence that the semantic-conceptual account of the noun-verb dissociation is not accurate. Specifically, the subjects' incorrect responses preserved the semantics of the target word. Lamb and Zhang (2002, 4) provided the following example: the target *jiao-hua* "to water flowers" elicited the response **hua-shui* (*hua* "flower", *shui* "water" (N)). This indicates that the subject understood the meaning of the target word, but was unable to access the correct expression to produce it. The evidence provided by Lamb and Zhang (2002) demonstrates that the verbal and nominal components of a compound word are represented separately from, and independently of, the node dedicated to the compound as a whole. Furthermore, Lamb and Zhang (2002) argue that this representation applies to well-established (heavily entrenched) compound words, as well as those that are not well-established (less entrenched). They then describe a relational network approach to the noun-verb dissociation, beginning with an explanation of the proximity principle. This principle proposes that areas in the brain sharing similar functions most likely are sited close to one another (Lamb, 1999, 217–223, 322–327, 352–362). The proximity principle provides an explanation for the possibility that verbs are represented in the frontal lobe, close to the motor cortex, whereas nouns are represented in the temporal lobe, close to the sensory cortices. Finally, Lamb and Zhang (2002) provide an excellent account of how simple the explanation is for Broca's aphasics' selective difficulty with the verb component of a compound noun by applying the relational network theory (see below). Through the proposed network explanation, they demonstrate the possibility of maintaining a lexical node dedicated to the compound word as a whole, in contra to the hypothesis forwarded by Bates et al. (1991), which posited that there is no independent lexical node for the compound word.

As evidenced by the research discussed above, it appears likely that nouns and verbs are discretely represented in the brain; however, I will now provide contrary evidence to this hypothesis.

4 Claims of common representations for nouns and verbs

Some experiments into the noun-verb dichotomy have concluded that nouns and verbs are not represented in anatomically distinct neural structures. This section will review four PET studies and two ERP studies, all purporting to have found widely distributed undifferentiated brain activation in response to both nouns and verbs. None of the studies presented here establish that nouns and verbs have separate local representations in addition to distributed representations.

In a PET study of six neurologically intact subjects, Wise et al. (1991) found anterior activation during a verb generation task, but argued that the activation was possibly due to factors including fluency control or inner speech, rather than verb retrieval. Therefore, it is uncertain whether the anterior activation is evidence of anterior representations of verbs or a result of other factors. The problem is, without investigating the activation during noun generation tasks, no valid conclusion can truly be drawn. More conclusive results could have been obtained from the performance of a noun generation task in conjunction with the verb generation task. This would provide insight into whether the anterior activation is due to verb retrieval or other factors, including fluency control or inner speech.

In a PET study of nine neurologically intact subjects, Warburton et al. (1996) found that, although noun and verb retrieval resulted in similar activation distributions, verb retrieval generated significantly stronger activations than noun retrieval in temporal, parietal and premotor/prefrontal areas. This evidence, though not indicative of an anatomical dissociation between nominal and verbal representations, demonstrates some sort of distinction between the processing of nouns and verbs.

It is noteworthy that the methodology of both Wise et al. (1991) and Warburton et al. (1996) may have affected their results. Both experiments employed a verb generation task in which the subjects were asked to silently produce verbs that came to mind in response to auditorily presented nouns. Of course this would result in widely distributed brain regions being activated! The brain is processing both nouns and verbs in this task such that any conclusions drawn from this task cannot be considered cogent evidence against discrete nominal and verbal representations in the brain.

A PET study of 14 neurologically intact individuals conducted by Perani et al. (1999) investigated the possibility of discrete neural representations of nouns and verbs. The subjects were given a lexical decision task in which the nouns and verbs were presented visually, requiring output in the form of silent reading. The activated areas common to both nouns and verbs were: left inferior frontal gyrus, superior temporal sulcus, posterior-superior temporal gyrus and inferior temporal gyrus. The areas with significantly more activation in response to verb processing than noun processing were: left dorsolateral frontal cortex and superior parietal, anterior temporal, middle temporal and occipital areas. No areas were significantly more activated by noun processing than verb processing. Though elevated activation specific to verb processing can be interpreted as further evidence that nouns and verbs are distinctly represented in the brain, Perani et al. argued that the evidence is insufficient. Specifically, they concluded that some of the verb-specific activation may be due to syntactic processing of verbs, particularly in the left dorsolateral frontal cortex. To reiterate, though Perani et al. (1999) concluded that their results failed to support the hypothesis of discrete representations of nouns and verbs, their results indicate some sort of distinction between the lexical-semantic representations of nouns and verbs in the brain.

Another PET study (Tyler et al., 2001) concluded that there are no discrete representations of nouns and verbs in the brain. Nine subjects performed a lexical decision task, while eight subjects performed a semantic categorization task. In the lexical decision task, the researchers measured reaction time to concrete and abstract nouns, concrete and abstract verbs, and non-words. In the semantic categorization task, reaction time was measured in response to low-frequency and high-frequency nouns and verbs. They found activation of a distributed network including the left prefrontal cortex and the inferior temporal lobe, with no distinction between word classes. Tyler et al. concluded that conceptual knowledge is represented within a distributed network with no anatomical divisions between nouns and verbs, but mentioned that their research investigated only the semantic level. This leaves open the possibility of syntactic/morphological or lexical accounts of the noun-verb dissociation.

Studies investigating the ERPs of neurologically intact subjects provide evidence of a difference in the processing of nouns and verbs, but not in the locations of their representations in the brain. Gomes et al. (1997) determined that, although there appeared to be anatomical differences in orthographic and phonological representations of words, no anatomical differences could be found between nouns and verbs. However, evidence of functionally distinct nominal and verbal lexical systems was discovered: temporal differences between the processing of nouns and verbs were found, indicating functional differences in nominal and verbal processing. Their results do not proscribe the possibility of anatomically distinct noun and verb representations, nor do they support such a distinction. Federmeier et al. (2000) examined ERPs in response to unambiguous nouns and verbs (e.g., *solution* and *carve*, respectively), and class-ambiguous nouns and verbs (e.g., *joke*) and pseudowords (e.g., *phream*) in noun- or verb-predicting contexts (p. 2555). They observed greater frontocentral negativity in response to ambiguous nouns used in noun-predicting contexts over ambiguous verbs used in verb-predicting contexts. Additionally, greater negativity over central-parietal loci in response to unambiguous nouns over unambiguous verbs, and left anterior positivity in response to unambiguous verbs were also discovered. Furthermore, they stressed that the processing of nouns and verbs is influenced by context. They concluded that different types of lexical items are represented in various ways, but specific word classes do not exist in a specific locus in the brain; rather, word classes emerge as a result of semantic and syntactic properties interacting at not only the lexical level, but also the discourse level.

Although the evidence provided in this section does not directly support the hypothesis of distinct representations of nouns and verbs in the brain, it is not sufficient to dismiss the possibility. Some of the studies presented here uncovered differences between the processing of nouns and verbs – though the differences do not evidence an anterior/posterior division of verbs and nouns, respectively.

5 Discussion

The majority of prior research bolsters the hypothesis of discrete representations of nouns and verbs in the mental lexicon. This section examines several accounts offering explanations for the double dissociation between nouns and verbs. These accounts, initially mentioned in the overview section of this paper, include syntactic/morphological, semantic-conceptual, and lexical accounts.

Proponents of syntactic/morphological accounts (Shapiro et al., 2001; Shapiro and Caramazza, 2003) strive to explain the noun-verb dissociation via the relative syntactic and/or morphological complexity of verbs versus nouns. It is true that nouns are syntactically 'simpler' than verbs, in that nouns can stand alone. Conversely, verbs can never be isolated from their arguments. While a noun carries meaning all by itself, a verb carries meaning only in relation to its arguments. As a result, verbs are inextricably associated with syntax. Some proponents of these accounts suggest that verbs carry more inflectional morphology than nouns. Although this is true of some languages, Chinese provides evidence that this is not always the case. Chinese verbs and nouns have virtually no inflectional morphology and, as discussed earlier, the noun-verb dissociation evidenced by Chinese-speaking Broca's and Wernicke's aphasics is still present (Bates et al., 1991). This evidence conclusively indicates that the noun-verb dissociation is not a result of the difference in morphological complexity of nouns and verbs. Additionally, it has been proposed that the relative verb deficit demonstrated by subjects with frontal lobe lesions may result in agrammatism (McCarthy and Warrington, 1985). This is not a viable explanation because not all subjects demonstrating verb deficits are agrammatic (Daniele et al., 1994). Therefore, it appears that syntactic/morphological accounts fail to explain the rationale for the noun-verb dissociation.

The semantic-conceptual account (Bates et al., 1991; McCarthy and Warrington, 1985; Daniele et al., 1994; Pulvermüller et al., 1996, 1999), attempts to explain the noun-verb dissociation as stemming from the semantic differences between verbs and nouns. Specifically, prototypical verbs are actions, whereas prototypical nouns are objects. Proponents of this theory suggest that verbs are represented in the frontal lobe because they signify actions and must therefore be processed close to the motor cortex. Conversely, nouns are represented in the temporal lobe because they signify objects that must be perceived, and are therefore processed near the sensory cortices. The proximity principle supports this idea, but the principle seems not to explain why non-action verbs and abstract nouns are represented in the frontal and temporal lobes, respectively. However, a possible explanation for the relative locations of non-action verbs in the frontal lobe and abstract nouns in the temporal lobe is that, during language acquisition, the first nouns and verbs learned are prototypical object nouns and action verbs. The proximity principle dictates that nouns become represented in the temporal lobe, whereas verbs become represented in the frontal lobe. At a later stage in the learning process, when non-action verbs and abstract nouns are learned, they join the already well-entrenched networks dedicated to verb and noun processing located in the frontal and temporal lobes, respectively. The semantic-conceptual account of the noun-verb dissociation is not easily dismissed, as it explains how, through the proximity principle, distinct representations of nouns and verbs are initially established. However, the semantic-conceptual account fails to explain how subjects such as ROX (McCarthy and Warrington, 1985) are able to mimic actions even when they are deficient in the comprehension and production of verbs. The ability to mimic actions demonstrates that the meaning of verbs remains intact and unaffected by the neurological damage. Subjects like ROX provide support for lexical accounts of the noun-verb dissociation in that their deficit appears to be at the level of the lexeme, rather than the conceptual representation. Lamb and Zhang (2002) also provide evidence in contra to the semantic-conceptual account. Their subjects' incorrect responses often carried the basic meaning of the target word (e.g., the target *jiao-hua* "to water flowers" elicited the response **hua-shui* (*hua* "flower", *shui* "water"(N)); Lamb & Zhang, p. 4). Furthermore, Miceli et al. (1984) concluded that the agrammatics in their study produced semantically relevant nominalizations when naming actions. As evidenced above, the semantic-conceptual account does not fully explain the noun-verb dissociation.

The lexical account sometimes overlaps with the semantic-conceptual account. Some of the previously discussed researchers (McCarthy and Warrington, 1985; Daniele et al., 1994) postulate that a lexical-semantic account provides a possible explanation for the noun-verb dissociation, indicating that conceptual and lexical representations of words are located together. Due to the contrary explanations to the semantic-conceptual account, it is logical that a lexical account of the noun-verb dissociation provides the best available explanation.

As shown by the above studies, the lexical account provides the best explanation for the noun-verb dissociation (Miceli et al., 1984; McCarthy and Warrington, 1985; Miceli et al., 1988; Caramazza and Hillis, 1991; Damasio and Tranel, 1993; Daniele et al., 1994; Hillis and Caramazza, 1995; Rapp and Caramazza, 1997; Lamb and Zhang, 2002; Laudanna et al., 2002). Much of the evidence provided above supports the probability that central nodes of verb lexemes are represented in the left frontal lobe, whereas those of nouns are represented in the left temporal lobe. Furthermore, it appears that nouns and verbs are differentially represented in the lexicon according to modality (written vs. spoken). Caramazza and Hillis (1991); Hillis and Caramazza (1995); Rapp and Caramazza (1997); Laudanna et al. (2002) have found evidence of not only separate orthographic and phonological lexicons, but also separate nominal and verbal lexicons within each modality's lexicon. Although Bates et al. (1991) favor the semantic-conceptual account of the noun-verb dissociation, their data also supports a lexical account. They disfavor the lexical account because it appears that in Chinese, a compound word is represented in the lexicon not as a whole, but rather by its components. Bates et al. (1991) concluded that this limits the applicability of the lexical account. However, it is clear that this does not pose the problem they suggest. Lamb and Zhang (2002) argue that the noun-verb dissociation within Chinese compound words is not sufficient to dismiss the possibility that the compound word has its own lexical representation (node). They designed a neurologically plausible network model of how the verb component of a compound word can be selectively impaired, even when the compound word is lexically represented by its own node as in the network model given in Figure 1.[1] Table 1 describes the features of this network representation.

Table 1. Description of Features in Figure 1

Feature	**Description**
wan-ju	"toy"
wan	"play"
ju	"instrument"
PLAY, TOY, INSTRUMENT	conceptual nodes
wan(M)	morphological node for wan
wan(PP)	phonological production node for wan
wan-ju(L)	lemma for wan-ju
ju(M)	morphological node for ju
dotted circle	damaged area in Broca's aphasia

Phonological production (PP) is located in the anterior portion of the cortex. The lemma representation (L) of *wan-ju* "toy," and the morphological representation (M) of *ju* "instrument," are located in the posterior region. This is consistent with prior research indicating representations of nouns in posterior portions of the cortex. The conceptual nodes for "toy" and "instrument" are also located

1 From "The mental representation of complex lexemes: Evidence from Chinese aphasics," by S. M. Lamb and X. Zhang, 2002, Unpublished manuscript, p. 13.

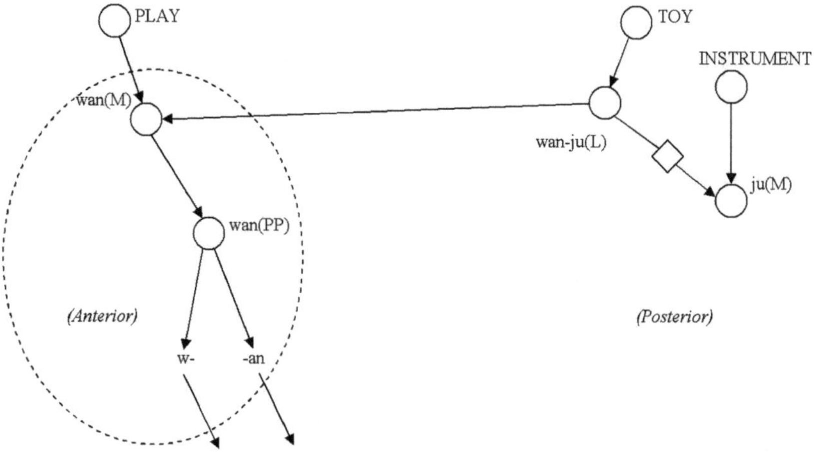

Figure 1. Network model representation of the Chinese compound wan-ju "toy"

in the posterior region. Consistent with prior research, they have situated the morphological representation (M) of the verbal element *wan* "play" in the anterior portion of the cortex. Notice that the conceptual node for "play" is also located in the anterior region. The arrows represent the flow of activation (this figure demonstrates production), and the small box between *wan-ju(L)* and *ju(M)* is a delay element (Lamb, 1999). The delay element is necessary because *ju* must be produced after *wan*. The delay element prevents the node dedicated to *ju(M)* from being activated before the node dedicated to *wan(M)*. The dotted circle represents an approximate area of damage in a Broca's aphasic. The damage affects the verbal component *wan* only; thus, the production of the compound noun *wan-ju* is deficient in the verbal component, but not the nominal component.

This network model demonstrates that the dissociation of nouns and verbs in Chinese compound words need not lead to the conclusion that the compound word is not represented as a whole, independent of its components, in the mental lexicon. The concern of Bates et al. (1991) over the lexical account is thus unwarranted. Therefore, for the reasons cited here, in addition to evidence opposing the syntactic-morphological accounts and the semantic-conceptual account, it is clear that the lexical account provides the best explanation of the noun-verb dissociation.

6 Conclusion

In conclusion, research supporting the hypothesis of discrete representations of nouns and verbs in the mental lexicon greatly exceeds research proposing the contrasting theory of a widely distributed lexicon without distinct nominal and verbal representations. It appears that nouns are represented in posterior regions of the left hemisphere (temporal lobe), whereas verbs are represented in anterior regions of the left hemisphere (frontal lobe). These differences between the representations of nouns and verbs pertain to their lexical representations, as opposed to their respective semantic-conceptual or syntactic/morphological representations. Furthermore, the lexicon appears to be organized by not only word class, but also modality. Additional research of nominal and verbal representations in the mental lexicon is warranted to further understand both the mental lexicon, as well as the human mind.

References

Bates, E., S. Chen, O. Tzeng, P. Li and M. Opie. 1991. The noun-verb problem in Chinese aphasia. *Brain and Language* 41: 203–233.

Caramazza, A. and A. E. Hillis. 1991. Lexical organization of nouns and verbs in the brain. *Nature* 349: 788–790.

Damasio, A. R. and D. Tranel. 1993. Nouns and verbs are retrieved with differently distributed neural systems. *Proceedings of the National Academy of Sciences of the United States of America* 90: 4957–4960.

Daniele, A., L. Giustolisi, M. C. Silveri, C. Colosimo and G. Gainotti. 1994. Evidence for a possible neuroanatomical basis for lexical processing of nouns and verbs. *Neuropsychologia* 32: 1325–1341.

Federmeier, K. D., J. B. Segal, T. Lombrozo and M. Kutas. 2000. Brain responses to nouns, verbs and class-ambiguous words in context. *Brain* 123: 2552–2566.

Gomes, H., W. Ritter, V. C. Tartter, H. G. Vaughan Jr. and J. J. Rosen. 1997. Lexical processing of visually and auditorily presented nouns and verbs: Evidence from reaction time and N400 priming data. *Cognitive Brain Research* 6: 121–134.

Hillis, A. E. and A. Caramazza. 1995. Representation of grammatical categories of words in the brain. *Journal of Cognitive Neuroscience* 7: 396–407.

Lamb, Sydney. 1999. *Pathways of the Brain: The Neurocognitive Basis of Language*. Amsterdam: John Benjamins.

Lamb, Sydney and X. Zhang. 2002. The mental representation of complex lexemes: Evidence from Chinese aphasics. Unpublished manuscript.

Laudanna, A., M. Voghera and S. Gazzellini. 2002. Lexical representations of written nouns and verbs in italian. *Brain and Language* 81: 250–263.

McCarthy, R. and E. K. Warrington. 1985. Category specificity in an agrammatic patient: The relative impairment of verb retrieval and comprehension. *Neuropsychologia* 23: 709–727.

Miceli, G., M. C. Silveri, U. Nocentini and A. Caramazza. 1988. Patterns of dissociation in comprehension and production of nouns and verbs. *Aphasiology* 2: 351–358.

Miceli, G., M. C. Silveri, G. Villa and A. Caramazza. 1984. On the basis for the agrammatic's difficulty in producing main verbs. *Cortex* 20: 207–220.

Perani, D., S. F. Cappa, T. Schnur, M. Tettamanti, S. Collina and et al. Rosa, M. M. 1999. The neural correlates of verb and noun processing: A pet study. *Brain* 122: 2337–2344.

Pulvermüller, F., W. Lutzenberger and H. Preissl. 1999. Nouns and verbs in the intact brain: Evidence from event-related potentials and high-frequency cortical responses. *Cerebral Cortex* 9: 497–506.

Pulvermüller, F., H. Preissl, W. Lutzenberger and N. Birbaumer. 1996. Brain rhythms of language: Nouns versus verbs. *European Journal of Neuroscience* 8: 937–941.

Rapp, B. and A. Caramazza. 1997. The modality-specific organization of grammatical categories: Evidence from impaired spoken and written sentence production. *Brain and Language* 56: 248–286.

Shapiro, K. and A. Caramazza. 2003. Grammatical processing of nouns and verbs in left frontal cortex? *Neuropsychologia* 41: 1189–1198.

Shapiro, K., A. Pascual-Leone, F. M. Mottaghy, M. Gangitano and A. Caramazza. 2001. Grammatical distinctions in the left frontal cortex. *Journal of Cognitive Neuroscience* 13: 713–720.

Tyler, L. K., R. Russell, J. Fadili and H. E. Moss. 2001. The neural representation of nouns and verbs: Pet studies. *Brain* 124: 1619–1634.

Warburton, E., R. J. S. Wise, C. J. Price, C. Weiller, U. Hadar and S. Ramsay. 1996. Noun and verb retrieval by normal subjects: Studies with pet. *Brain* 119: 159–179.

Wise, R., F. Chollet, U. Hadar, K. Friston, E. Hoffner and R. Frackowiak. 1991. Distribution of cortical neural networks involved in word comprehension and word retrieval. *Brain* 114: 1803–1817.

Zingeser, L. B. and R. S. Berndt. 1990. Retrieval of nouns and verbs in agrammatism and anomia. *Brain and Language* 39: 14–32.

Towards a language-based account on verbal working memory

Ralf Rummer and Johannes Engelkamp

1 Introduction

Many cognitive tasks require short-term storage of verbal information. Thus, it is not surprising that short-term memory for verbal information is an important field of interest for cognitive psychologists. Even though a lot of research was conducted to provide and test models of working memory and short-term retention, there are still problems with applying these models to cognitive tasks relevant in every-day life. An example of such a task is language processing.

We suggest that one of the reasons for this unsatisfying situation is that most of the models referring to the storage of linguistic information focus on the investigation of cognitive mechanisms relevant for the storage of phonological information. In our opinion, there are two main reasons for this reductionist view on working memory: one of them being of historical, the other one being of methodological nature.

Firstly, since Conrad (1964) it has been a basic assumption of cognitive psychology that short-term storage uses a phonological code (e.g. Atikinson and Shiffrin, 1968). Secondly, for methodological reasons, experimental psychologists try to reduce the complexity of their materials as much as possible. Thus, most of the research on verbal short-term memory was (and is still) based on experiments with lists of unrelated characters, digits, pseudowords, or words. With regard to the immediate retention of unrelated lists, phonological information indeed plays a very important role (e.g., Conrad 1964; for an overview cf. Baddeley 1986). However, it is questionable whether the mechanisms relevant for the storage of unrelated lists are the same as those that are relevant for the storage of verbal information in everyday tasks. Before we discuss this objection against the reductionist view in detail, we will sketch the most prominent model of verbal working memory, the phonological loop model proposed by Baddely and Hitch (1974, cf. also Baddeley 1986, 1999).

Baddeley's working memory model, which has been revised several times, as in his recent version (Baddeley, 2000), suggests that short-term retention of linguistic information takes place in a phonological 'slave system,' the phonological loop (PL). The PL includes two mechanisms: first, a passive store, which retains phonological information for about two seconds, and second, a subvocal rehearsal mechanism, which can refresh the phonological information so that it is available for another two seconds. If we hear a word list, a phonological trace of the list is immediately stored in the phonological store. If the words are presented visually, the rehearsal mechanism transfers the list into the phonological store. After the last word of the list has been presented, participants start subvocal rehearsal. That is, an inner speech mechanism repeats the list in the same order in which it has been presented. This prevents the phonological traces from decaying for another two seconds. Together, the two subsystems – phonological store and rehearsal mechanism – can retain as much information as can be rehearsed within two seconds. If the rehearsal process takes longer than two seconds (e.g., because the list includes too many words, the words are too long, or the articulation rate of a participant is not fast enough), the item(s) presented in the first list position(s) has (have) already decayed in the phonological store. In this case, recall will not be successful.

The PL model is supported by many studies using immediate serial recall of lists containing unrelated words or syllables. In such studies, it has been shown that word length – in terms of articulation time – is critical for retention (e.g. Baddeley et al., 1975) and that the phonological similarity of the presented stimuli decreases recall performance, which is referred to as phonological similarity effect (cf. e.g. Baddeley 1986, 1999).

In sum, the PL model explains quite well how unrelated lists of words, characters, or digits (e.g., telephone numbers) are retained in short-term memory. As predicted by Baddeley's model, the capacity of verbal short-term memory depends on many factors related to the material (e.g., length of the items in terms of articulation time or the phonological similarity of the words) and the subjects' individual characteristics, particularly their articulation rate. The capacity of most individuals' PL system is not higher than about seven short words.

During the last 25 years approximately, it has been shown in several studies that the PL is involved in many tasks like problem solving, reasoning, elementary arithmetic, and language processing. Most of these studies used interference tasks that selectively interfered with either the PL's rehearsal or storage component. Interference was interpreted as evidence in favor of PL involvement; in contrast, the fact that no interference was observed has been interpreted as evidence against PL involvement. Our objection against some of these studies concerns the conclusion drawn on the basis of these results. Some of the researchers did not differentiate between PL and verbal storage in general. That is, if the result of an experiment implied that the PL was not involved in the particular cognitive task, the researchers suggested that verbal short-term memory in general was not involved in this task. As suggested by studies on sentence processing (particularly by studies on sentence recall), such an overgeneralization is not adequate. If the goal consists in obtaining information about the involvement of linguistic short-term representations in general, another kind of model is necessary.

In the 1980ies, researchers investigated how the PL system supports sentence comprehension. However, the results of these studies were inconsistent: some studies demonstrated a contribution of the PL (e.g. Baddeley et al., 1984) while others did not (e.g. Martin 1993). One explanation for these inconsistent results is that sentence comprehension (like most cognitive tasks) requires processing of syntactically structured materials rather than processing of unrelated word lists. The fact that the processes involved in sentence processing differ from those involved in the processing of unrelated word lists is demonstrated, for instance, by a neuropsychological patient study published by Nespoulous et al. (1988). When their patient was asked to read sentences written vertically, one word below the other, he read the words appropriately up to the point of realizing that it was a sentence. At the point where he started to read it 'as a sentence,' he failed. Obviously, the cognitive processes involved in list and sentence processing differ from each other. Assuming that there is a close relation between the representations and processes involved in word perception and those involved in short-term memory (cf. e.g. Barnard, 1985; Martin et al., 1999), the dissociation reported by Nespoulous et al. (1988) suggests that short-term storage of word lists and of sentences might be based on different cognitive mechanisms. Potter and Lombardi (1990) demonstrated that this is indeed the case. Given these results (and the observation that recall of sentences is much better than recall of unrelated word lists), even Baddeley himself states that short-term recall of verbal material does not exclusively rely on the PL (cf. Baddeley, 2000; Gathercole and Baddeley, 1993). To our knowledge, no convincing model of short-term sentence retention is available up to now.

The present paper provides a framework for such a model. As a first step, a model of sentence recall has to address the question which type of information is potentially involved and, as a second step, the model has to predict under which conditions these representations contribute to sentence recall. The primary goal of the research sketched here is not to replace reductionist models like Baddeley's PL model but to show that sentence recall involves more than phonological information.

2 A model of verbal working memory

The basic idea of our model stems from 'language-based' models of short-term memory. "These [...] models [...] have emphasized the close relation between the representations and processes involved in word perception and production and those involved in short-term memory" (Martin et al., 1999, 3). In line with this approach, we assume that short-term memory for verbal materials is based on the same cognitive mechanisms involved in comprehending and producing these materials.

Taking into account this assumption, an appropriate model of verbal short-term memory has to be based on psycholinguistic theories of sentence processing. These models predict which type of information is encoded during presentation and might be available in short-term retention. In connection with findings concerning the decay functions of these types of information, this framework allows for detailed predictions.

Our model is based on the serial approach of sentence comprehension proposed by (Friederici 2002, cf. Figure 1). According to this model, sentence comprehension starts with the representation of the sensory information of the stimulus. This kind of sensory information is stored even for non-linguistic stimuli. Depending on the modality of presentation, pre-linguistic representations are stored for both auditory and visual stimuli.[1] Based on this type of information, a phonological representation is generated. The phonological code is assumed to be an abstract (i.e., modality unspecific) code which is provided by both auditory and visual presentations (cf. Baddeley, 1986). However, auditorily presented items activate a phonological code directly, whereas visually presented items have to be phonologically recoded. This recoding process can be conceptualized in analogy to Baddeley (1986), who assumes that visual representations are recoded by the rehearsal component of the PL. The next processing step concerns the activation of morpho-syntactic information – for instance, gender information or other information relevant for building a syntactic structure. Immediately afterwards, the syntactic structure is established. Models of sentence processing suggest that the syntactic structure is predicted on the basis of morpho-syntactic representations. That is, after the first word of a sentence has been presented to a participant, he or she starts predicting a syntactic structure. In some models, the predictive process reflects economic principles (e.g., minimal attachment, Frazier and Rayner 1982), others are frequency based (e.g. MacDonald and Christiansen, 2002). The predicted syntactic structure is updated by the process-

[1] It is important to note that visual-sensory information decays rather quickly, whereas acoustic-sensory information is available for a longer period of time. This difference is the precondition of the modality effect which suggests that retention of auditorily presented linguistic materials is better than retention of visually presented linguistic information.

ing system whenever new information is provided to the participants. Thereafter, lexico-semantic representations are activated, and finally, lexico-semantic representations are integrated in the syntactic frame, and the propositional meaning of the sentence is constructed.

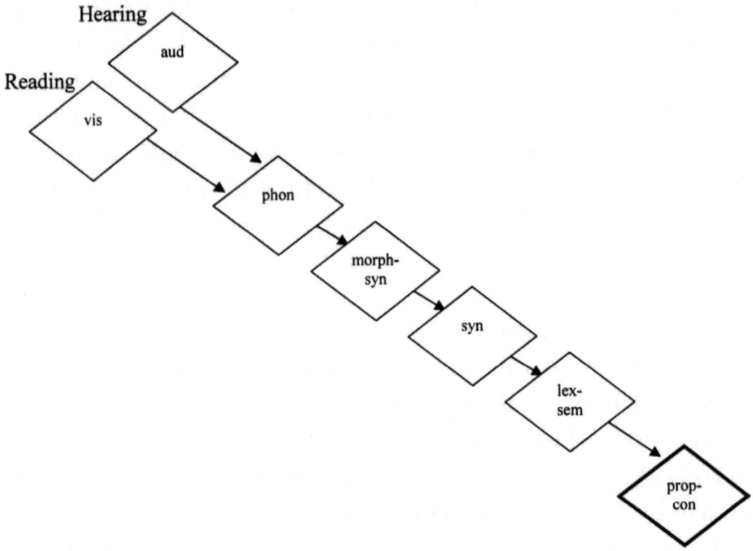

Figure 1. Model of sentence comprehension (after Friederici, 2002)

This model can be adopted to explain immediate retention of verbal information. The general idea is that any kind of information that is the result of a processing step is stored in a buffer system specialized for the representation of the respective type of information (Barnard, 1985). In line with Friederici (2002), we assume that the following types of information are stored during sentence processing: modality specific *visual* or *auditory* word representations, modality unspecific *phonological* representations, *morpho-syntactic* representations, *syntactic* representations, *lexico-semantic* representations, and *conceptual-propositional* representations. This first part of our model predicts that any of these representations can contribute to sentence retention under specific circumstances.

In order to predict under which conditions these representations do contribute to sentence recall, and under which conditions they do not, it is necessary to include basic findings of elementary memory research in our model. In particular, we are interested in the following two questions: how long can each type of information be retained in short-term memory (given that is has been provided during presentation), and which task accesses which kind of information (given the respective type of information is available)? This second part of our model has not yet been developed to completion.

A direct way to test this model is to instruct participants to *recall* sentences. With Potter and Lombardi (1990), we suggest that sentence recall is based on a *regeneration* process, in which the message of the sentence (i.e., its conceptual propositional meaning) plays a very important role. According to Potter and Lombardi's *conceptual regeneration hypothesis*, sentences are regenerated on the basis of their conceptual message (i.e., the conceptual-propositional representation of the sentence). This (re)generative nature of sentence recall is one of the central suggestions of our model as well. Therefore, our model has to incorporate assumptions about the (re)production process. To model the reproduction process, we adopt the language production model proposed by Levelt (1989; cf. also Levelt et al. 1999).

Levelt's serial and modular approach states that a sentence is produced based on the message which is equivalent with conceptual-propositional information. The message activates abstract semantic entries, termed lemmata, which also include morpho-syntactic information. On the basis of this information, a syntactic frame is established. The next processing step is the activation of a specific word form (which implies the activation of phonological information) and, finally, an articulatory program is started. Levelt's model differs from our assumptions with respect to the segmentation of the processes involved in language processing. However, he assumes that language production follows the inverse time course proposed by Friederici's comprehension model. Therefore, his model can be easily applied to our working memory account. We connect information represented during sentence comprehension in the storage units of the processing system with these stages of sentence production. This connection suggests that information represented in the processing system can be used during sentence regeneration. In terms of our model, sentence recall is a kind of specific sentence production with the particular feature that the production process is based on information stored in the comprehension system. Figure 2 illustrates the complete model of sentence recall.

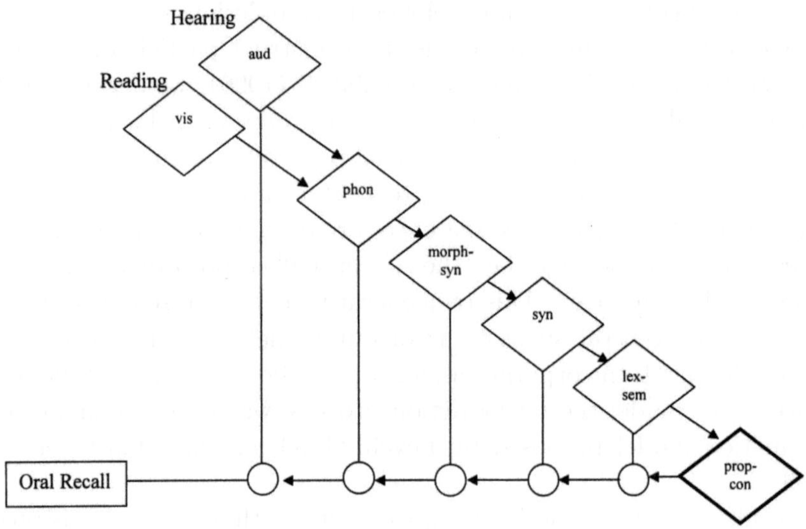

Figure 2. Model of sentence regeneration

The current version of the model includes a specification for phonological information: that is, we predict under which circumstances phonological information is recoded and stored during sentence processing, and we predict under which circumstances it is accessible during recall. With respect to the first point, we suggest that the presentation technique plays an important role. For instance, we assume that rapid serial visual presentation (RSVP) leads to weaker phonological traces than slow visual presentation or auditory presentation. The second point concerns the assumption that not any type of information stored during sentence processing is available during recall. We assume that whether a specific type of representation is available or not depends on the characteristics of the respective type of information. Hence, we assume that phonological information decays after two seconds (Baddeley et al., 1975), whereas lexico-semantic representations should be rather long-lived. Based on such considerations, we can predict under which conditions phonological information does contribute to recall and under which conditions it does not.

In the subsequent section, we describe a series of experiments supporting the proposed model of sentence recall. First, these experiments demonstrate that – under specific circumstances – any kind of information stored in the various processing units can contribute to sentence recall; second, the experiments show under which circumstances the respective types of information do contribute to sentence recall and under which circumstances they do not. Most of these experiments are based on Potter and Lombardi's (1990) intrusion paradigm.

3 Empirical evidence for the model

In this section, we will first report a study which demonstrates that (propositional and lexical) conceptual representations contribute to sentence recall. Subsequently, we will report experiments which demonstrate that acoustic-sensory, phonological, morpho-syntactic, and syntactic representations contribute to sentence recall as well.

3.1 Evidence for the contribution of conceptual-propositional and lexico-semantic information

The most convincing results supporting the assumption that both conceptual-propositional and lexico-semantic information contribute to sentence recall are based on Potter and Lombardi's (1990) intrusion paradigm which combines verbatim recall of sentences with a lexico-semantic interference task. In most of Potter and Lombardi's experiments, participants were presented with a sentence that was followed by a short list of unrelated nouns. Half of these word lists included a word with a meaning similar to a target word in the sentence (i.e., a lure word) while the other half of the lists included a word that was conceptually and phonologically unrelated to the target word (i.e., a control word). The sentences were constructed such that the lure word fitted the sentence better than the target word. Both the sentences and the word lists were presented using the rapid serial visual presentation technique (RSVP, cf. Forster 1970). That is, the words constituting the sentences and the lists were presented serially in the center of the computer screen with a presentation rate of 200 ms per word for the sentences and 250 ms per word for the word lists. To ensure that the words in the list were actively processed, the participants were additionally presented with a probe word for which they had to decide whether it was part of the word list or not. The target word and the lure word were conceptually similar but differed with respect to their phonological representation. Thus, if phonological information was used in sentence recall, it was to prevent the lure word from replacing the target word. The subsequent example illustrates the trial structure of the experiment.

Sentence presentation:	*The knight rode around the* ***palace*** *searching for a place to enter.*
Distractor list with lure word:	*turtle recipe booth* ***castle*** *medal*
Distractor list without lure word:	*turtle recipe booth* ***vowel*** *medal*
Probe word:	*SHOWER*
Sentence recall:	*The knight rode around the* ***castle*** *searching for a place to enter.*

Potter and Lombardi (1990) observed a lure intrusion effect: the lure word replaced the target word to-be-remembered more often in instances where the target word was included in the list than in instances where the control word was included in the list. That is, participants more often produced sentences like *The knight rode around the* ***castle*** *searching for a place to enter* if the list included the word *castle*. This effect demonstrates that both conceptual-propositional and lexico-semantic information contribute to sentence recall. The sentences are regenerated on the basis of the propositional conceptual message of the sentence. This is demonstrated by the finding of spontaneous intrusions. The assumption that, in addition, lexico-semantic information contributes to sentence recall is supported by the finding that the presentation of the lure word in the word list increases the proportion of lure intrusions. These results support Potter and Lombardi's conceptual regeneration hypothesis: a "sentence is generated in immediate recall from a representation of its meaning using recently activated words" (Potter and Lombardi, 1990, 633). In addition, these findings support the assumption that the cognitive mechanisms involved in sentence regeneration differ from those involved in list recall.

However, in our opinion, Potter and Lombardi go too far with their interpretation when taking their results as evidence against the contribution of phonological information to sentence recall in general. Their statement that lure words and target words differ with respect to their phonological surface and that the contribution of phonological representations should prevent the substitution of the target by the lure word is correct. However, it is questionable whether phonological information is available during recall in Potter and Lombardi's experiments. Phonological information is assumed to decay after two seconds. If a word list has to be processed between sentence presentation and sentence recall, no phonological information should be available during recall. In addition, there is evidence that RSVP leads to weak phonological memory traces (Potter, 1999). As Potter and Lombardi presented their materials via RSVP, the fact that the authors did not find any phonological contribution hardly comes as a surprise. In the following paragraph, we will report experimental data that provide evidence for a contribution of phonological information.

3.2 Evidence for the contribution of phonological information

First evidence for the contribution of phonological information stems from neuropsychological patient studies. For instance, Martin et al. (1994, see also Martin 1993) described a neuropsychological patient with a considerable impairment of her phonological short-term memory (span < 2 items) but intact semantic short-term memory. This patient was able to understand sentences quite well, but her recall performance (for comparable sentences) was extremely decreased. Another patient with a considerable impairment of his semantic short-term memory, but only a slight impairment of his phonological short-term memory, showed the complementary pattern of data. These findings show that an intact phonological short-term memory is a prerequisite for verbatim sentence retention.

The contribution of phonological information to sentence recall was tested by Park and Martin (2002). Basically, the idea of their experiment was to manipulate the relation between lure and target word so that a phonological contribution could be tested. While Potter and Lombardi (1990) presented their participants with lure and target words which were semantically related but phonologically dissimilar, Park and Martin (2002) used either lure-target combinations that were solely semantically related or such that were related both semantically and phonologically. If phonological information did contribute to recall, the number of intrusions was to increase when lure and target words were phonologically and semantically similar. The following sentence and word lists give an example of a semantically and phonologically related lure-target combination.

In a sentence completion study, Park and Martin (2002) made sure that there was no general advantage for phonological-semantic lures over semantic lures. The lure words were also controlled for word frequency and semantic similarity to the target words. The authors found a substantially higher degree of lure intrusions if the lure and the target words were semantically and phonologically related. This finding (among others: e.g. Willis and Gathercole, 2000; Alloway and Gathercole, 2005) demonstrates that besides lexical and propositional-conceptual information, phonological information also contributes to short-term recall of sentences.

Sentence presentation:	*Asian countries are not a good* ***market*** *for automobiles due to lack of demand.*
Distractor list with lure word:	*bottle pencil trousers* ***market*** *theatre*
Distractor list without lure word:	*bottle pencil trousers* ***window*** *theatre*
Probe word:	*PENCIL*
Sentence recall:	*Asian countries are not a good* ***market*** *for automobiles due to lack of demand.*

Another aspect of our model concerns the circumstances under which phonological information is provided in the presentation phase and the circumstances under which it is still available during recall. Rummer and Engelkamp (2003) addressed these two concerns using the Potter-Lombardi intrusion paradigm. First, they changed the order of list and sentence presentation such that an immediate recall condition was created. That is, the sequence of events was: presentation of word list, presentation of sentence, recall of sentence, response to probe word. Under this condition, phonological information was to be available during recall. Rummer and Engelkamp (2003) contrasted this condition with a delayed recall condition as used by Potter and Lombardi (1990). In this condition, no phonological information was to be available during recall. Second, they presented the sentences either via RSVP or auditorily. As expected, the intrusion effect was restricted to delayed recall with auditory presentation. The intrusion effect disappeared if immediate recall was utilized. With RSVP, the intrusion effect was found in both the immediate and the delayed condition, because little phonological information was provided in either case. The lack of an intrusion effect in the auditory immediate recall condition demonstrates that phonological information plays an important role in sentence recall. Figure 3 depicts the differences between induced intrusions (i.e., the lure word was included in the word list) and spontaneous intrusions (i.e., a control word was included in the word list instead) as a function of the modality of presentation and the delay between sentence presentation and sentence recall.

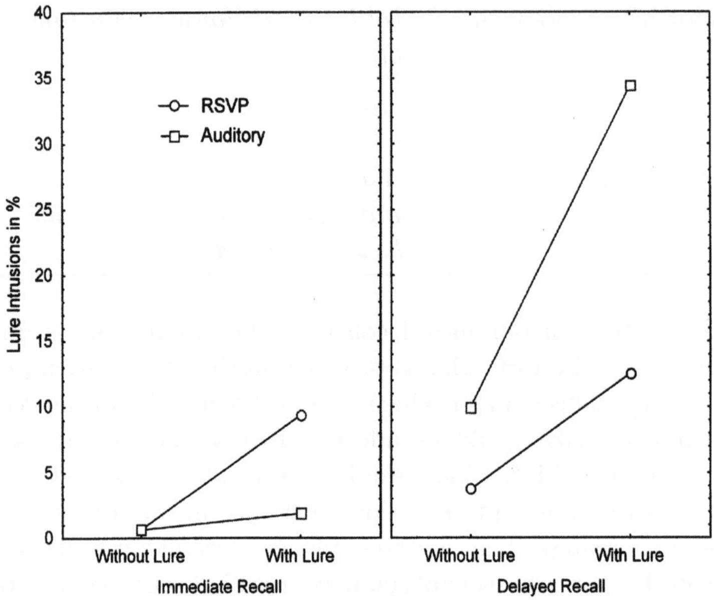

Figure 3. Results of Rummer and Engelkamp (2003). Figure includes mean proportions of lure intrusions as a function of delay (immediate vs. delayed recall), modality of presentation (auditory presentation vs. RSVP), and lure condition (list without vs. with lure word).

As predicted, Rummer and Engelkamp's (2003) results show that the phonological traces provided by RSVP are weaker than those provided by auditory presentation and that phonological information is only available for a short period of time. Lure intrusion effects are restricted to those conditions that do not provide phonological information. If phonological information is available during recall, namely in the auditory immediate recall condition, there is no difference between the two lure conditions (list without lure vs. with lure).

In sum, these findings suggest that phonological information contributes to short-term recall of sentences if available. However, it is worth noting that recall performance is still very good, even if the phonological traces are comparably weak.

3.3 Evidence for the contribution of acoustic-sensory information

We know from studies with unrelated word lists that – at least with unimpaired subjects – performance in immediate recall or recognition tasks is better if the lists are presented in an auditory than in a visual modality (e.g. Conrad and Hull 1968; Crowder 1967; a comprehensive overview is given by Penney 1989). This effect, which is restricted to the most recent item positions, is explained by the assumption that acoustic-sensory information can be used more efficiently and is longer-lasting than visual-sensory representations. Our model predicts that such an advantage for auditory presentation should also be observed with sentence recall. Rummer and Schweppe (2005) tested this hypothesis by means of the Potter-Lombardi intrusion paradigm. They contrasted silent reading and reading aloud. It was assumed that, in addition to the types of information provided by silent reading (i.e., visual-sensory, phonological, morpho-syntactic, syntactic, lexico-semantic, and propositional-conceptual information), reading aloud would provide an acoustic-sensory code.

The experiment used a short-delay version of the intrusion paradigm. That is, the list was presented before the sentence, then the probe word appeared, and finally, participants had to recall the sentence. In addition, this experiment differed in two more aspects from the experiments described above: first, the sentences were presented simultaneously to enable normal reading; that is, phonological recoding was possible under all conditions. Second, as the modality effect is restricted to the most recent item positions, the target words were located at the end of the sentences (i.e., one of the three most recent positions). A further important aspect of the experiment is that the word lists and the probe words were read silently in both the silent reading and the reading aloud condition. The authors expected that, if acoustic-sensory information would contribute to short-term sentence recall, this should lead to a smaller intrusion effect in the reading aloud than in the silent reading condition.

However, a possible objection against this interpretation is that silent reading and reading aloud differ from one another not only with respect to acoustic-sensory information but also with respect to articulatory information. To exclude this alternative interpretation, Rummer and Schweppe's experiment included a silent mouthing condition. Finally, the reading aloud and the silent reading conditions differ from each other in how they relate to the word list: under silent reading conditions, both the word list and the sentence are read silently; in contrast, under reading aloud conditions, the word list and the sentence are read differently. This might help to discriminate the target from the lure word. To exclude this objection, a second reading aloud condition in which both word lists and sentences were read aloud was introduced. Participants in the silent reading condition were instructed to read the sentence and the word lists silently. Participants in the mouthing condition had to move their lips and tongues as though they were speaking, but without voicing the sentence (Cheng, 1974). In the first reading aloud condition, participants had to read the sentence aloud and the distractor list silently, and in the second reading aloud condition, both sentence and distractor list had to be read aloud.

The assumption that acoustic-sensory information contributes to sentence recall predicts a smaller intrusion effect in those conditions providing acoustic-sensory information than in those conditions that do not provide an acoustic-sensory code. In addition, there should be no difference between the two reading aloud conditions on the one hand and the silent reading and mouthing on the other hand. Rummer and Engelkamp's (2005) experiment confirmed just that.

The findings of this experiment suggest that besides propositional-conceptual information, lexico-semantic information, and phonological information, acoustic sensory information also contributes to sentence recall. Then again, the findings contradict the assumption of a contribution of articulatory information.

3.4 Evidence for the contribution of morpho-syntactic information

The model of linguistic short-term memory proposed in this article assumes that morpho-syntactic representations also contribute to short-term sentence recall. Schweppe and Rummer (2004) used a modified version of the Potter-Lombardi paradigm to test this hypothesis. In their experiment, they manipulated grammatical gender to demonstrate such a contribution.

In German, there is no systematic correspondence between the conceptual representation of a noun and its grammatical gender (e.g., ***das*** *Messer* "the [NEUT] knife", ***die*** *Gabel* "the [FEM] fork", ***der*** *Löffel* "the [MASC] spoon"). Given that the assumption of morpho-syntactic contribution to sentence recall is correct, participants should demonstrate a higher intrusion effect (i.e., the difference between induced and spontaneous intrusions) if the gender of the lure word is congruent with the gender of the target word than if it has a different grammatical gender. The example below illustrates how the intrusion paradigm was modified to test this assumption.

The data of the experiment were as expected; that is, congruency between target and lure gender increased the intrusion effect. The materials were controlled for cloze probability, word frequency, word length, and semantic similarity of the lure to the target words. Even more convincingly, subjects did not produce more congruent than incongruent spontaneous intrusions, which demonstrates that participants do not have a general preference for the congruent lure word. In sum, Schweppe and Rummer's data support the assumption that morpho-syntactic information is involved in sentence regeneration. The findings thus do support our model of sentence regeneration.

Sentence presentation:	*Die Kollegen hatten ihn mehrfach aufgefordert, sie abends in das* [NEUT.] *Café am Stadtrand zu begleiten.* "The colleagues had often asked him to accompany them to the [NEUT.] cafe on the outskirts in the evening."
Distractor list with congruent lure:	*Land* ***Restaurant*** [NEUT.] *Automobil Fehlen Forderung Philosoph* "country *restaurant* [NEUT.] automobile lack demand philosopher"
Distractor list with incongruent lure:	*Land* ***Kneipe*** [FEM.] *Automobil Fehlen Forderung Philosoph* "country *pub* [FEM.] automobile lack demand philosopher"
Distractor list without lure:	*Land* ***Tasse*** *Automobil Fehlen Forderung Philosoph* "country *cup* automobile lack demand philosopher"
Probe word:	*TELEFON* "telephone"
Sentence recall:	*Die Kollegen hatten ihn mehrfach aufgefordert, sie abends in das* [NEUT.] *Restaurant am Stadtrand zu begleiten.*

3.5 Evidence for the contribution of syntactic information

According to our model, after extracting morpho-syntactic information, a syntactic frame is built up by the readers or hearers of the sentence. Syntactic representations include information concerning the sentence's phrase structure. This syntactic representation should also contribute to short-term sentence recall. As a change of the syntactic structure usually changes the sentences' meaning, as well as the number of words or syllables, it is quite difficult to look separately at the influence of syntactic structure on sentence recall. Evidence for syntactic involvement stems from Engelkamp and Rummer (2002) and Rummer et al. (2003), who tested whether subordination vs. coordination would influence short-term recall. They varied the syntactic structure and kept other relevant aspects (i.e., the sentences' propositional-conceptual structure and the number of syllables) constant. The task was immediate serial recall. Participants were presented with either two subordinate or two coordinate causal structures. The following sentences give an example of the sentences presented in these experiments.

Coordinate structure:	*Er öffnete das Fenster, deshalb wurde die Kerze ausgeblasen.* "He opened the window; therefore, the candle was blown out."
Subordinate structure:	*Weil er das Fenster öffnete, wurde die Kerze ausgeblasen.* "Since he opened the window, the candle was blown out."

In order to test whether or not a possible syntax effect is independent from phonological short-term memory, the length of the nouns was manipulated (monosyllabic vs. three-syllabic nouns) within the sentences in addition to the manipulation of the sentences' syntactic structure (Engelkamp and Rummer, 1999; Willis and Gathercole, 2000). A subordination effect, which was not linked to the word-length effect, was found independently from whether the sentences were presented auditorily (Engelkamp and Rummer, 2002) or via self-paced reading (Rummer et al., 2003). This subordination effect states that recall accuracy was better for subordinate than for coordinate structures. This advantage for subordinate structures goes back to the second clause. While recall performance did not vary between the first and the second clause with subordinate structures, there was a significant decrease from clause 1 to clause 2 for coordinate structures. This syntax effect did not interact with word length. In sum, the results of this experiment are in line with our model of sentence recall: the fact that recall performance for sentences with monosyllabic nouns was better than recall for sentences including three-syllabic nouns is further support for the assumption that phonological representations contribute to recall; in addition, the syntax effect demonstrates that syntactic information also contributes to sentence recall.

4 General discussion

The studies reported above support the three basic assumptions of our model. First, the results demonstrate that sentence recall is the result of a conceptually driven regeneration process, which is based on the propositional-conceptual message of the sentence. Second (and most importantly), the results of the studies reported above demonstrate that lexico-semantic, phonological, acoustic-sensory, morpho-syntactic, and syntactic information may contribute to short-term sentence recall. Third, the phonological studies exemplarily demonstrate how the specific characteristics of the presentation procedure and the delay between sentence presentation and recall constrain the use of a particular type of information. Based on these three assumptions, it is possible to predict which type of information contributes to oral verbatim short-term sentence recall. Given that we know about the modality of presentation and the delay between presentation and recall, we can predict which representations contribute to the regeneration process.

In addition, the findings reported above strictly argue against a theoretical approach that treats linguistic short-term memory and phonological short-term memory (e.g., the phonological loop) as equivalent. Verbal short-term storage cannot be reduced to the use of one isolated cognitive mechanism (like the PL). Instead, we postulate various language-related cognitive mechanisms that together produce what is usually termed short-term memory performance. We do not rule out that these cognitive mechanisms can be modeled in terms of small scale theories such as the PL model, for instance.

Until now, our model has only been specified for oral verbatim recall. We expect that the characteristics of the task (i.e., oral vs. written recall, recall of content vs. verbatim recall, etc.) modulate the access of available information. Thus, the specification of a fourth dimension is necessary in order to extend our model to sentence retention in general. It has to be investigated how the characteristics of the tasks influence which type of (potentially available) information is selected for regeneration. Thereby, the regeneration process can be overt (as with recall) or covert (as with other retention tasks). To illustrate this, we will give an example of different overt recall tasks: recall for content may be particularly based on the conceptual-propositional message of the sentence, whereas lexical and sensory representations should contribute to a lesser degree. In contrast, participants instructed to recall a sentence as accurately as possible should focus much more on phonological information than those who read or hear a sentence under the instruction to recall its content.

Finally, we would like to readdress the studies on working memory and sentence processing. The results of these studies suggest that working memory, as it has been conceptualized by cognitive psychologists, does not contribute to the online processing of sentences. Caplan and Waters (1999) distinguish interpretive and post-interpretive processes. The processes that take place during first path reading or hearing are termed interpretive processes; those processes that take place in order to correct the results of first path processing (e.g., syntactic reanalysis in garden path structures) are termed post-interpretive processes. While interpretive processes depend on a particular online working memory system specialized on syntactic online processing, post-interpretive processes depend on an offline working memory system. The latter system is what is usually termed working memory. When focusing on syntactic reanalysis, it becomes obvious that, even in this restricted field, the data are not unambiguous. That is, there are some studies that demonstrate a contribution of the PL and there are others that do not. In our opinion, the question of working memory involvement in syntactic reanalysis of (local) ambiguous sentences should be reformulated. According to our model, the question should be which kind of information is provided, retained, and regenerated during second path processing. We would expect that a research program addressing these questions should lead to clearer results.

References

Alloway, T. P. and Susan E. Gathercole. 2005. Working memory and short-term sentence recall in young children. *European Journal of Cognitive Pychology* 17: 207–220.

Atikinson, R. C. and R. M. Shiffrin. 1968. Human memory: A proposed system and its control processes. In: K. W. Spence and J. T. Spence (eds.), *The Psychology of Learning and Motivation: Advances in Research and Theory*, volume 2. New York: Academic Press, 89–195.

Baddeley, Alan D. 1986. *Working Memory*. Oxford: University Press.

Baddeley, Alan D. 1999. *Essentials of Human Memory*. Howe: Psychology Press.

Baddeley, Alan D. 2000. The episodic buffer: a new component of working memory? *Trends in Cognitive Sciences* 4: 417–423.

Baddeley, Alan D. and Graham J. Hitch. 1974. Working memory. In: G. H. Bower (ed.), *The Psychology of Learning and Motivation*, volume 8. New York: Academic Press, 47–90.

Baddeley, Alan D., V. J. Lewis and G. Vallar. 1984. Exploring the articulatory loop. *Quarterly Journal of Experimental Psychology* 36: 233–252.

Baddeley, Alan D., N. Thomson and M. Buchanan. 1975. Word length and the structure of short-term memory. *Journal of Verbal Learning and Verbal Behavior* 14: 575–589.

Barnard, P. J. 1985. Interacting cognitive subsystems: A psycholinguistic approach to short term memory. In: A. Ellis (ed.), *Progress in the Psychology of Language*, volume 2. London: Erlbaum, 197–258.

Caplan, D. and G. Waters. 1999. Verbal working memory and sentence comprehension. *Behavioral and Brain Sciences* 22: 114–126.

Cheng, C. 1974. Different roles of acoustic and articulatory information in short-term memory. *Journal of Experimental Psychology* 103: 614–618.

Conrad, R. 1964. Acoustic confusions in immediate memory. *British Journal of Psychology* 55: 75–84.

Conrad, R. and A. J. Hull. 1968. Input modality and the serial position curve in short-term memory. *Psychonomic Science* 10: 135–136.

Crowder, R. G. 1967. Prefix effect in immediate memory. *Canadian Journal of Psychology* 21: 450–461.

Engelkamp, Johannes and Ralf Rummer. 1999. Syntaktische Struktur und Wortlänge im Satzrecall. *Zeitschrift für Experimentelle Psychologie* 46: 1–15.

Engelkamp, Johannes and Ralf Rummer. 2002. Subordinating conjunctions as device for unifying sentences in memory. *European Journal of Cognitive Psychology* 14: 353–369.

Forster, Kenneth I. 1970. Visual perception of rapidly presented word sequences of varying complexity. *Perception and Psychophysics* 8: 215–221.

Frazier, L. and K. Rayner. 1982. Making and correcting errors during sentence comprehension: Eye movements in the analysis of structurally ambiguous sentences. *Cognitive Psychology* 14: 178–210.

Friederici, A. D. 2002. Towards a neural basis of auditory sentence processing. *Trends in Cognitive Sciences* 6: 78–84.

Gathercole, Susan E. and Alan D. Baddeley. 1993. *Working Memory and Language*. Hove: Lawrence Erlbaum.

Levelt, Willem J. M. 1989. *Speaking: From Intention to Articulation.* Cambridge, MA: MIT Press.

Levelt, Willem J. M., A. P. A. Roelofs and A. S. Meyer. 1999. A theory of lexical access in speech production. *Behavioral and Brain Sciences* 22(1): 1–37.

MacDonald, M. C. and M. H. Christiansen. 2002. Reassessing working memory: A comment on Just and Carpenter (1992) and Waters and Caplan (1996). *Psychological Review* 109: 35–54.

Martin, R. C. 1993. Short-term memory and sentence processing: Evidence from neuropsychology. *Memory & Cognition* 21: 176–183.

Martin, R. C., M. Lesch and M. Bartha. 1999. Independence of input and output phonology in word processing and short-term memory. *Journal of Memory and Language* 41: 3–29.

Martin, R. C., J. R. Shelton and L. S. Yaffee. 1994. Language processing and working memory: Neuropsychological evidence for separate phonological and semantic capacities. *Journal of Memory and Language* 33: 83–111.

Nespoulous, Jean-Luc, Dordain Monique, Cecile Perron, Bernadette Ska, Daniel Bub, David Caplan, Jacques Mehler and Andre Roch Lecours. 1988. Agrammatism in sentence production without comprehension deficits: Reduced availability of syntactic structures and/or of grammatical morphemes? A case study. *Brain and Language* 33(2): 273–295.

Park, N. and R. C. Martin. 2002. A contribution of phonological representations to immediate sentence recall. Poster presented at the 15th Annual CUNY Conference on Human Sentence Processing, New York City.

Penney, C. G. 1989. Modality effects in the structure of short-term verbal memory. *Memory & Cognition* 17: 398–422.

Potter, M. C. 1999. Understanding sentences and scenes: The role of conceptual short-term memory. In: V. Coltheart (ed.), *Fleeting Memories: Cognition of Brief Visual Stimuli*. Cambridge, MA: MIT Press, 13–46.

Potter, M. C. and L. Lombardi. 1990. Regeneration in the short-term recall of sentences. *Journal of Memory and Language* 29: 633–654.

Rummer, Ralf and Johannes Engelkamp. 2003. Phonological information in immediate and delayed sentence recall. *The Quarterly Journal of Experimental Psychology* 56(A): 83–95.

Rummer, Ralf, Johannes Engelkamp and L. Konieczny. 2003. The subordination effect: Evidence from self-paced reading and recall. *European Journal of Cognitive Psychology* 15: 539–566.

Rummer, Ralf and J. Schweppe. 2005. Evidence for a modality effect in sentence retention. *Psychonomic Bulletin and Review* 12: 1094–1099.

Schweppe, J. and Ralf Rummer. 2004. Morpho-syntactic information contributes to short-term memory for sentences. Paper presented at the 17th Annual CUNY Conference on Human Sentence Processing.

Willis, C. S. and Susan E. Gathercole. 2000. Phonological short-term memory contributions to sentence processing in young children. *Memory* 9: 349–363.

Mental models and noun-phrase anaphora

Alan Garnham and H. Wind Cowles

1 Introduction

When people are talking or writing they often refer to the same person or thing or event more than once. Typically, a second, *anaphoric*, reference uses a linguistic expression of a different form from that used the first time. For example, someone referred to initially as *John* might later be referred to as *he* or, in a context where he is being contrasted with someone younger, as *the older man*. Notably, direct repetition of the same linguistic expression (*... John.... John....*) can seem stilted, or even infelicitous, if the two occurrences of the expression are not separated by some distance. Traditional accounts of anaphoric reference attempted to analyse the phenomenon at the textual level, often taking the anaphoric expression to stand in for a repetition of the original expression (see, Bosch (1983), chapter 1 for a historical overview). However, more recent accounts, based in cognitive science (Garnham, 1987; Cornish, 1999), recognize that the phenomenon must be explained, at least in part, in terms of mental representations of what is referred to anaphorically. The case for this type of approach can be made most clearly when the use of what is naturally analysed as an anaphoric expression occurs without a linguistic antecedent, or at least without a linguistic antecedent with the same meaning.

For example, in (1) *them* refers to the dreams that John had, but the explicit reference in the first clause is to the activity of dreaming, rather than the dreams themselves.

(1) *John used to dream a lot, but he never remembered them.*

Cornish (1999) refers to the verb *dream* in this example as the *antecedent trigger*. This antecedent trigger is not the antecedent itself, as specified in traditional analysis. A standard antecedent for a definite pronoun such as *them* would refer to the same thing (or set of things) as the pronouns, for example in (2).

(2) *John used to have a lot of dreams, but he never remembered them.*

The antecedent trigger is what causes the representation of what would be referred to in a standard antecedent phrase to be introduced into the mental representation of the text. However, it is an open question whether dreams are represented when the activity of dreaming is mentioned in the first sentence above, or only when the pronoun *them* is encountered.

2 Mental models theory

The mental models theory (Johnson-Laird, 1983; Garnham, 1981, 1987) provides a natural framework in which to develop this kind of approach to anaphoric reference. According to the mental models account of language understanding, a listener or reader creates a mental representation of the situation in the real world, imaginary world, or abstract domain that the text is about. The primary constituents of such models are representations of the people, animals, objects, properties, events and so on that the discourse or text is about. These constituents are introduced, either directly or indirectly, into mental models by the (understanding of) linguistic expressions. However, because there is not necessarily a direct one-to-one mapping between linguistic expressions and elements of a mental model, it is possible for a seemingly anaphoric expression to refer to something that was introduced into the model indirectly. Hence that expression need not have an 'antecedent' in the standard linguistic sense, though it is likely to have an antecedent trigger.

There are many types of anaphoric expression. English, for example, is particularly rich in verbal anaphors, such as verb phrase ellipsis (*John went to see the new Harry Potter movie, and Sally did, too*), gapping (*Rachel likes ice-cream and Jenny frozen yoghurt*), and sluicing (*Sonia thinks someone has been looking through her personal possessions, but she doesn't know who*). In this chapter, however, we will be concerned primarily with noun phrase anaphors. This class of anaphoric expressions includes definite pronouns (e.g., in English, *he, she, it, they*), bare demonstratives (*this, that, these, those*), demonstrative noun phrases (e.g. *that woman, those shoes*), and many types of definite noun phrases (*the man, the red tablecloth, the car I was driving last night*). In their standard uses, though not in all of their uses, noun phrase anaphors are identity of reference anaphors. They refer back to something that has already been referred to in the discourse or text, most typically by an explicit antecedent expression. So, in a text that introduces someone as *George* and goes on to talk about what *he* did, *he* refers to the same person as George. In this respect it differs from, for example, an indefinite anaphoric pronoun such as *one*. In *George has a new Mercedes and I want one, too*, *one* means a Mercedes, but not the same Mercedes that George has. Such indefinites are called identity of sense anaphors. They have the same meaning in the sense of same sense as their antecedents, but they do not refer to the same object.

As we have already said, because mental models represent things that have already been referred to in the text, it is natural to take identity of reference anaphors as referring to elements of mental models. However, as we have seen, there are various types of definite noun phrase anaphors. The existence of these different anaphor types raises questions about how such anaphors are differentiated and why they exist at all. For example, why do repeated noun phrase anaphors sometimes appear to be problematic? After all, in many ways, repeating a noun phrase would seem logically to be the least problematic method of re-referring, as it would be the least likely to generate referential 'ambiguities' (or indeterminacies).

3 Linguistic theories on anaphoric reference

In the theoretical linguistics literature, these kinds of issues have been addressed in discussions about the connection of referential form to underlying representations (Ariel, 1988, 1990; Gundel et al., 1993). Gundel et al. proposed the *givenness hierarchy*: a set of implicationally related cognitive statuses. They propose that the form of a referring expression is tied to the givenness of the corresponding referent, with the use of different determiners and pronominal forms signalling different cognitive statuses. This hierarchy ranges from *type identifiable* referents that are referred to using indefinite noun phrase anaphors (e.g. *a cat*), in which the hearer must be able to identify a representation of the type of object that is indicated by the reference, to referents that are *in focus* and referred to using unaccented third person pronouns (e.g. *it*). A referent that is in focus is one that the hearer has in working memory and is currently at the centre of attention. Ariel's (1988; 1990) *accessibility hierarchy* is a similar notion, with the accessibility of a referent determining its appropriate reference form.

Other studies have suggested that the choice of reference form for a given anaphor helps structure the discourse. For example, fuller forms of reference, such as definite NP anaphors, may mark episode transitions (Fox, 1984; Marslen-Wilson et al., 1982; Fletcher, 1984; Vonk et al., 1992). In two written sentence/discourse production tasks, Vonk et al. (1992) found that participants tended to produce shifts in topics more often when they were prompted to use an over-specified form of anaphor rather than a pronoun. Conversely, participants also produced fuller forms of reference more often when they produced a shift in topic compared to when they continued it. Further, in a probe recognition task, Vonk et al. found that reaction times for content word targets that were in the same clause as the antecedent of either over-specified (name plus modifier) or non-overspecified (pronoun) anaphors took longer when the anaphor was over-specified. This finding suggested that the anaphor caused a decrease in the availability of the surrounding antecedent context, and in a further study they found that this was an immediate effect, found shortly after the anaphor.

These proposals, and the empirical evidence on which they are based, support the casual observation that different types of NP anaphor are used in different circumstances – they are not just free variants. Very crudely, the less semantic content an anaphoric form has itself, the closer, in some sense, it needs to be to its antecedent. Definite pronouns, for example, which have little semantic content other than gender and number, typically occur very close to their antecedents, or in a string of pronominal references to the same person or thing. What, then, determines when one form should be used in preference to another? One important notion in accounting for the variation in the form of anaphoric noun phrases is *focusing* (in a psychological sense – the term 'focus' has a related, but separate, sense as compared to the one used within linguistics). From the perspective of mental model theory, focusing can be regarded as a device for dividing mental models into parts (or the entities represented in mental models into subsets), and these divisions play a role in determining which anaphoric form or forms are appropriate for referring back to particular entities.

4 Psychological models of anaphoric reference

Within psychology an early, and influential, view of focusing is that of Sanford and Garrod (1981) – part of their scenario-mapping hypothesis, revised later in works such as Sanford and Garrod (1998). For the purposes of text comprehension, Sanford and Garrod (1981) distinguished between two memory partitions, implicit and explicit focus. Explicit focus contains representations of those things explicitly mentioned in the text or discourse. Implicit focus contains information related to things explicitly mentioned, and activated by the current scenario. According to Sanford and Garrod, only items in explicit focus can be referred to by pronouns. It is possible to refer to items in implicit focus, but fuller noun phrase anaphors are needed. An example of reference to something in implicit focus would be in cases where a definite NP reference has to be linked into the text representation by the kind of bridging inference discussed by Clark and Haviland (1975) and Clark (1977). For example, in the text below, there is no mention in the first sentence of the car's fuel pipe. However, because each car has a fuel pipe it is possible to refer felicitously to the fuel pipe of the car mentioned in the first sentence, as in (3). It is not, however, possible to do so using a pronoun.

(3) *Our car broke down on the way to Edinburgh.*
Its fuel pipe had become blocked.

Once the fuel pipe has been mentioned (in the second sentence) it will then be in explicit focus. There are, nevertheless, some cases where pronouns can be used to refer to implicit referents (Cornish et al., 2005) but only if those referents are central or nuclear, as in (4).

(4) *Speaker A: Did you know that Marie is six-months' pregnant again?*
Speaker B: Yes, she's already knitted a cardigan for it.

The simple distinction between implicit and explicit focus does not explain why some things that have been explicitly mentioned can be referred to pronominally and why other things cannot. A more detailed approach to focusing derives from the literature of computational linguistics. Barbara Grosz (1981), in her work on the comprehension of dialogues that accompanied goal-directed tasks, suggested the notion of focus spaces that were structured in a way similar to the task itself. So, for example, in a dialogue accompanying the assembly of a complex mechanism, there would be focus spaces corresponding to subtasks, such as finding a tool or putting together a subassembly. Once a subtask was completed, the dialogue would move onto another subtask, and the focus space would change accordingly. Because of the relation it proposes between the structure of the representation and the structure of the 'world', this notion meshes well with mental models theory.

Sidner (1983) distinguished between discourse focus and focused agent, and emphasized the role of (subsequent) pronominalization in determining focus. She also suggested that previous foci were held on a focus stack (a last-in, first-out memory). Grosz and Sidner (1986) combined and modified their ideas in a theoretical framework that placed emphasis on the psychological notions of attention and intention. They distinguished between global, or discourse, focus and local focus. Grosz and Sidner claim that discourses are linguistically structured into discourse segments, which are related to one another by a set of coherence relations. Global coherence and the overall or global focus of the discourse are determined by the intentions of the speaker or writer. Transitions from one segment to another could be signalled by the form of referring expression chosen for a particular entity (see above). Within a segment, local coherence must be maintained and local focusing depends on a continually shifting focus of attention.

Grosz later developed, with others (Grosz et al., 1995), a more detailed theory of local focus, *Centering Theory.* Centering Theory is a theory of how attention shifts within a discourse segment. The theory claims that each utterance has a set of (potential) foci of attention associated with it, the set of forward-looking *centers.* These centers are things that are likely to be talked about in the upcoming discourse, and they are ordered, or at least partially ordered, in terms of how likely they are to be talked about. Other things being equal, the subject of a sentence is its highest ranked forward looking center, but other factors, such an animacy, can also affect the ordering of the forward looking centers. Each utterance also has one backward-looking center, which should be a member of the set of forward-looking centers of the previous utterance. Centers can be continued, retained or shifted. Shifts can be smooth or rough. In a continuation, the highest ranked forward-looking center remains the centre of attention over a sequence of utterances. In retention, the same thing is talked about, even though it is not always the highest-ranked forward-looking center. In a shift, the backward-looking center changes from one utterance to the next. Since Centering Theory is couched in terms of things that are referred to, it is compatible with a conception of focusing as the partitioning of mental models.

Centering Theory incorporates the notion that the local focus is likely to be referred to (on second and subsequent mentions) pronominally. However, in its later versions it does not claim, because of empirical evidence to the contrary, that the highest-ranked forward-looking center of an utterance will be pronominalized if it is referred to in the next utterance. Rather, it makes the weaker claim that if any of the forward-looking centers of the previous utterance are pronominalized in the present utterance, the backward looking center of the present utterance must be.

As has been hinted, earlier versions of centering theory suggested that where a center was continued, the second reference should be pronominal. This claim suggests that a fuller noun phrase is somehow inappropriate, and might cause problems of interpretation. This claim was investigated empirically by Peter Gordon and his colleagues, who suggested that there would be a processing penalty for repeating a name – either a proper name or a common name – instead of using a pronoun. Gordon called this phenomenon, which he did find in his empirical data, the *repeated name penalty*. Gordon et al. (1993) demonstrated the phenomenon for repeated proper names. They showed it was particularly associated with repetition as the syntactic subject of the second utterance. They also found that the repeated name penalty was much reduced following a center shift, which may be related to the phenomenon of more specific noun phrase anaphors being related to changes of topic or perspective (see above).

Within the psycholinguistic literature, Greene et al. (1992) made a stronger claim than that made in Centering Theory, namely that at any point in a well-formed discourse there should be just one (focused) entity that a pronoun can refer to. Greene et al. claimed to have shown empirically that when texts contained pronouns that had more than one possible referent, people failed to resolve them. It has, however, been suggested (Gordon and Scearce, 1995) that the participants in Greene et al.'s study did not engage in the normal processes of comprehension, because the experimental task discouraged them from doing so. It is certainly widely assumed, for example in the literature on implicit causality, that a pronoun can readily refer to more than one entity in the preceding clause, even where gender does not resolve the issue. Both (5) and (6) are perfectly comprehensible in either version.

(5) *John confessed to Jill/Bill because he wanted a reduced sentence.*

(6) *John/Jane confessed to Bill because he offered a reduced sentence.*

Nevertheless, at any point in a discourse there are only a very small number of entities that can successfully be referred to pronominally, and one of these entities is usually preferred above the others. The full range of factors that determine membership of this set is not fully understood. However, it is clear that the set can be regarded as a subset of the entities in the overall mental model for a text.

Centering Theory is primarily an account of what anaphoric references are possible. It can also be taken to be making the implicit claim that anaphoric references that do not satisfy the criteria it lays down will be difficult to comprehend. However, in so far as its proponents make specific psychological claims, those claims appear to rest on additional assumptions.

A different, and more uniform, approach to explaining when and why different types of noun phrase anaphor are easy or difficult to understand is found in Almor's (1999) *informational load hypothesis.* Although Grosz and Sidner make use of psychological concepts, such as attention and intention, in their account of focusing, their theory is clearly grounded in computational linguistics, rather than psychology. Almor's approach is more firmly based in standard psychological notions and empirical methodology. And Almor's principal question is: what makes an NP anaphor more or less difficult to interpret?

Almor assumes that anaphoric expressions typically make contact with their antecedent expressions (or, rather, representations of the entities referred to by those expressions) in working memory. Almor assumes that working memory has a limited capacity, but remains otherwise agnostic as to which particular working memory theory is correct. Almor calls the process by which an anaphor makes contact with its antecedent *identification.* However, this term is a misleading one and its use highlights one particular, and we believe major, weakness of Almor's theory. The term is misleading because anaphoric expressions typically have several possible antecedents, as shown in the 'implicit causality' sentences mentioned above, one of which is repeated here, as (7).

(7) *John confessed to Bill because he wanted a reduced sentence.*

Although *he* refers to John, at the point where it is encountered it could also refer to Bill. The term identification, as applied to an anaphoric expression of this kind, might be thought to describe the process by which its antecedent is selected from a pool of candidates. However, Almor does not appear to refer to this process by his term identification. In fact he tries to side-step the issue of selecting an antecedent from a pool of candidates by using experimental materials in which there is only one antecedent that has a large degree of semantic overlap with the anaphor. However, although it may be obvious to the reader that there is only one 'possible' antecedent in such passages, it is only by making an explicit comparison between an anaphor and a potential antecedent that the lack of overlap can be established. Almor does not consider the process of comparison to see which possible antecedent gives the best fit, or the contribution of this process to the selection of a particular antecedent, and hence to the difficulty of understanding an anaphoric expression. As a result, we do not know how the ILH might explain this selection process. Instead, by identification, Almor means the process by which the anaphor and the actual antecedent are determined to be (possibly) coreferential expressions. His discussion is always of cases where the identification is successful, whereas the interplay of cases where it is successful and cases where it is not undoubtedly contributes to the difficulty of understanding anaphoric references.

Almor describes identification, or at least a crucial part of it, as a "matter of reactivating the representation of the antecedent in working memory" (1999, 750). Representations decay over time, and reactivation depends on semantic (and possibly phonological) overlap between the anaphor and its antecedent. The greater the textual distance between the two, the more decay of the representation of the antecedent will have taken place and, hence, the greater the overlap required for successful reactivation. Hence the often-made observation that more reduced anaphoric forms (such as pronouns) typically occur close to their antecedents, whereas fuller forms occur when the antecedent is further away.

One of the most novel aspects of Almor's account is that another property of working memory counteracts the tendency just described.

It is well known (Baddeley, 1992) that phonological similarity causes disruption to the performance of working memory tasks. Remember a list of rhyming words in order (e.g. cat, rat, bat, mat, hat, sat) is more difficult than remembering a list of non-rhyming words of similar length and frequency. Similarly, according to Almor, semantic overlap causes interference in working memory. So, given a reference to *the cobra*, a second reference to *the snake* is potentially more problematic than a second reference to *it*, because there is greater semantic overlap between *cobra* and *snake* than between *it* and *snake*. This *cost* to using a semantically more loaded expression must be justified, for example by the aid it gives to carrying out the identification process (*snake* will reactivate *cobra* more successfully than *it*). So, when the representation of the antecedent is weak, perhaps because the antecedent is distant, or out of focus, the cost of the semantic overlap in working memory might be justified. However, when the antecedent is close and focused, the cost cannot be justified, and the semantically more specific anaphoric expression might be not only no better than the less specified expression, it might be more difficult to process.

However, this kind of functional justification for the form of an anaphoric expression actually further underlines the weakness in Almor's account that is introduced by his failure to consider nonantecedents. For a distant antecedent, it might be thought that nearer potential antecedents would have to be considered and rejected before the actual antecedent was considered (or at least that a set of potential antecedents would have to be considered in parallel). One consideration on the form of an anaphoric expression is that it must discourage any match (i.e. successful identification) with a nonantecedent. This is one reason why pronouns often cannot be used with distant antecedents – because they would match with other potential antecedents that were mentioned more recently.

One interesting consequence of Almor's account is that the repeated name penalty reported by Gordon and his colleagues is not a penalty for failing to pronominalize, as Centering Theory seems to say. Rather, it is a penalty for using an overspecific anaphoric expression when a less specific one would have performed the identification (reactivation) function equally well. Thus, Almor's ILH predicts that there should be a penalty for using *the snake* as an anaphor for *the cobra* in cases where *the cobra* remains in focus, and can be readily identified with *it.* We have made some preliminary attempts to investigate this claim, but we do not yet have any definitive evidence that bears on it.

Almor's informational load hypothesis claims that there are three principal factors that determine, in interaction, the difficulty of processing an anaphoric expression: discourse focus, the amount of new information added by the anaphor, and the informational load of the anaphor-antecedent pair. Almor does not provide a detailed account of focus, unlike proponents of Centering Theory. For the purpose of his experimental work, he operationalizes focus as clefted elements in it-clefts and wh-clefts (pseudoclefts), which are well known in the linguistics literature to mark focus, and in particular contrastive focus (Kiss, 1998). He does not, of course, claim that only clefted elements are focused. What he does imply is that, at any point in a discourse, there is a single most highly focused element, which is the default referent for any anaphoric expression. This element is highly activated, and so identification (in Almor's sense) is always easy with such an element. In many ways, this element has a similar status to the highest ranked forward-looking center in Centering Theory.

Informational load is defined in terms of the conceptual distance between the anaphor and its antecedent. Informational load is positive when the anaphor has more conceptual content than its antecedent, and hence adds information about the referent (e.g. ... *the bird... the robin...*). However, when the antecedent is more general than the anaphor – the more typical case – informational load is negative, and hence greater conceptual distance produces a smaller (more negative) informational load. The informational load of ... *the robin... the bird...* is greater (less negative) than the informational load of ... *the robin... it....* As Almor rightly points out, he cannot make predictions about cases in which the anaphor adds new information about the referent because he does not specify a metric for comparing (and hence generating a trade-off function for) increases in informational load with increases in the amount of new information provided by an anaphoric expression.

Almor's informational load hypothesis makes one further novel, and surprising, prediction about noun phrase anaphors. When an anaphor's antecedent is in focus, there is no benefit from semantic overlap between the anaphor and the antecedent, because the purpose of that overlap would be to help identification (reactivation) of the representation of the antecedent and, in this case, no reactivation is necessary. Semantic overlap does, however, still produce a cost, because of interference in working memory. So informational load is not justified, and an anaphor that has less overlap with the antecedent will be preferred. The novel prediction is that, for example, a category anaphor will be easier to understand when it follows an atypical instance antecedent (*... the ostrich... the bird...*) than when *it* follows a typical instance antecedent (*... the robin... the bird...*) – an *inverse typicality effect*. Typicality effects are very common in a variety of domains, and have been reported for anaphor comprehension (Garrod and Sanford, 1977; Duffy and Rayner, 1990; Rayner et al., 2000; Myers et al., 2000). Almor's (1999) Experiment 5 appears to be the first study to report an inverse typicality effect, which he takes as support for his informational load hypothesis. For unfocused antecedents, the benefit of semantic overlap will be felt, because the representation of the antecedent does need to be reactivated. However, interference will also occur, according to Almor's hypothesis, particularly once the antecedent has become reactivated. It is difficult to gauge the relative strength of these two effects, so it is not absolutely clear that the informational load hypothesis predicts a typicality effect, even though such effects are empirically established in the literature, and Almor reports them for his own studies.

The inverse typicality effect is the main prediction of the informational load hypothesis that clearly differentiates it from other theories of anaphor resolution. It is, therefore, important for Almor that he should be able to explain apparent inconsistencies with previous results, and also that it should be replicable and generalizable to other cases of semantic distance effects other than typicality. Looking at previous results first, it appears that in most cases where a standard typicality effect was found, the antecedent was not in focus, and so an inverse effect would not be expected. Rayner et al. (2000) used antecedents embedded in predicates, rather than in subject position, as did Duffy and Rayner (1990). In Myers et al.'s (2000) study antecedents were not in a syntactically prominent position, and their primary dependent measure was for a repetition of the antecedent following the category anaphor, rather than at the anaphor itself.

Thus, the only study that appears to contradict Almor is the original Garrod and Sanford (1977) study. In the example materials in that paper, the antecedent is in subject position, which should be focused. Almor suggests that subject position may simply not be focusing enough to trigger inverse effects. However, as we shall see below, other work (Cowles and Garnham, 2005) has shown an inverted semantic distance effect (albeit with category hierarchies, rather than typicality) when the antecedent is in subject position. Thus, the issue of why Garrod and Sanford (1977) did not find an inverse effect remains unresolved.

Turning to attempts to replicate Almor's findings, Cowles and Garnham (2011) had mixed success in attempting to replicate Almor's basic inverse typicality effect, for reasons that we did not fully succeed in identifying. In an eye-tracking study, Gompel et al. (2004) did partially replicate Almor's results, however the time course of the effects they found led them to propose a two-stage model, in contrast to Almor's. The difficulty in cleanly replicating Almor's results could be partially explained by Almor's theory itself: the measured effect is a result of competing tendencies of facilitation and interference from semantic overlap, and so the exact predictions are not clear. In a more recent set of experiments (Cowles and Garnham, 2005) using category hierarchies (e.g. *reptile, snake, cobra*), we looked at what we considered to be clearer semantic distance effects (*... the snake... the reptile...* vs. *... the cobra... the reptile...*). In these studies we did find a clear pattern of inverse semantic distance effects for focused antecedents (clefted or syntactic subject) and normal semantic distance effects for nonfocused antecedents (the nonclefted elements in cleft sentences, or elements in the 'by' phrase of a passive sentence). A further attempt to replicate Almor's results by using adjectives to modify semantic distance (*...the oak...the tree...* vs. *...the gnarled oak...the tree...*) produced quite different results, which we will return to below. Almor's original paper contains examples of category hierarchies and of adjectival modification, and it is clear that his predictions are based on a general notion of semantic overlap and not on a notion that is restricted to typicality effects. Thus, Almor's account would be best supported if all cases in which semantic overlap is manipulated produced the effects predicted by the ILH. So far the results are mixed.

Another issue for Almor is whether it is possible to demonstrate more directly the semantic interference effects in working memory that underpin his theoretical position. Almor likens these effects to the well-established phonological interference effects in working memory. However, parallel semantic effects are not easy to find. They do not occur in immediate memory for semantically related words in the same way that they do for phonologically similar words. Baddeley (1966) reports a 6% reduction in performance in immediate memory for semantically related words as compared to controls, compared with a 72% effect for phonologically related words. We replicated Baddeley's original study (though with different stimuli) and performed a second experiment in which the word lists were embedded in passages such as (8).

(8) *Steve went to a jumble sale at the weekend. He spied a glove and a belt, and then noticed a coat and a shirt next to a shoe.*
OR
He spied a tape and a tent, and then noticed a tray and a stool next to a phone.

Here, the first version of the second sentence contains five semantically related words from the domain of CLOTHING, whereas the second version contains five (comparatively) unrelated words. In both studies we found large effects of phonological similarity (18% reduction in correct recall of words in their correct serial positions for lists and 25% for texts), but no effects of semantic similarity (<2% in the wrong direction vs. <1% in the wrong direction).

One reason for this lack of an effect may be that immediate memory is not semantically based. Indeed, this would be the traditional view. For example, in the Baddeley and Hitch (1974) working memory model, phonological interference occurs because words are held briefly in the phonological loop. And generally speaking, people find little difference in immediate memory for lists of semantically related words and list of unrelated words. An alternative view would be that the interference effects are counteracted by facilitation effects – remembering one word helps memory for a related word. Recent reports of semantic effects in immediate memory (Haarman and Usher, 2001) are reports of facilitatory effects. However, Haarmann and Usher, and others, believe that there are separate phonologically-based and semantically-based short-term stores. Interestingly, but perhaps not surprisingly, Haarmann et al. (2003) suggest that semantic working memory is more important in text comprehension than the phonological loop. Overall, there seems to be little support for the idea of semantic interference in working memory, and hence Almor's account of NP-anaphor comprehension must be challenged.

While Almor's informational load hypothesis represents a bold attempt to provide a unified and psychologically based attempt to account for factors that make noun phrase anaphors easy or difficult to understand, we believe it to suffer from both conceptual and empirical problems. We agree that working memory, a relatively short-term storage and processing system, is vitally important in the comprehension of anaphoric expressions. Like Almor, we are not committed to any particular model of working memory. However, unlike Almor, we do not believe that interference in working memory between semantically similar items is a likely mechanism for problems in resolving anaphoric noun phrases. Furthermore, we believe that there are important factors neglected by Almor.

First, as we mentioned previously, it seems odd to talk about 'identifying' the referent of an anaphoric expression without explicitly discussing the choice between possible antecedents as part of that identification process. Indeed, there is a wealth of empirical evidence that nonantecedents affect the interpretation of noun phrase anaphors (Corbett and Chang (1983), and many later papers). Almor does not consider this issue, and the only way it could have an effect in his system is if alternative referents somehow interfere with the reactivation of the actual antecedent. By not considering this issue, Almor overlooks the fact that the choice of an anaphoric expression may be determined by what possible referents, other than the actual referent, are available. To take an extreme case, there is no problem in following *John came into the room and...* with *he...*, but *he...* following *John and Bill came into the room and...* is uninterpretable. In this particular case it might be possible to argue that John (as an individual) is not in focus in the second case, whereas he is in the first. However, cases such as (9) and (10) are more problematic.

(9) *June blamed Bill because he...*

(10) *John blamed Bill because he...*

Bill is not in focus in either case, but *he* is Bill in the first instance, whereas in the second it is more likely (at this point) to be John, until the ending disambiguates (*...needed a scapegoat* vs. *...had been very careless*). In fact, in such cases, it is not possible to interpret the pronoun definitively until later material has been processed. This raises further questions about the process that identifies the anaphor and its antecedent.

Second, it is well known (Vonk et al., 1992) that anaphoric expressions play roles other than simply making contact with previous referents. For example, a noun phrase anaphor that is more specific than required for the purposes of identifying its referent, may signal a thematic shift.

One possible way of incorporating this idea into a framework similar to Almor's is to analyse the notion of thematic shift in terms of focusing. As has been mentioned, Almor's discussion of focusing is rather limited. He talks about the discourse focus and seems to assume that it is one person or thing that is currently at the centre of attention. This idea might work in the very brief texts he uses in his experimental studies, but more generally there is a distinction between global and local focus, as discussed, for example, by Grosz and Sidner (1986). Describing an object in a particular way may not only allow it to be identified with something previously mentioned, it might also suggest a particular (perhaps new) perspective on that object.

Another issue that requires further investigation is the relationship between adjectival modification and focus. In (11) the hiker is focused by being in cleft position.

(11) *It was the hiker that saw the (frightened) cobra.*

Correspondingly, the (frightened) cobra is not focused by structural means. However, the results of our empirical work (Cowles and Garnham, 2003b,a) showed that references back to the frightened cobra or simply the cobra in the above sentence or in (12) were only difficult in the case where *cobra* was both not focused by the cleft structure and not modified.

(12) *What the hiker saw was the (frightened) cobra.*

This finding suggested that modification of *cobra*, in this case by *frightened*, served to add focus to cobra. One way of thinking about this effect is that there seems to be no reason to modify *cobra*, certainly none provided by the passages we used, other than to bring attention to it. This idea relates to the idea discussed earlier that overspecified noun phrases signal a discourse function, in this case a possible shift of (local) topic to an entity not focused by syntactic structure.

A further complication in interpreting our results on modification derives from a consideration of the relation between the clefted sentences and the context in which they occurred. For the sentences above, the context was (13).

(13) *A hiker and his dog were startled after they sat down to rest.*

Clefting is associated not only with focus, but with *contrastive* focus (Kiss, 1998). Thus, when the hiker is focused, in the *it* cleft, there is an implicit contrast with some other person or animal that might have been doing something. In this case the context clearly introduces two individuals, the hiker and the dog, and the implied contrast is that it was the hiker rather than the dog that saw the snake. The pseudocleft, however, focuses the (frightened) cobra. Here the context does not provide another entity with which the cobra is naturally contrasted. Hence, the pseudocleft is less felicitous in this context than the *it* cleft. It is possible that this difference between the two types of cleft has an effect on the subsequent interpretation of an anaphoric phrase, such as *the snake* referring back to the (frightened) cobra. In future experiments, we intend to explore this possibility by creating contexts that make the two types of cleft equally felicitous.

In the experiment described above, the adjectives modified a nondefining feature of the antecedent. For example, being frightened (or not) is not a feature that is part of the identity of snakes. In a second experiment, we used adjectives that caused a typical or defining feature of the antecedent to no longer have a typical value, for example as in (14).

(14) *A keeper and her intern needed to move some injured animals at the zoo.*
It was the intern that didn't want to touch the (toothless) cobra.
What the intern didn't want to touch was the (toothless) cobra.

Snakes typically have fangs/teeth, but the particular snake described here does not. In this experiment we found an inverse semantic distance effect for both *it* clefts and pseudoclefts, though it was more pronounced (and only statistically significant) for the pseudoclefts. *The snake* as the subject of a following sentence was read more quickly following *the toothless cobra* than following *the cobra.* Our explanation of this finding was that the most important effect of the adjectival modification, particularly in this case where the modification produced an atypical result in terms of the properties of the modified object, was to increase the focus on, for example, the cobra. Focused antecedents produce inverse semantic distance effects.

It is clear that the effects of adjectival modification are more complex than would be predicted by the simple application of Almor's ILH. Almor (1999, 751) gives the example of *crippled robin* as being semantically more distant from *bird* than the unmodified *robin.* This was the basis of our prediction of semantic distance and inverse semantic distance effects for adjectival modification. However, there appears to be a difference between deciding to call something a cobra rather than a snake and deciding to call something a frightened (or toothless) cobra rather than a cobra. This may be because adjectival modification makes it clearer that the bare noun could have been used and that, therefore, there should be some justification for the adjective.

5 Conclusions

Noun phrase anaphora is most commonly identity of reference anaphora in which a second or later reference is made to an entity that has been previously introduced, either explicitly or implicitly in a text. Mental models theory provides a natural context in which to describe such anaphora, since mental models contain representations of entities mentioned explicitly in text and can, via inference making, usually based on real world knowledge, contain representations of related entities (regarded as mentioned implicitly). However, if noun phrase anaphora were that simple, the standard case would be anaphora by direct repetition of the phrase originally used to introduce the entity referred to by the anaphoric noun phrase. In fact, this type of case is relatively rare and can often sound infelicitous. At a descriptive level, entities that remain salient, or focused, or available in some sense can be referred to by noun phrase anaphors that have relatively little semantic content of their own, in particular definite pronouns. Less accessible entities require fuller anaphoric forms.

There is no general consensus on how these facts should be explained, though it is clear that notions such as accessibility are psychological ones. For complex texts, focusing is a relatively complex phenomenon, and its operation is not fully understood. Centering Theory attempts to order, or partially order, recently mentioned entities in terms of how likely they are to be mentioned again – it deals with local aspects of focusing, while acknowledging that there are global aspects that must be dealt with separately. Almor's Informational Load Hypothesis is a much more thorough psychological attempt to explain when an anaphoric noun phrase will be easy to process and when it will be difficult. Almor acknowledges the importance of focus, though he does not give a detailed account of how focusing works. He also suggests a role for semantic or conceptual distance between an anaphoric noun phrase and its antecedent phrase. Or rather he suggests two roles. On the one hand semantic overlap tends of confirm coreferentiality. On the other hand, it causes interference in working memory, the system in which semantic overlap is established. Semantic interference effects in working memory are hard to establish. This may be because the well-established facilitatory effects of semantic overlap tend to overwhelm them. Or it may be because they do not exist. Nevertheless, semantic overlap does play a role in resolving NP anaphors, and Almor is right to point to its importance.

The other point in the ILH's favour is that it attempts to account for apparent differences in processing among different types of non-pronominal anaphors, such as repeated (proper) names, and category NPs, a matter on which other theories have had relatively little systematic to say.

Two major shortcomings in the ILH are, first, its failure to be clear about what happens when there are two or more potential antecedents for an anaphoric expression or, more generally, how it is established whether something is a potential antecedent, and, second, its failure to consider the discourse function of the form of an anaphoric noun phrase. In the first case, Almor writes as if all that matters in 'identifying' the referent of an anaphoric expression were the relation between it and its antecedent. However, whether the search for a referent is a serial or a parallel process, it seems more than likely that the other potential referents, the way they are described, and their semantic relations with the anaphoric expression, will affect how easy it is to establish the link between the anaphor and its actual antecedent (or referent).

On the second issue, Almor considers only two possible functions of an anaphoric expression: to make contact with the antecedent and so establish coreference and to add information about the referent. However, there is evidence that the form of an anaphoric expression can serve other functions. For example, anaphors that are more specific than they need be for establishing coreference, but which do not add any new information, may signal a change in perspective on the referent or a shift in the general direction of a discourse.

More generally, the mental models theory provides a sensible framework within which theories of noun phrase anaphor interpretation can be developed. Models contain representations of entities, and it is to these represented entities that anaphoric noun phrases refer. However, it is only a framework that the theory provides. Detailed accounts of the psychological processes underlying anaphor resolution must be developed.

This account may need to drawn on the insights of linguistically oriented accounts, such as Centering Theory and account of the Accessibility Hierarchy. What is more important, however, in psycholinguistics is a detailed account of the underlying psychological processes. Thus, while we have criticized the details of Almor's Informational Load Hypothesis, we believe it is a good example of the kind of account, firmly based in basic psychological theorizing, that is needed in this domain.

Acknowledgements

Our research on the informational load hypothesis was supported by ESRC Grant R000239362 'Local focus and NP interpretation: Testing the informational load hypothesis' awarded to Alan Garnham.

References

Almor, Amit. 1999. Noun-phrase anaphora and focus: The informational load hypothesis. *Psychological Review* 106: 748–765.

Ariel, Mira. 1988. Referring and accessibility. *Journal of Linguistics* 24: 65–87.

Ariel, Mira. 1990. *Accessing Noun-Phrase Antecedents*. London: Routledge.

Baddeley, Alan D. 1966. Short-term memory for word sequences as a function of acoustic, semantic and formal similarity. *Quarterly Journal of Experimental Psychology* 18: 362–365.

Baddeley, Alan D. 1992. Working memory. *Science* 255: 556–559.

Baddeley, Alan D. and Graham J. Hitch. 1974. Working memory. In: G. H. Bower (ed.), *The Psychology of Learning and Motivation*, volume 8. New York: Academic Press, 47–90.

Bosch, Peter. 1983. *Agreement and Anaphora: A Study of the Role of Pronouns in Syntax and Discourse*. London: Academic Press.

Clark, Herbert H. 1977. Bridging. In: P. N. Johnson-Laird and P. C. Wason (eds.), *Thinking: Readings in Cognitive Science*. Cambridge: Cambridge University Press, 411–420.

Clark, Herbert H. and Susan E. Haviland. 1975. Comprehension and the given-new contract. In: R. Freedle (ed.), *Discourse Production and Comprehension*. Norwood, NJ: Ablex, 1–40.

Corbett, Albert T. and Frederick R. Chang. 1983. Pronoun disambiguation: Accessing potential antecedents. *Memory & Cognition* 11: 283–294.

Cornish, Francis. 1999. *Anaphora, Discourse, and Understanding: Evidence from English and French*. Oxford: Oxford University Press.

Cornish, Francis, Alan Garnham, H. Wind Cowles, Marion Fossard and Virginie Andre. 2005. Indirect anaphora in English and French: A cross-linguistic study of pronoun resolution. *Journal of Memory and Language* 52(3): 363–376.

Cowles, H. Wind and Alan Garnham. 2003a. Antecedent focus and conceptual distance in NP anaphor resolution. Poster presented at the 9th Annual Conference on Architectures and Mechanisms for Language Processing (AMLaP-2003).

Cowles, H. Wind and Alan Garnham. 2003b. Effects of antecedent focus, specificity, and adjective modification in NP anaphor resolution. Paper presented at the 16th Annual CUNY Conference on Human Sentence Processing.

Cowles, H. Wind and Alan Garnham. 2005. Antecedent focus and conceptual distance effects in category noun-phrase anaphora. *Language and Cognitive Processes* 20(6): 725–750.

Cowles, H. Wind and Alan Garnham. 2011. The role of focus, semantic overlap and discourse function in noun-phrase anaphor resolution. In: Edward Gibson and Neal J. Perlmutter (eds.), *The Processing and Acquisition of Reference*. Cambridge, MA: MIT Press.

Duffy, Susan A. and Keith Rayner. 1990. Eye movements and anaphor resolution: Effects of antecedent typicality and distance. *Language and Speech* 33: 103–119.

Fletcher, Charles R. 1984. Markedness and topic continuity in discourse processing. *Journal of Verbal Learning and Verbal Behavior* 23: 487–493.

Fox, Barbara A. 1984. Anaphora in popular written English narratives. In: R. S. Tomlin (ed.), *Coherence and Grounding in Discourse, Vol 11: Typological Studies in Language*. Amsterdam: Benjamins, 157–174.

Garnham, Alan. 1981. Mental models as representations of text. *Memory and Cognition* 9: 560–565.

Garnham, Alan. 1987. *Mental Models as Representations of Discourse and Text*. Chichester: Ellis Horwood.

Garrod, Simon C. and Anthony J. Sanford. 1977. Interpreting anaphoric relations: The integration of semantic information while reading. *Journal of Verbal Learning and Verbal Behavior* 16: 77–90.

Gompel, Roger P. G. Van, Simon P. Liversedge and Jamie Pearson. 2004. Antecedent typicality effects in the processing of noun phrase anaphors. In: M. Carreiras and C. Clifton Jr. (eds.), *The On-line Study of Sentence Comprehension: Eyetracking, ERP and Beyond*. Psychology Press, 119–137.

Gordon, Peter C., Barbara J. Grosz and Laura A. Gilliom. 1993. Pronouns, names, and the centering of attention in discourse. *Cognitive Science* 17: 311–347.

Gordon, Peter C. and Kimberly A. Scearce. 1995. Pronominalization and discourse coherence, discourse structure and pronoun interpretation. *Memory & Cognition* 23: 131–323.

Greene, Steven B., Gail McKoon and Roger Ratcliff. 1992. Pronoun resolution and discourse models. *Journal of Experimental Psychology: Learning Memory and Cognition* 18: 266–283.

Grosz, Barbara J. 1981. Focusing and description in natural language dialogs. In: A. Joshi, B. L. Webber and I. A. Sag (eds.), *Elements of Discourse Understanding*. Cambridge: Cambridge University Press, 84–105.

Grosz, Barbara J., Aravind Joshi and Scott Weinberg. 1995. Centering: A framework for modelling the local coherence of discourse. *Computational Linguistics* 21: 203–226.

Grosz, Barbara J. and Candace L. Sidner. 1986. Attention, intentions and the structure of discourse. *Computational Linguistics* 12: 175–204.

Gundel, Jeanette, Nancy Hedberg and Ron Zacharski. 1993. Cognitive status and the form of referring expressions in discourse. *Language* 69(2): 274–307.

Haarman, Henk and Marius Usher. 2001. Maintenance of semantic information in capacity-limited item short-term memory. *Psychonomic Bulletin & Review* 8: 568–578.

Haarmann, Henk J., Eddy J. Davelaar and Marius Usher. 2003. Individual differences in semantic short-term memory capacity and reading comprehension. *Journal of Memory and Language* 48: 320–345.

Johnson-Laird, Philip N. 1983. *Mental Models. Towards a Cognitive Science of Language, Inference, and Consciousness*. Cambridge, Mass.: Cambridge University Press.

Kiss, Katalin. 1998. Identificational focus versus informational focus. *Language* 74: 245–283.

Marslen-Wilson, William, Elena Levy and Lorraine K. Tyler. 1982. Producing interpretable discourse: The establishment and maintenance of reference. In: R.J. Jarvella and W. Klein (eds.), *Speech, Place and Action: Studies in Deixis and Related Topics*. Chichester: John Wiley, 339–378.

Myers, Jerome L., Anne E. Cook, Gretchen Kambe, Robert A. Mason and Edward J. O'Brien. 2000. Semantic and episodic effects on bridging inferences. *Discourse Processes* 29: 179–200.

Rayner, Keith, Gretchen Kambe and Susan A. Duffy. 2000. The effect of clause wrap-up on eye movements during reading. *The Quarterly Journal of Experimental Psychology* 53(A): 1061–1080.

Sanford, Anthony J. and Simon C. Garrod. 1981. *Understanding Written Language: Explorations in Comprehension Beyond the Sentence*. Chichester, West Sussex: John Wiley & Sons.

Sanford, Anthony J. and Simon C. Garrod. 1998. The role of scenario mapping in text comprehension. *Discourse Processes* 26: 159–190.

Sidner, Candace L. 1983. Focusing in comprehension of definite anaphora. In: M. Brady and R. C. Berwick (eds.), *Computational Models of Discourse*. Cambridge, MA: MIT Press, 267–330.

Vonk, Wietske, Lettica G. M. M. Hustinx and Wim H. G. Simons. 1992. The use of referential expressions in structuring discourse. *Language and Cognitive Processes* 7: 301–333.

Text comprehension as the interface between verbal structures and cognitive memory processes: The case of resolving direct and indirect anaphora

Monika Schwarz-Friesel

1 Introduction

Text comprehension can best be described as a complex cognitive process which is dependent on both the surface structure of the text and on the mental activity of the reader. By using different kinds of information from long-term memory in a highly flexible way, the reader is able to construct a text-world model in working memory. The text-world model of a specific text is based on the information of the text itself but elaborated by the readers cognitive processing in order to get to a coherent mental representation. Using data from natural texts dealing with underspecified verbal structures involving anaphoric expressions of different kinds, it is illustrated that the resolution of many direct anaphors often involves much more than a simple search-and-match-procedure and that the comprehension of indirect anaphors may involve more cognitive processing than merely activating an appropriate script from long-term memory. Besides, it is argued, that the traditional view of anaphora as a means of referential continuity with topical function and the availability of given information has to be revised. Taking a procedural perspective concerning the thematic development and information distribution in text, I will show that both direct and indirect anaphors may add new information to the mental files of the referents in the text-world model. Furthermore, a proposal for the general treatment of these textual phenomena is presented within a cognitive theory of coherence. The principle of conceptual plausibility will be shown to be the dominant constraint which determines the reconstruction of coherence within which resolving anaphors occurs. In this respect, explaining coherence means at the same time finding an explanation for the interaction between language structures and memory processes within the exemplary realm of text comprehension.

2 Text, mind, and world: basic assumptions about text comprehension

A text consists of linguistic information which refers to a non-linguistic (part of the) world. It depends on the text function whether the reference is to the real world or some kind of fictional, imaginative or otherwise mental world. *Text* is used here in a textlinguistic sense of a complex (written) linguistic structure which performs a communicative function and which consists of at least two sentences. Although a text can consist of one sentence or just one word, this definition of text is chosen because there is no cohesion and/or coherence in a word. Connective ties of interest for text linguistics are to be found only in utterances longer than one sentence.

To fully understand a text, a reader must integrate information in one sentence with information in another. And explaining how people do so, is one of the main tasks of modern text linguistics. On the grammatical surface of the text particular expressions serve as cohesive ties to relate different parts of the text: The sentences of the text are usually (either explicitly and/or implicitly) connected with each other. These connective relations tie together the referents, events, and so on, that are described in the text. The text, as a consequence, is perceived as a coherent structure, rather than as an assembly of disjointed referential information.

One of the central assumptions in modern text linguistics, however, is that the explicit grammatical structure of the text is to be regarded as just one part or level of textual coherence. Accordingly, recent developments in text research suggest that the implicit conceptual relations in text are of vital importance and deserve particular attention (cf. Gernsbacher and Givon, 1995; Bublitz et al., 1999; Spooren, 1999; Sanders and Spooren, 2001). At the same time, many researchers have realized that no serious analysis of coherence can be carried out without appealing to its cognitive aspects (cf. Hobbs, 1979; Dahl, 1995; Sanford and Moxey, 1995; Cornish, 1999; Schwarz, 2000a; Zelinsky-Wibbelt, 2003).

This position, however, should not lead to the assumption that coherence is some non-textual phenomenon explainable solely in cognitive terms. Although coherence can best be described as conceptual linkage, as relations between the states of affairs which are expressed in the text, this should not lead to the conclusion that coherence is "not an inherent property of a... text" (Gernsbacher and Givon 1995, vi; for a similar view see Bublitz et al. 1999, 1).

Conceptual linkage is dependent on surface structure and in this respect bound to the explicit information given in the text. It is the surface structure which helps to activate semantic and conceptual representations and to stimulate building up a mental model of the state-of-affairs.

In order to fully describe and explain coherence as part of the comprehension process, three different levels of textual representation have to be distinguished, as is illustrated in the model below (for similar conceptions of multiple text representations see Dijk and Kintsch, 1983; Kamp and Reyle, 1993; Fauconnier, 1994; Kintsch, 1998).

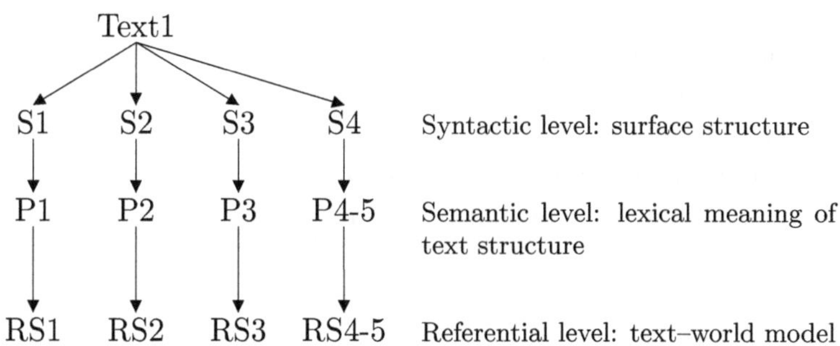

Figure 1. Levels of text representation

The surface structure of a text1 involves the sentences S1, S2 etc. with their grammatical structure (and sometimes with cohesive ties). At this level we find the representation of the exact linguistic material in the text. Second, there is the semantic representation which can best be described as a set of propositions P1, P2 etc. These representations form the lexical meaning of the text and are based on the explicit information of the surface structure. The semantic form is compositionally derivable from the lexical means of the sentences. The propositions depict referential state-of-affairs. These referential states-of-affairs (RS1, RS2 etc.) can be described in terms of conceptual constellations which form the text-world model of the text including all participating referents, their relations among each other and the events and situations in which they are performing.

There is no isomorphic relation between the informational representations of the three levels: a complex sentence may include several propositions (as depicted in the model by S4), and a proposition may refer to a more elaborated conceptual representation (within the text-world model). In most cases, thus, texts do not give us enough information on surface structure to build up an appropriate text-world model, since they are underspecified (cf. Spooren, 1997; Schwarz, 2000a; Carston, 2002). A text T is referentially underspecified if there is either no explicit link between the propositions P1 and P2 etc. of the sentences S1 and S2 etc. and/or the syntactically bound meaning representation does not provide the specific referential values which belong to the complete conceptual representation of the RS1 and RS2 etc.

In example (1), the vehicles involved in the accidents are not mentioned. In order to establish the full conceptual representation of the text structure, the reader has to activate knowledge of the world and insert the appropriate referents into the mental text model (the capital letters indicate conceptual information which does not occur explicitly in the text).

(1) *Wegen Glatteis musste die Zoobrücke...vorübergehend gesperrt werden. Auf spiegelglatter Fahrbahn hatten sich...mehrere Unfälle* (MIT FAHRZEUGEN) *ereignet. Dabei entstand Blechschaden.* (Kölner Stadtanzeiger (KSTA) 54, 4.3.96, 10)
"The Zoo-Bridge-road had to be closed down because of slippery ice. Several accidents (WITH VEHICLES) had caused a lot of damage."

Thus, the reader will elaborate the semantic form by a slot-filling activity with a referential default value such as VEHICLES. The result of such an activation is quite predictable because it is based on common and shared default assumptions which are part of our conceptual knowledge in long-term memory. No reader of (1) would make an elaboration filling the referential slot with BOOKS or KEYS. Completing the propositional form in order to get to the underlying referential representation becomes necessary quite frequently and often involves some kind of semantic-thematic decomposition as can be seen in (2):

(2) *She dug a hole into the frozen ground.*

In order to get to the complete conceptual representation, some slot-filling or referent-recreating operation involving WITH AN INSTRUMENT, TYPICALLY A SHOVEL has to be performed (see Singer 1994; Broek 1994, for a detailed discussion of the procedural aspects of these elaborations). In (3) it can be seen that these default elaborations play an important role in establishing and accepting coherence:

(3) *She opened the door reluctantly.*

a. *When she turned the key...* /

b. ?? *When she turned the spoon...* /

c. ?? *When she turned the shovel...*

The continuation with *key* in (a) is accepted as coherent without any cognitive effort, whereas in (b) and (c) the reader would have to make an extra inference to establish some kind of (strange or unusual) continuity relation.

Another type of underspecification can be seen in (4): text-internally expressed actions or events are not always linked together by explicit means which indicate a continuity (e.g. in the sense of causality; see for causal relations in text Keenan et al., 1984; Dahl, 1995; Noordman and Vonk, 1998):

(4) *I was stuck in traffic for almost two hours.* (BECAUSE OF MY BEING LATE) *My boss was mad as hell and threw a book at me* (WHEN I ARRIVED AT WORK).

Although the two events described in (4) are not connected in any way at the surface structure, the reader relates them conceptually in the sense that the first event is the cause of the second event. Furthermore, the reader will establish a text-world model for the first sentence which includes the conceptual representation (IN TRAFFIC: IN A VEHICLE ON A ROAD).

Underspecification is an essential feature of the relation between verbal expressions and the conceptual representations they are intended to express. Therefore, underspecification and implicitness in text should by no means be regarded as some kind of textual deviance (as it is implied in many accounts). On the contrary, systematic underspecification is to be regarded as default. It is the result of applying the principle of relevance to the production process by leaving out superfluous information (see Sperber and Wilson, 1992). In accordance with some principle of cognitive economy, underspecification is achieved by selecting only the really relevant information and thereby avoiding redundancy (Schwarz 2000a, 83, Sanders and Spooren 2001, 4).

In order to complete the semantic form of the text, the reader automatically assigns a mental text-world model to the surface structure, which incorporates both information from the text and information activated through conceptual instantiation and inferential processing. Thus, the text-world model represents a referential constellation of states-of-affairs in working and in episodic memory which is (in most cases) more complex and elaborated than the semantic text basis. From a procedural perspective, semantic enrichment and conceptual elaboration (as part of text world model building) occur spontaneously and have to be considered as part of our textual competence. The readers' elaborative capacity is based on their memory structures and the ability to activate parts of these knowledge structures or to draw inferences.

Hence, text comprehension implies both decoding the surface structure of the text and at the same time constructing a mental text-world model which is a cognitive conceptualisation of the world depicted in the text. The term *text-world model* refers to the assumption that readers create a mental model of the world described in a specific text and store it in episodic memory.

The general idea behind this is that verbal expressions serve as mental processing instructions for the reader (Givon, 1992, 1995; Fauconnier, 1994). As already pointed out, the text-world model of a text is based on the information of the text itself but elaborated by the readers' cognitive processing. It is the result of applying knowledge representations to the text base. Building up a text-world model is an automatic process which always takes place in the comprehension process (for slightly different conceptions of text-worlds or mental models see Beaugrande and Dressler, 1981; Dijk and Kintsch, 1983; Johnson-Laird, 1983; Garnham and Oakhill, 1992; Givon, 1995; Cornish, 1999).

The text-world model, however, does not include a representation of the speaker`s hypothesized communicative goals, as Cornish (2002) has postulated it for his mental discourse model, since to my view the mental reconstruction of such goals is not part of the model of conceptual continuity. This belongs to the interpretation process beyond the establishment of coherence (see Schwarz, 2001a, 20f.). The ability to establish coherence is part of our textual competence based on both our linguistic and conceptual knowledge and is not to be equated with the process or result of general text interpretation. Every text can be interpreted with some kind of cognitive effort, even if it is a non-coherent text. Hence, the set of coherent texts is not identical with the set of interpretable texts. The task of text linguistics, however, is to describe and explain the constraints and principles which govern conceptual continuity and help to distinguish between coherent and non-coherent texts (see Reinhart, 1980; Schwarz-Friesel, 2006, for a more detailed account of this).

Once a text-world model has been developed during reading, all subsequently encoded information will be integrated into the configurations of the model. These configurations or mental files, which are stored in working memory, are constantly being updated as the reading process progresses. For instance, the conceptual file of the text referent introduced in the first sentence of (5) includes the information (YOUNG MAN IN COLOGNE) in short-term memory.

(5) *Köln. Ein junger Mann wurde gestern Abend Opfer eines brutalen Überfalls. Als der 25jährige Vizedirektor des Kaufparks in Nippes die Tür öffnete...Joachim H. sah plötzlich eine Kanone vor seinen Augen...Der Vater von 2 kleinen Kindern...*(KSTA, 11.3.04)
"Cologne. A young man has been brutally assaulted yesterday evening. When the 25-year-old assistant director of the shopping center in Nippes opened the door. . . .Joachim H. saw a gun right before his eyes. . . The father of 2 little kids. . .)"

With each sentence new information is added to the conceptual knot (which functions as a file address in working memory), and the end result of the referential movement is a file which includes the following information: (YOUNG MAN JOACHIM H. IS 25-YEARS-OLD, HAS 2 LITTLE CHILDREN AND WORKS IN COLOGNE AS ASSISTANT DIRECTOR).

3 Coherence and the principle of plausibility: building up conceptual continuity within text-world models

It is a common assumption in all cognitive sciences, that conceptual representations of the world are stored in long-term memory which function as background knowledge for all kinds of mental tasks people have to perform in daily life. Many cognitive accounts and empirical investigations have shown the influence of complex mental schemata on text comprehension, too (Sanford and Garrod, 1981; Brown and Yule, 1983; Singer, 1990; Sanford and Garrod, 1994a,b; Kintsch, 1998, cf.). Formally, frames and scripts can best be described as conceptual networks representing referential information as knots which are linked to each other by different kinds of relations (e.g. part-of, attribute-of, location-of etc.). Information stored in frame-structures is taken to be prototypical knowledge of the world. These prototypical constellations of states-of-affairs are taken as default cases which serve as an orientation system that governs the evaluation process concerning the normality of a state-of-affairs. For instance, the knowledge stored with the expression *zoo* includes (A

ZOO IS A PLACE WHERE YOU CAN SEE ALL KINDS OF ANIMALS), but it does not include (IS A PLACE WHERE TEACHERS GIVE TALKS TO STUDENTS). Reading the word *zoo*, thus, triggers certain predictable expectations.

These general kinds of knowledge frames regarding predictable co-occurrences of entities in text supply the grounds for the accessibility of text referents: after a previous linguistic mention of *zoo*, the speaker can immediately talk of *the lions, the fences*, and so on. Accordingly, having read *restaurant* the reader is not surprised to encounter the definite NPs *the waiter, the cook, the food.* All members of the linguistic community know that the set of things which make up a restaurant typically include these (see Hawkins 1991, 409, Givon 1992, 32, Barsalou 1992, 21f.).

Thus, reading a text always involves a matching-process in which the constellations described by the explicit information of the text are compared with the prototypical mental world constellations. In (6) this matching process results in finding a plausible continuity relation, whereas in (7) the reader finds himself confronted with a state-of-affairs which does not fall into the category of "normality". Hence, applying the principle of plausibility in the matching process to (7) leads to the conclusion that (7) is neither coherent nor makes any sense.

(6) *The man went to the shop. He wanted to buy some flowers for his wife.*

(7) *The lion went to the flower. The waitress wanted to discuss atomic energy with the chicken.*

Coherence in text may be expressed explicitly or implicitly. (8) is an example of a text in which the sentences are both connected by cohesive ties and at the same time are conceptually related.

(8) *A man arrived at the station in the middle of the night. He was tired and hungry. The man looked around. He wanted to order some good food. But he couldn't find any restaurant.*

The anaphoric expressions indicate referential identity which is an important form of continuity. Further continuity relations are, for instance, causality, identity of time and place, identity of goals and motivations, global themes, results etc. (see Hobbs, 1979, 1983; Broek, 1994; Hellmann, 1995; Dahl, 1995; Zelinsky-Wibbelt, 2000). Following Sanders et al., it should be pointed out that the concept of conceptual continuity does not only take into account the semantic and referential source of coherence relations but also pragmatic and general encyclopaedic knowledge (cf. Sanders et al., 1992; Sanders and Spooren, 1999, 2001).

In many accounts, the direct form of anaphoric reference has been described as the fundamental referential means which serves to facilitate text comprehension, since there is a direct linking of the anaphor to its antecedent. Considering (9), however, we see a text which is perfectly coherent, although it lacks explicit cohesive means:

(9) *The man arrived at the station in the middle of the night. The clock stroke midnight. The train had been two hours late. The shops were all closed and there was no taxi available on the street.*

Cohesion, then, is not a necessary condition for a text to be coherent (see Lundquist, 1985; Hellmann, 1995; Cornish, 1999; Schwarz, 2001b,a).

According to many linguists, texts which are implicitly coherent have a special status among the class of coherent texts in the sense that the recipient has to apply special procedures in order to impose coherence (see, for instance Reinhart, 1980, 163). I do not conform to this assumption: Readers accept and understand texts implicitly connected with the same ease as texts explicitly connected.

The missing overt connectedness is made up by a plausible conceptual interrelationship between the events described in the sentences. The states-of-affairs described in the text are compatible with the readers' mental representations in memory. Hence, there is a plausibility assumption leading the comprehension process which plays an important role in establishing coherence.

Further, there need not be a local coherence relation between each adjacent pair of sentences if a common conceptual integrator exists. Considering the case of global coherence in text, a common theme or connector may integrate seemingly disconnected events into a continuity relation, as in (10):

(10) *Children were yelling on the street. A dog was barking furiously. The radio of my neighbour was playing. Two men were engaged in a discussion on taxes. I could not stand this noise any longer.*

The different events described in the four sentences are summarized and taken up by the complex anaphor *this noise* which at the same time creates a conceptual knot in text-world model representing an abstract referent of a higher semantic level (see section 5.1 for complex anaphors; for other cases of global coherence see Schwarz-Friesel 2006).

In (11) no conceptual relationship can be seen, although we find cohesive means on the surface structure. There is no compatibility found by using a matching process in which the semantic representations of the sentences are mapped into an appropriate world-model.

(11) *A man crossed the street. His dad danced with the pink journal on the moon. Hence, linguistics will be interesting.*

Therefore, it is difficult if not impossible for the reader to establish plausible conceptual relations between the sentences. Only by applying several interpretive inferences one might get to some overall sense of (11). Without any other information (stimulated, for instance, by the fact that the sentences are part of a science-fiction-novel or a modern fairy tale) which could help as a clue to integrate the seemingly absurd events described into some kind of a text-world-model, this task, however, will turn out to be quite difficult.

Conceptual plausibility is more dominant than cohesion and may even overrule the function of cohesive ties as it is illustrated in (12) and (13):

(12) *Evyatar has been ill. He could not go to the exams.*

(13) ?? *Evyatar has been ill. Therefore, he is extremely happy.*

Even though a connector links the state-of-affairs described in (13), the reader will find the causality relation expressed highly unlikely since there is no plausible congruence between the causal continuity in the text and the default causal continuities found in or inferred from memory. In (12), there is no explicit connector expressing causality, yet the reader will find it easy and highly plausible to relate the events.

A text, then, is considered to be coherent if its state-of-affairs representation in short-term or working memory is congruent or matching with any plausible continuity constellation derivable from the readers long-term memory representations. In this respect, explaining coherence means at the same time finding an explanation for the interaction between language structures and cognitive structures in text comprehension.

Thus, conceptual plausibility which is fundamentally grounded on prototypical world knowledge stored in long-term memory, is the most dominant principle in establishing continuity in text. This principle of plausibility should be understood as some kind of preference rule: If there is no information to the contrary, the default values of the world model in long-term memory are to be taken as standard in understanding the states-of-affairs in text.

Plausibility, however, is dependent on the specific text-world model of the text. What is considered normal varies with the text at hand. Conceptual plausibility, thus, is also governed by the global pattern of the mental text-world in working memory and its specific ontology with which the reader finds himself confronted and which functions as the overall framework in which he/she has to incorporate all further information. The complexity of the problem stands out much more clearly when looking at real texts rather than constructed examples.

(14) is an example of a text sequence in which the state-of-affairs described is not compatible with our model about the real world but it is perfectly reasonable within the text-world model.

(14) *After a while she remembered that she still held the pieces of mushroom in her hands, and she set to work very carefully, nibbling first at one and then at the other,... until she had succeeded in bringing herself down to her usual height.* (L. Carroll, Alice in Wonderland, 47)

The event described in the first clause is interpreted as the cause of the event in the second clause. The causal relation between eating from a mushroom and changing ones height is plausible only because it can be incorporated in the pre-established conceptual representation of the states-of-affairs of the fictional text-world. Similar examples can be found in other fairy tales. For instance, within the text-world model of the fairy tale "Das Feuerzeug" by H.C. Anderson we accept the otherwise highly unusual causal relation between the event of lighting a fire and the appearance of three dogs (see Schwarz, 2001a, for a more detailed discussion of these examples). The comprehension of the following joke illustrates very nicely the dependency of establishing conceptual continuity in the ontology of the specific text-world.

(15) *Ein Snob ist auf Kreuzfahrt den Nil herunter. Das Schiff kentert. Sofort kommen einige Krokodile angeschwommen. "Oh, wie edel", ruft er entzückt, "sogar die Rettungsboote sind von Lacoste."* (Bäckerblume 9, 1995, 6)
"A snob is on a cruise on the Nile. The boat capsizes. Within a second, some crocodiles get near the boat. 'Oh, how noble', the snob shouts delightedly, 'even the lifeboats are made by Lacoste.' "

In this example we find a very specific and highly unusual kind of referential identity, namely that between crocodiles and lifeboats. This specific identity which exists only in the perspective of the snob is established uniquely within the internal text-world model of the text at hand. In this perspective, *some crocodiles* serves as antecedent and *the lifeboats* as anaphor establishing coreference. The acceptance of this coreference (which is usually regarded as bizarre) is dependent on how the reader is able, on the basis of his knowledge on text functions and types (in particular jokes) and his encyclopaedic knowledge on the crocodile-label from Lacoste, to accept the relationship within the cognitive state of the text-world. Building up coherence and, at the same time, understanding the joke is building up a text-world model representing the entities on two different conceptual level: on the normal, ontological level in which there is no identity between boats and crocodiles and on the level of text-world-model including the mental perspective of the snob in which there is identity between the different entities.

4 Mental accessibility of referents and information distribution in text: a cognitive conception of the given-new-distinction

One of the most important aspects of explaining coherence in text involves the division between old (or given) and new information. Different cognitive accounts concerning the information distribution and thematic development, have been proposed in the last years (cf. Prince, 1981; Grosz, 1981; Givon, 1992; Gordon et al., 1993; Chafe, 1994; Lambrecht, 1994). *Old* or *given* information refers to entities assumed to be accessible in text/discourse, new information refers to entities to be assumed inaccessible to the reader. Usually, definite referential expressions indicate given information and topic continuity, whereas indefinite expressions are taken as labels for new information.

Concern with the resolution of (definite) referential expressions which connect sentences and serve as signals for topic continuity leads to the question how readers access and recover the referents of these expressions in text comprehension and what information has to be available in order to establish continuity.

The notion of accessibility is of particular interest here. This notion refers to the degree of activation of information in long or short-term memory (see Givon, 1995, on grounding). It is assumed that highly accessible mental entities (those which are most active in consciousness) require less processing effort to be retrieved than do entities of low accessibility (cf. Gundel et al., 1993; Ariel, 1988; Gundel, 1996). Ariel (1990, 22ff.) mentions four factors that affect accessibility: recency of mention (the more recent the last mention of an entity, the more accessible it will be); saliency (either physical or textual salience); competition (salience of an entity compared to other entities of the same type that may also be present in the context); unity (whether an antecedent is within the same paragraph or point of view as an anaphor). One of the main functions of referring expressions is to indicate the degree of accessibility of the mental representations of their referents in a given context (Ariel 1990, 16; Heusinger for formal aspects of accessibility theory see 2000, 2003). Accessibility theory has generally treated accessible text referents as mental entities that are retrievable from memory. In this sense, accessible referents constitute given information.

Linking accessibility and givenness within the account of our text-world model proposal, referential movement in text comprehension can best be described as a sequence of the following three transitional states: Activation, re-activation and de-activation (see Givon, 1992; Chafe, 1994); similar states have been postulated by centering theory, i.e. continuing, retaining and shifting; (cf. Grosz, 1981; Gordon et al., 1993; Maes, 1997).

Activation of a text referent takes place when a new mental file (formally represented as a knot in a network) is opened. The referent is activated and stored as a conceptual label, and incoming information about the same referent may be filed under this label. This process is to be characterised as reactivation, since the already established knot in the text-world model is called up again in short-term or in working memory. If a new referent is mentioned in the text, the referent in current focus is de-activated while at the same time a file for the new referent is opened and stored as an additional conceptual knot in the text-world model. In this regard, *given* means that the referent is mentally accessible in text-world model, *new* means that this is not the case. This can be illustrated with the following example from a newspaper text (concentrating on the protagonist entity):

(16) *Ein qualmender Hinterreifen hat sich in der Nacht zum Donnerstag als verräterisch für eine angetrunkene Autofahrerin* (AKTIVIERUNG) *erwiesen. Die 37-jährige Frau* (REAKTIVIERUNG) *hatte auf der Fahrt von Erfurt nach Elxleben Brandgeruch bemerkt, gestoppt und das Auto in Augenschein genommen. Ein Mann* (DEAKTIVIERUNG UND GLEICHZEITIG AKTIVIERUNG EINES NEUEN REFERENZKNOTENS), *dem dies aufge-*

fallen war, alarmierte die Polizei. (TLZ 4, 2003)
"A burning tyre has been treacherous for a drunken car driver (activation). The 37-years-old woman (reactivation) noticed smoke and stopped to check the car. A man (de-activation and activation of new referential file) who had observed this, called the police."

The distributive flow of information in text comprehension, then, is to be described as an interplay of retaining continuity and moving/progressive development. Traditionally, definite NPs serving as anaphors are regarded as the main grammatical means to indicate continuity by referring to accessible, given entities. In the following section, however, I shall present a number of definite anaphoric NPs whose referents are seen as accessible even though they would procedurally be viewed as constituting new instead of given information.

5 The case of resolving direct and indirect anaphora: conceptual continuity and "given-new-entities" within referential development

5.1 Anaphora in text

The traditional view in text linguistics has been that anaphora are used to continue a pre-established reference in text, that they point back to a specific antecedent, usually an NP already introduced, and thereby sustain the current focus. Their main function is topic continuity: "The anaphoric procedure is a linguistic instrument for having the hearer continue (sustain) a previously established focus." (Ehlich 1982; see also Clark 1978; Murphy 1985; Carter 1987; Bosch 1988; Givon 1992). In this respect, "anaphoric elements tell the reader where to search for the topic in the existing storage structure of episodic memory" (Givon, 1992, 5). Hence, the classical and prototypical anaphoric case can be seen in example (17):

(17) *A man* (referent 1_1) *entered the room. He/The man* (referent 2_1) *looked around.*

The referential relationship between anaphor and antecedent is based on coreference (indicated by the subscript), and the link between the expressions denoting coreference can be described in terms of grammatical congruence and semantic compatibility. In this respect, anaphors have been described as retrieval cues or echoes of their antecedents (Hintzman 1987, 412; Gernsbacher 1989, 100). According to this view, anaphor resolution is seen as some kind of search procedure which aims at discovering the best matching antecedent in textual structure.

This mental checking in resolving anaphors in text comprehension always leads to the conclusion that R(EFERENT)2 IS IDENTICAL WITH R(EFERENT)1. Our distinction between referent 1 (the text referent first encountered in reading) and referent 2 (and accordingly, referent 3 etc. in longer reference chains) takes into account that in on-line processing the reader must decide in each case of definite reference whether there is referential identity or not. Considering (18), one can see that referent 2 in (a) is identical with referent 1, whereas in (b) this is not the case.

(18) a. *Klaus K.* ($R1_1$) *hat seine Frau umgebracht. Der Mann* ($R2_1$) *kennt keine Skrupel.*
"Klaus K. ($R1_1$) murdered his wife. The man ($R2_1$) is quite unscrupulous."

b. *Klaus K.* ($R1_1$) *hat seine Frau umgebracht.. Der Mann* ($R2_2$), *der gegenüber wohnt, hat alles beobachtet.*
"Klaus K. ($R1_1$) murdered his wife. The man ($R2_2$) who lives across the street, saw everything."

Anaphors which establish topic continuity by merely reactivating the information knot of their antecedent involve pronouns, NPs with the same head noun, hyperonyms, synonyms and certain general expressions. The analysis of anaphors, however, calls for a more flexible description. Establishing the relationship of identity (R2 IS IDENTICAL WITH R1) which is necessary for successful anaphoric processing, very often demands more than just checking semantic compatibility. Reference chains in natural language texts reveal a lot more types of anaphora which do not fall into the category "echo of their antecedent". The establishment of co-reference and continuity relies much more both on the context and constructive mental activity of the reader than on the grammatical devices in the text.

We are going to discuss now a number of anaphora with explicit antecedents which do not only reactivate old files in text-world model constellations, but activate at the same time new information about the referent in focus. It should be noted that these types of anaphors occur quite frequently in natural language texts and are by no means to be evaluated as some kind of textual deviance.

To illustrate these *progressive* or *moving anaphors*, consider example (19) which depicts specifying anaphors ("Spezifikationsanaphern" in German). I am concentrating on the referential chain for the protagonist referential entity in focus and leave out all the other entities mentioned in the text.

(19) *Ein qualmender Hinterreifen hat sich in der Nacht zum Donnerstag als verräterisch für eine angetrunkene Autofahrerin erwiesen. Die 37-jährige Frau hatte auf der Fahrt von Erfurt nach Elxleben Brandgeruch bemerkt, gestoppt und das Auto in Augenschein genommen. Ein Mann, dem dies aufgefallen war, alarmierte die Polizei. Die Blutprobe ließ die Beamten staunen: Die Mutter von 3 Kindern hatte 3,16 Promille intus. Den Führerschein musste die Verkehrssünderin abliefern.* (TLZ 4, 2003)

"A burning has been treacherous for a drunken car driver (activation of R1). The 37-years-old woman (R2 is identical with R1: reactivation and specification of R1 by activation) noticed smoke and stopped to check the car. A man who had observed this, called the police....The mother of 3 children (R3 is identical with R1: reactivation and further specification of R1 by activation) had a lot of blood alcohol. The traffic offender (R4 is identical with R1: reactivation and specifying evaluation of R1) had to submit her drivers' licence."

In (19), the anaphoric expressions are much more than a mere semantic echo of their antecedent. Several new information chunks are filed successively in the same conceptual node. Hence, continued elaboration through activation processes of the current open file is the case. In on-line comprehension, specifying anaphors include both reactivation and activation in working memory. In cognitive terms, their informational status is both given and new, since the text-world model constellation changes (see example (5) for a similar case; see as well Schwarz 2000b).

Further, anaphors (with explicit antecedents) may not only introduce new information about the textual referent, they may even trigger new referents into the text-world model. Examples (20) and (21) show that referents can change dramatically in the course of time (or more precisely in the text world; cf. Stenning 1992).

(20) *Johannes hat sein altes Auto endlich doch noch zum Schrottplatz gebracht. Als er dann aber später das zusammengepresste Eisenpaket sah, wurde ihm weh um's Herz.*
"John brought his old car (R1) to the scrap yard. But when later he saw the little iron package (R2=CHANGED R1), he felt very bad."

(21) *Ich muss wohl zwei oder drei Raupen aushalten, wenn ich die Schmetterlinge kennen lernen will.* (Saint-Exupery, Der kleine Prinz, Dt. Übersetzung, 26)
"Well, I have to cope with two or three caterpillars (R1), if I want to see the butterflies (R2=FUTURE R1)."

To identify and retrieve the matching antecedent in (20) means to realize that (R2 IS IDENTICAL WITH R1, BUT R1 HAS CHANGED DRASTICALLY), in (21) (R2 IS IDENTICAL WITH R1, BUT R1 WILL HAVE CHANGED DRASTICALLY). In both examples, the anaphor contains new information about the referent. In fact, in both examples the anaphoric expression refers to an entity with a different ontological status than that of the antecedent referent. The reader has to infer that some change has taken place (in 20) or, as in (21), will take place in order to interpret the anaphor properly and thus get to a coherent representation.

In both cases, the semantic representation of the text and the conceptual representation of the text-world model is a completely different one if we use pronouns as anaphors instead of the definite NPs. This is to be seen as a clear grammatical hint that (although there is a co-reference relation) in the text-world model two nodes (linked by the relation IS IDENTICAL WITH) have been established.

In accordance with our conception of coherence, felicity of all those anaphors depends crucially on the plausibility criterion which is dependent both on long-term memory knowledge and on the text-world model at hand. This is quite evident in (22):

(22) *John brought his old car, which had served him well for many years, to the scrap yard. But when he later saw the little iron package #the cheese/#the flower/#the dog/#/the ice cream, he felt very bad.*

On the basis of world knowledge (ON SCRAP YARDS, CARS ARE SOMETIMES PRESSED INTO IRON PACKAGES), the definite NP *the iron package* is regarded as an anaphoric device although the anaphor and the antecedent *car* are not semantically equivalent or compatible. Drawing the plausible inference, however, that the car has been crushed by a steel press, continuity and co-reference can be established. Obviously, this does not work with definite NPs (as indicated by the #) whose referents do not fit into the text-world model constellation.

In (23) and (24) we see *combining anaphors* ("Kombinationsanaphern" in German) combing mixable entities into a new referent with different ontological status (for similar examples see Brown and Yule, 1983; Stenning, 1992; Freitas and Lopes, 1996).

(23) *Das Pulver* $(R1)_1$ *in das Wasser* $(R2)_2$ *einrühren. Die Lösung* $(R3)_3$ *in einem Zug trinken, denn sie* $(R3)_3$ *schmeckt scheußlich.* "Mix the powder $(R1)_1$ with the water $(R2)_2$ and stir well. Drink the solution $(R3)_{1+2=3}$ in one go. It (R3) has a nasty taste."

(24) *Butter und Mehl gut verrühren, bis keine Klümpchen mehr da sind. Milch dazugeben. Die Mehlschwitze dann in eine Schüssel schütten.*
"Stir butter $(R1)_1$ and flour $(R2)_2$, until there are no more lumps. Add some milk $(R3)_3$. Pour the/this mixture $(R4)_{1+2+3=4}$ into a bowl."

A new text referent (*solution* in (23) and *mixture* in (24)) is created on the basis of old information. In contrast to (20) and (21) where we already have individual entities as referents which are coded by the anaphors as transformed entities, and the reader has to mentally reconstruct this transformation, in (23 and 24) the new referent comes out as the result of a process which is presented before the very eyes of the reader. In both cases, resolving the anaphors means activating a new file for a new referent in the text-world model. If the anaphors were replaced by a pronoun, the result would be awkward.

Turning to *complex anaphors*, now, referent-creating mechanisms can be seen, as well.

(25) *Am Donnerstag stürzte in H. ein Einfamilienhaus in sich zusammen* (RS1). DAS EREIGNIS ($R2_{RS}$) *geschah in den frühen Morgenstunden ... Das Unglück* ($R3_{RS}$) *veränderte das Leben aller Bewohner. Es* ($R3_{RS}$) ... (TLZ, 2003)
"Thursday, a house broke down in H. (RS1). The incident ($R2_{RS}$) happened in the early morning. The disaster ($R3_{RS}$) affected the life of all inhabitants."

(26) *Mein zweites Zeugnis war bereits von mehreren genügend verunstaltet* (RS1)....*So geht das nicht, kommentierte mein Großvater die Misere* ($R2_{RS}$). (Bernhard, Ein Kind, 95)
"My school report included some bad marks (RS1)...This is not be accepted, was my grandfathers remark about this plight ($R2_{RS}$)." (Note that in German the definite article is used.)

In both examples, it is not a single word or phrase functioning as antecedent, but a clause or several clauses (see Halliday and Hasan 1976 for "extended reference" and "reference to fact", Fraurud 1992, Dahl and Hellmann 1995 for "situational anaphora", Asher 1993 for "abstract object anaphora", Francis 1986 for "labelling", Webber 1991 for "discourse deixis"; Conte 1996).

Accordingly, the referential status is described by RS (indicating that it is a referential state-of-affair and not an individual). Referents of the anaphoric NPs, then, are not individual entities (although coded by an NP) but second-order or third-order entities (see Lyons, 1989, for aspects of semantic ascent) like states-of affair, facts, events or propositions (indicated by R_{RS}). A higher level in the semantic hierarchy of the text is produced. Functioning as a paraphrase for a preceding part in the text, a hypostatisation takes place denoted by the anaphoric expression. On the basis of old information, a new referent is created in the dynamics of the text. In other words, the anaphoric NP establishes a node for the contents of the proposition. Further, complex anaphors do not only include a categorisation (e.g. *the incident*) but also very often give an evaluation of the contents of the preceding co-text (e.g. *the tragedy*). Hence, two main functions can be made out: Complex anaphors give a classification (in the sense ($X \leftarrow Y$); this Event is A Disaster) and a new conceptual file node (DISASTER) is established in the text-world model. In cognitive terms of the given-new-distinction, both reactivation and activation takes place at the same time (for further discussion of complex anaphors see Schwarz-Friesel et al., 2004).

So far we have seen, that in many cases the processing of anaphoric devices is not only constrained by their lexical content, but strongly by the activation of conceptual knowledge representations and the performance of referent-creating operations. Besides, the examples discussed show that the resolution of many direct anaphors involves much more than a simple search-and-match-procedure. Their full interpretation requires a more complex cognitive process. Resolving anaphors with the strategy (R2 IS IDENTICAL WITH R1) may involve specification, combination, classification, and/or evaluation mechanisms. From a procedural perspective, many anaphors combine given and new information for the reader, and therefore can be characterized as given-and-new-entities in the text.

5.2 *Indirect Anaphora: combining activation and re-activation in referential assignment*

That definite NPs may introduce new referents into the text-world model and at the same time signal topic continuity, can be most clearly illustrated with the phenomenon of indirect anaphora. Corpus-based and text-linguistic studies have shown that definite NPs commonly occur as *indirect anaphors*, that is without explicit antecedents in text or discourse (Schwarz 2000a; Consten 2004, see for a detailed account of indirect anaphora as a form of domain-bound reference.) The passage in (27) is perfectly coherent although there is no textual antecedent for the definite NP *the tyres.*

(27) *The car was found in the ditch. The tyres were punched.*

Indirect anaphora fall under the heading of anaphora because the interpretation of the definite NPs depends on the existence of an adequate textual element in the preceding text (as in (27) where *car* functions as anchor). Further, they establish referential continuity just like direct anaphora. Adopting the terminology of Fraurud (1990, 1992), we will call such elements *anchors* and the process of linking indirect anaphors to these expressions *anchoring* (Hawkins 1978 calls them "trigger" and Cornish 1999 "antecedent trigger").

In text comprehension, the resolution of indirect anaphors confronts the cognitive system of the reader with the problem of identifying and localizing the referent to which the definite description refers in the text. The definite article signals accessibility of the referent, but in the text structure no such referent can be found. Thus, we are concerned with the accessibility of implicit referents in the text world. The prevailing assumption is that there is an associative relationship between trigger and anaphor which helps to establish some link between the two expressions. Thus, these referential instances are often called associative anaphors (e.g. Hawkins, 1978; Heim, 1991; Löbner, 1996). However, since only a small amount of indirect reference relations can be explained through the activation of associations we prefer to use the more general term indirect anaphor (cf. Erkü and Gundel, 1987). According to most theories, the relation between anchor and indirect anaphor can best be explained in terms of associability, and the anchoring always involves some kind of inferential linking or bridging (cf. Clark, 1977; Fraurud, 1992; Sanford and Garrod, 1994b; Gundel, 1996; Cornish, 1999).

Example (28), however, illustrates that even a strong association between two items is sometimes not a sufficient criterion for the use of an indirect anaphor.

(28) *Es floss viel Blut in diesem Kampf. #Das Rot/#Die Röte stach den Kriegern in die Augen.*
"A lot of blood was shed in the battle. #The red thrust the warriors in the eyes."

Although we strongly associate blood with the colour red (in fact, this relation is stored in our mental lexicon as part of our semantic-conceptual knowledge), it is not possible or at least awkward to use *blood* as an anchor and *red* as an indirect anaphor in this example. Interestingly, this constraint does not hold for all mass nouns as anchors and/or colour terms as anaphors. Consider, for instance (29):

(29) *Als wir erwachten, lag alles voller Schnee. Das Weiß blendete unsere Augen.*
"When we got up, there was snow all over. The white was simply overwhelming."

In the text-world model of (29), the conceptual image of the scene depicted in the text implies the overall impression of the whiteness. Thus, the mental image or visualisation of the state-of-affairs which is part of the text-world model allows coding the appropriate colour term as an indirect anaphor.

According to another popular view, indirect anaphora are explained as frame-evoked entities in implicit focus. In this respect, Sanford and Garrod (1981, 1994a,b) and Garrod (1995) distinguish direct and indirect anaphors with the help of explicit and implicit focus. Explicit focus is the current focus of attention, the highly activated part of workspace where incoming information is temporarily held, that is short-term memory which contains representations of active referents explicitly introduced. Implicit focus is the representation of entities evoked implicitly as they form part of a frame retrieved from memory. Whereas the referents of direct anaphora are accessible in explicit focus, the referents of indirect anaphora have to be available in implicit focus, that is as default values of a frame or script.

But not all indirect anaphora in a text refer to particular parts of a frame. Besides, we have seen that the resolution of many direct anaphora demands more than a search-and-match in short term memory. Here, too, mental configurations are build up which exceed the explicit information in the text.

Therefore, we will argue for a more complex cognitive approach. Taking a procedural perspective, we want to demonstrate that there are different types of indirect anaphora. A distinction will be drawn between indirect anaphora which are based on the activation of default knowledge in long-term memory and indirect anaphora which require a more refined cognitive process for their resolution. Further, we are going to explain why all kinds of indirect anaphora have to be seen as given-and-new-entities.

Four main types of indirect anaphora can be distinguished. The criteria established for distinguishing these different types are based on the linguistic expressions used as anchor and on the different knowledge structures involved in interpreting the mental relationship between anchor and indirect anaphor. The examples (which are taken from natural language texts in German) concern the most frequent and prototypical types of textual indirect anaphora.

In example (30) the NP *a blue Mercedes* provides an anchor for the indirect anaphor *the wheel*, the anchor for the indirect anaphor *the temples* is provided by the NP *the man.*

(30) *Alphons Clenin...fand einen blauen Mercedes...Es war ihm, als sei der Fahrer auf das Steuer gesunken....Er bemerkte jedoch im gleichen Augenblick, dass der Mann tot war. Die Schläfen waren durchschossen.* (Dürrenmatt: Der Richter und sein Henker, 5)

"Alphons Clenin noticed a blue Mercedes.... It looked as if the driver was lying on the wheel...He saw that the man was dead. His temples (in German the definite article!) were shot through."

This type of indirect anaphor is established by the semantic relation between the anchor and the indirect anaphor, there is a part-whole-relationship between them. The knowledge structures needed for the interpretation of the anaphoric expressions are stored in our mental lexicon as part of our semantic knowledge (that is in the form of meronymy relations).

Example (31) shows an indirect anaphor based on lexical knowledge, too, more precisely on the thematic roles of the verb in the preceding sentence.

(31) *Ich wollte rasch die Haustür aufschließen, weil ich das Telefon klingeln hörte. Der Schlüssel war aber tief unten im Einkaufswagen vergraben.* (Evanovich, Einmal ist keinmal, 123)
"I wanted to unlock the door quickly, because I could hear the telephone ringing. But the key was nowhere to be found in my bag."

The definite NP *the key* used as indirect anaphor represents the instrument role which is part of the semantic representation of the verb *unlock* which serves as the anchor. Referential anchoring is established through the assignment of the indirect anaphor to a specific verb role in the verb frame of *unlock.*

In examples (32) and (33), script-based types are seen. The anchoring of the indirect anaphor is based on the activation of the appropriate default values in long-term memory.

(32) *In jenen letzten Augusttagen des Jahres 1961 erwacht in einem kleinen Krankenhauszimmer (Anker) das Mädchen Rita Seidel...Die Krankenschwester tritt an das Bett... als morgens der Arzt...* (Wolf, Der geteilte Himmel, 9).
"In those last days of august 1961, a girl named Rita Seidel awakens in a hospital room. The nurse comes to the bed... the doctor..."

(33) *Wenn Sie ein wirklich exzellentes Restaurant suchen: Gehen Sie ins LaCaverna. Das Essen ist köstlich, und die Bedienung ganz besonders nett.* (OTZ 24, 2003)
"If you look for a really thrilling restaurant: Visit Lacaverna. The food is excellent and the waiter is an extremely nice guy."

Establishing a coherent link between the sentences in (33) is to treat *the waiter* and *the food* as fulfilling typical roles or default values of the script RESTAURANT in long-term memory which is activated in a top-down-process by the anchor-expression *restaurant.* Accordingly, *hospital* serves as anchor for *the nurse* and *the doctor.* The recipient has to localize the referents of the indirect anaphora in the mental structure of the script.

Thus, resolving indirect anaphora involves an elaboration which extends the explicit representation of the text. Comprehension depends on the extension of the current representation, taking into account more than textual information.

It is a common view that all indirect anaphora are based on some kind of inference or linking. This claim, however, neglects the difference between indirect anaphors which are based on a cognitive process involving the activation of semantic roles or default values and indirect anaphors which are truly based on an inference process. The term *inference* should not be used for all kinds of memory processes involved in text comprehension in the sense of "any piece of information that is not explicitly stated in the text" (McKoon and Ratcliff, 1992, 440), but only for problem-solving activities, that is the constructive use of world knowledge. Otherwise, it is impossible to describe cognitive processes more precisely and in explicit detail. Lexical decomposition, slot-filling or spreading activation, belong to a type of semantic activation processes which should not be equated with using knowledge in inferential problem-solving activities. An indirect anaphor which is resolved not merely by activating a semantic role or default value, but by drawing an inference is exemplified in (34):

(34) *Nachts stürzt ein Mann auf die Polizeiwache und berichtet erregt, dass er soeben im Dunkeln an seiner Gartenpforte nieder-*

geschlagen worden sei. Ein Polizist wird beauftragt, am Ort des Überfalls Spuren zu sichern. Kurz darauf kommt er mit einer Riesenbeule am Kopf zurück: "Ich habe den Fall aufgeklärt." "Bravo", sagt sein Chef, "und wie?" "Ich bin auch auf die Harke getreten!" (Hörzu, 19.4.96, 17)
"A man rushes into the police station at night and tells the policemen that he has just been knocked down in the dark in his garden. One policeman is asked to go and look for traces at the place of the assault. After a short time he returns with a huge swelling at his head and says 'I solved the case'. 'Bravo', says his chef, 'and how did you do that?' 'I stepped on the rake, too.' "

The NP *the rake* is a typical example of an indirect anaphor based on inference. It can only be understood if the reader/listener draws some complex inferences about what has been going on in the text world. These inferences are triggered by the expression *too*: *there never has been any assault. the man, just like the policeman, stepped on some rake which could not be seen in the dark.*

This process of inferential anchoring does not necessarily involve the activation of one specific frame or script. However, a lot of inferences are based on script knowledge. Besides, inferential processing does occur within the configuration (and constraints) of the text-world model. Hence, the referents of inference-based indirect anaphors have to be integrated into the text-world model of the specific text and are governed like all other types of direct and indirect anaphors by the principle of plausibility.

(35) *Der britische Agent Dobbs wird auf den angeblich abtrünnigen Regierungsbeamten Fennan angesetzt. Kurz darauf ist der tot. Trotz des Abschiedsbriefs/#des Eierkuchens zweifelt Dobbs am Selbstmord.* (Hörzu 27.12.96, 65)
"The British secret service man Dobbs has orders to survey the activities of the civil servant man Fennan. Shortly after that, Fennan is dead. In spite of the farewell-letter/# the pancake, Dobbs does not believe in suicide."

The conclusion (A FAREWELL LETTER WITH DOBBS' SIGNATURE WAS FOUND WITH THE CORPSE) fits into the mental representation, and can plausibly be integrated into the text-world model, whereas *the pancake* does not make any sense. Thus, plausibility of the inference within the anchoring domain is needed for an indirect anaphor to be appropriate.

The examples so far discussed, show that within the group of indirect anaphors, different types can be made out which rely both on different knowledge structures and processing operations for their anchoring (Schwarz, 2000a).Indirect anaphora which rely on the activation of semantic or conceptual knowledge, are resolved within the immediate mental scope of the anchor expression comprising the prototypical information of the cognitive domain. Resolving inferrable indirect anaphors involves the expansion of this scope.

In general, anchoring conditions of referents for indirect anaphors can be formulated in the following way: The referent of an indirect anaphor must be either an identifiable part of the implicit semantic structure of the preceding sentences, or it must be a default value of a specific frame or script activated by the anchor expression, or it must be inferrable on the basis of cognitive plausibility determined by prototypical world knowledge.

The definite NP denoting an indirect anaphor, refers to an entity being introduced into the text for the very first time. In this respect, indirect anaphora carry new information into the text-world model. Even more, a new node for the new referent has to be established in an activation process in working memory. On the other hand, at the semantic level of the text the definite article signals that (given) information is easily accessible and, thus, demands a re-activation process. Seen as grammatical means with processing instructions, indirect anaphora signal accessibility of the text referent while a new referent is introduced to the text-world model.

From a given-new-perspective, thus, indirect anaphora combine both referential continuity and elaborative development in information processing. An activation process is taking place by establishing a new file in short-term memory, while at the same time we have reactivation in long-term memory. More precisely, the cognitive domain of the anchor expression has been in the status of semi-activation (for aspects of activation levels and the status of semi-activation in long-term memory representations of the anchors, see Schwarz, 2000a, 136ff.). Hence, re-activation of the semi-activated domain accounts for the ease of processing and the acceptability of indirect anaphora as continuity markers. In this respect, indirect anaphora serve as means to establish coherence in the same way as direct anaphora.

To sum up: The anchoring of indirect anaphora is neither solely determined by the principle of associability nor by the activation of a script. It turns out, that both associability and inferrability are restricted by the conceptual constraint of plausibility. A strong semantic link between anchor and indirect anaphor does not per se guarantee proper and successful anchoring. Rather, the plausibility within the specific text-world model governs the anchoring process. The immediate resolution of indirect anaphors comes about through an interaction between the information in the anchor and the anaphor, the mental accessibility of the implied referent within a specific context and the focus state of the prior and current textual representation. From a perspective of referential movement, indirect anaphora have to be regarded as given-and-new-entities. Combining both easy accessibility and the establishment of new nodes in text-world models, they serve as *progressive continuity markers.*

To establish coherence, a mental representation for the textual referent must be either available in the conceptual text representation or inferrable from memory at the time the anaphoric item is processed. Given this similarity between direct and indirect anaphors, the interpretation of direct and indirect anaphors seems to obey similar rules (cf. Schwarz, 2000a; Consten, 2003).

In both cases, the semantics of these expressions only provides a minimal framework, which needs being complemented by different cognitive mechanisms at the conceptual level of the text-world model. In all anaphoric instances of both explicit and implicit types, the definite article is characterized as a grammatical instruction to the reader to access or construct the referents needed in order to establish a coherent representation. The definite article itself does not spell out the precise connections that have to be constructed in the progress of resolving any individual NP. A unified theory of anaphora has to specify the conditions under which the various uses of anaphora can be resolved and how the resolution depends on the meaning of the antecedents/anchors. In order to provide a full account of how indirect and direct anaphors are processed, a cognitive theory of reference resolution must include both representational and procedural factors of short-term and long-term memory in more detail.

6 Conclusion

Building up coherence and resolving anaphoric expressions in text comprehension are two processes which go hand in hand. Focussing on the role of the text-world model and the leading principle of conceptual plausibility in understanding and constructing coherent representations of texts, the interface between verbal structures and memory representations has been illustrated. Coherence has been described as conceptual continuity, in the sense that the states-of-affairs expressed by parts of the text can be connected and integrated into the text-world model automatically and without effort on the basis of our linguistic and conceptual competence. The maintenance of continuity can best be described as a process of mapping referential representations onto conceptual representations evoked by prior text.

It has been shown that the range of possible mental configurations in a text-world model is constrained both by linguistic and cognitive factors: the grammatical expressions at the surface structure serve as processing hints, leading the reader in activating specific knowledge representations. However, surface structure very often does not give enough information to enable the reader to reconstruct the referential representation. Thus, elaboration processes are needed. Considering the knowledge structures used for the interpretation of direct and indirect anaphora as the basis for a more general explanation of how people process definite referring expressions, different types of anaphora have been distinguished. Some cognitive processes are required in all cases, but the type of mental operation needed differs in a number of ways. All types, however, are interpreted according to the preference rule of plausibility which is governed by the prototypical knowledge stored and activated from long-term memory. From a procedural perspective which takes the given-new-development into account, indirect anaphora and many cases of direct anaphora have to be regarded as given-and-new-entities, combining both activation and re-activation processes.

We have further shown that there is no clear-cut distinction between direct and indirect anaphora in texts, thereby weakening the claim for a strict distinction between the two types. This leads to a plea for a more unified account of anaphora in text within a cognitive theory of coherence.

References

Ariel, Mira. 1988. Referring and accessibility. *Journal of Linguistics* 24: 65–87.

Ariel, Mira. 1990. *Accessing Noun-Phrase Antecedents*. London: Routledge.

Asher, N. 1993. *Reference to Abstract Objects in Discourse*. Dordrecht: Kluwer.

Barsalou, Lawrence. 1992. *Cognitive Psychology: An Overview for Cognitive Scientists*. Hillsdale, N.J.: Erlbaum.

Beaugrande, Robert-Alain de and Wolfgang Ulrich Dressler. 1981. *Einführung in die Textlinguistik*. Tübingen: Niemeyer.

Bosch, Peter. 1988. Representing and accessing focussed referents. *Language and Cognitive Processes* 3: 207–231.

Broek, P. van den. 1994. Comprehension and memory of narrative texts. In: M. A. Gernsbacher (ed.), *Handbook of Psycholinguistics*. San Diego: Academic Press, 539–588.

Brown, G. and G. Yule. 1983. *Discourse Analysis*. Cambridge: Cambridge University Press.

Bublitz, W., U. Lenk and E. Ventola (eds.). 1999. *Coherence in Spoken and Written Discourse*. Amsterdam & Philadelphia: Benjamins.

Carston, R. 2002. *Thoughts and Utterances: The Pragmatics of Explicit Communication*. Malden: Blackwell.

Carter, P. 1987. *Interpreting Anaphors in Natural Language Texts*. Chichester: Ellis Horwood.

Chafe, W. L. 1994. *Discourse, Consciousness, and Time. The Flow and Displacement of Conscious Experience in Speaking and Writing*. Chicago: Chicago University Press.

Clark, Eve V. 1978. Awareness of language: Some evidence from what children say and do. In: Anne Sinclair, Robert J. Jarvella and Willem J. Levelt (eds.), *The Child's Conception of Language*. Berlin: Springer Verlag, 17–43.

Clark, Herbert H. 1977. Bridging. In: P. N. Johnson-Laird and P. C. Wason (eds.), *Thinking: Readings in Cognitive Science*. Cambridge: Cambridge University Press, 411–420.

Consten, M. 2003. Towards a unified model of domain-bound reference. In: F. Lenz (ed.), *Deictic Conceptualisation of Space, Time and Person*. Amsterdam & Philadelphia: Benjamins, 223–248.

Consten, M. 2004. *Anaphorisch oder deiktisch? Zu einem integrativen Modell domänengebundener Referenz*. Tübingen: Niemeyer.

Conte, M. E. 1996. Facts, events, propositions in anaphoric encapsulation Paper read at the Workshop "Indirect Anaphors" in Lancaster.

Cornish, F. 2002. Indirect anaphora: the discourse-referential scope of unaccented pronouns and zero anaphors. Paper read at the 4th International Conference on Discourse Anaphora and Anaphor Resolution, Lisbon.

Cornish, Francis. 1999. *Anaphora, Discourse, and Understanding: Evidence from English and French*. Oxford: Oxford University Press.

Dahl, Östen. 1995. Causality in discourse. In: Gerd Rickheit and Christopher Habel (eds.), *Focus and Coherence in Discourse Processing*. Berlin: de Gruyter, 251–260.

Dahl, Östen and C. Hellmann. 1995. What happens when we use an anaphor? Ph.D. thesis, University, Dept. of Linguistics, Stockholm.

Dijk, Teun A. van and Walter Kintsch. 1983. *Strategies of Discourse Comprehension*. New York: Academic Press.

Ehlich, K. 1982. Anaphora and deixis: Same, similar or different? In: R. J. Jarvella and W. Klein (eds.), *Speech, Place and Action: Studies in Deixis and Related Topics*. Chichester: Wiley, 315–339.

Erkü, F. and J. K. Gundel. 1987. The pragmatics of indirect anaphors. In: J. Verschueren and M. Bertucelli-Papi (eds.), *The Pragmatic Perspective*. Amsterdam & Philadelphia: Benjamins, 533–545.

Fauconnier, G. 1994. *Mental Spaces: Aspects of Meaning Construction in Natural Language*. 2nd edition. Cambridge, MA: Bradford.

Francis, Gill. 1986. *Anaphoric Nouns*. Birmingham: University of Birmingham.

Fraurud, K. 1990. Definiteness and the processing of NPs in natural discourse. *Journal of Semantics* 7: 395–434.

Fraurud, K. 1992. *Processing Noun Phrases in Natural Discourse*. Stockholm: Stockholm University, Dept. of Linguistics.

Freitas, S. and J. G. Lopes. 1996. Solving the reference to mixable entities. Paper read at the Workshop "Indirect Anaphors", Lancaster.

Garnham, Alan and J. Oakhill. 1992. *Discourse Representation and Text Processing: A Special Issue of Language and Cognitive Processes*. Hove: Lawrence Erlbaum Associates.

Garrod, Simon. 1995. Distinguishing between explicit and implicit focus during text comprehension. In: G. Rickheit and Ch. Habel (eds.), *Focus and Coherence in Discourse Processing*. Berlin & New York: de Gruyter, 3–17.

Gernsbacher, M. A. 1989. Mechanisms that improve referential access. *Cognition* 32: 99–156.

Gernsbacher, M. A. and T. Givon. 1995. Introduction: Coherence as a mental entity. In: M. A. Gernsbacher and T. Givon (eds.), *Coherence in Spontaneous Text*. Amsterdam & Philadelphia: Benjamins.

Givon, T. 1992. The grammar of referential coherence as mental processing instructions. *Linguistics* 30: 5–55.

Givon, T. 1995. Coherence in text vs. coherence in mind. In: M. A. Gernsbacher and T. Givon (eds.), *Coherence in Spontaneous Text*. Amsterdam & Philadelphia: Benjamins, 59–115.

Gordon, Peter C., Barbara J. Grosz and Laura A. Gilliom. 1993. Pronouns, names, and the centering of attention in discourse. *Cognitive Science* 17: 311–347.

Grosz, Barbara J. 1981. Focusing and description in natural language dialogs. In: A. Joshi, B. L. Webber and I. A. Sag (eds.), *Elements of Discourse Understanding*. Cambridge: Cambridge University Press, 84–105.

Gundel, J. K. 1996. The form of indirect anaphora. Paper read at the Workshop "Indirect Anaphors", Lancaster.

Gundel, Jeanette, Nancy Hedberg and Ron Zacharski. 1993. Cognitive status and the form of referring expressions in discourse. *Language* 69(2): 274–307.

Halliday, Michael A. K. and Ruqaiya Hasan. 1976. *Cohesion in English*. London: Longman.

Hawkins, John. 1991. On (in)definite articles: implicatures and (un)grammaticality prediction. *Journal of Linguistics* 27: 405–442.

Hawkins, John A. 1978. *Definiteness and Indefiniteness: A Study in Reference and Grammaticality Prediction*. London: Croom Helm.

Heim, I. 1991. Artikel und Definitheit. In: A. von Stechow and D. Wunderlich (eds.), *Semantik. Ein internationales Handbuch der zeitgenössischen Forschung*. Berlin & New York: de Gruyter, 487–535.

Hellmann, Ch. 1995. The notion of coherence in discourse. In: G. Rickheit and Ch. Habel (eds.), *Focus and Coherence in Discourse Processing*. Berlin: de Gruyter, 190–202.

Heusinger, K. von. 2000. Anaphora, antecedents, and accessibility. *Theoretical Linguistics* 26: 75–93.

Heusinger, K. von. 2003. The double dynamics of definite descriptions. In: J. Peregrin (ed.), *Meaning in the Dynamic Turn*. Amsterdam: Elsevier, 150–168.

Hintzman, D. L. 1987. Schema abstraction in a multiple-trace model. *Psychological Review* 93: 411–428.

Hobbs, J. R. 1979. Coherence and coreference. *Cognitive Science* 3: 67–90.

Hobbs, J. R. 1983. Why is discourse coherent? In: F. Neubauer (ed.), *Coherence in Natural Language Texts*. Hamburg: Buske, 29–70.

Johnson-Laird, Philip N. 1983. *Mental Models. Towards a Cognitive Science of Language, Inference, and Consciousness*. Cambridge, Mass.: Cambridge University Press.

Kamp, H. and U. Reyle. 1993. *From Discourse to Logic*. Dordrecht: Kluver.

Keenan, J. M., S. D. Baillet and P. Brown. 1984. The effects of causal cohesion on comprehension and memory. *Journal of Verbal Learning and Verbal Behavior* 23: 115–126.

Kintsch, Walter. 1998. *Comprehension. A Paradigm for Cognition*. Cambridge: Cambridge University Press.

Lambrecht, K. 1994. *Information Structure and Sentence Form: Topic, Focus and the Mental Representation of Discourse Referents.* Cambridge: Cambridge University Press.

Löbner, S. 1996. *Associative Anaphors.* Düsseldorf: University of Düsseldorf.

Lundquist, L. 1985. Coherence: From structure to processes. In: E. Sözer (ed.), *Text Connexity, Text Coherence. Aspects, Methods, Results.* Hamburg: Buske, 151–175.

Lyons, J. 1989. Semantic ascent: A neglected aspect of syntactic typology. In: D. Arnold, C. Grover and L. Sadler (eds.), *Essays on Grammatical Theory and Universal Grammar.* Oxford: Clarendon Press, 153–186.

Maes, A. 1997. Referent ontology and centering in discourse. *Journal of Semantics* 14: 207–235.

McKoon, G. and R. Ratcliff. 1992. Inference during reading. *Psychological Review* 99: 440–466.

Murphy, Gregory L. 1985. Processes of understanding anaphora. *Journal of Memory and Language* 24: 290–303.

Noordman, L. G. and W. Vonk. 1998. Memory-based processing in understanding causal information. *Discourse Processes* 26: 191–212.

Prince, E. 1981. Toward a taxonomy of given–new–information. In: P. Cole (ed.), *Radical Pragmatics.* New York: Academic Press, 223–255.

Reinhart, T. 1980. Conditions of coherence. *Poetics Today* 1: 161–180.

Sanders, T. and W. Spooren. 1999. Communicative intentions and coherence relations. In: W. Bublitz, U. Lenk and E. Ventola (eds.), *Coherence in Text and Discourse.* Amsterdam & Philadelphia: Benjamins, 235–250.

Sanders, T. and W. Spooren. 2001. Text representation as an interface between language and its users. In: T. Sanders, J. Schiperoord and W. Spooren (eds.), *Text Representation: Linguistic and Psycholinguistic Aspects.* Amsterdam & Philadelphia: Benjamins, 1–25.

Sanders, T., W. Spooren and L. G. Noordman. 1992. Toward a taxonomy of coherence relations. *Discourse Processes* 15: 1–35.

Sanford, Anthony J. and Simon C. Garrod. 1981. *Understanding Written Language: Explorations in Comprehension Beyond the Sentence.* Chichester, West Sussex: John Wiley & Sons.

Sanford, Anthony J. and Simon C. Garrod. 1994a. Resolving sentences in a discourse context. In: M. A. Gernsbacher (ed.), *Handbook of Psycholinguistics*. San Diego: Academic Press, 675–698.

Sanford, Anthony J. and Simon C. Garrod. 1994b. Selective processing in text understanding. In: M. A. Gernsbacher (ed.), *Handbook of Psycholinguistics*. Academic Press, 699–719.

Sanford, Anthony J. and L. M. Moxey. 1995. Aspects of coherence in written language: A psychological perspective. In: M. A. Gernsbacher and T. Givon (eds.), *Coherence in Spontaneous Text*. Amsterdam & Philadelphia: Benjamins, 161–187.

Schwarz, Monika. 2000a. *Indirekte Anaphern in Texten. Studien zur domänengebundenen Referenz und Kohärenz im Deutschen.* Tübingen: Niemeyer.

Schwarz, Monika. 2000b. Textuelle Progression durch Anaphern - Aspekte einer prozeduralen Thema-Rhema-Analyse. *Linguistische Arbeitsberichte* 74: 111–126.

Schwarz, Monika. 2001a. Establishing coherence in text. Conceptual continuity within the domain of text–world models. *Logos and Language* : 15–23.

Schwarz, Monika. 2001b. Kohärenz - Auf den materiellen Spuren eines mentalen Phänomens. In: M. Bräunlich, B. Neuber and B. Rues (eds.), *Gesprochene Sprache - transdisziplinär. Festschrift für Gottfried Meinhold*. Frankfurt am Main: Peter Lang, 151–160.

Schwarz-Friesel, Monika. 2006. Kohärenz versus Textsinn. Didaktische Facetten einer linguistischen Theorie der textuellen Kontinuität. In: M. Scherner and A. Ziegler (eds.), *Angewandte Textlinguistik. Perspektiven für den Deutsch- und Fremdsprachenunterricht*. Tübingen: Narr, 63–75.

Schwarz-Friesel, Monika, Manfred Consten and Konstanze Marx. 2004. Komplexanaphern. In: Kl. P. Konerding and I. Pohl (eds.), *Stabilität und Flexibilität in der Semantik*. Frankfurt: Peter Lang, 67–86.

Singer, M. 1990. *Psychology of Language. An Introduction to Sentence and Discourse Processes*. Hillsdale, N.J.: Lawrence Erlbaum Associates.

Singer, M. 1994. Discourse inference processes. In: M. A. Gernsbacher (ed.), *Handbook of Psycholinguistics*. San Diego: Academic Press, 479–515.

Sperber, Dan and Deirdre Wilson. 1992. *Relevance: Communication and Cognition*. 2nd edition. Oxford: Basil Blackwell.

Spooren, W. 1997. The processing of underspecified coherence relations. *Discourse Processes* 24: 149–168.

Spooren, W. 1999. Textlinguistik. In: R. Pörings and U. Schmitz (eds.), *Sprache und Sprachwissenschaft*. Tübingen: Narr, 187–210.

Stenning, K. 1992. Representations of individuals and the processing of reference change. *Quarterly Journal of Experimental Psychology. Human Experimental Psychology* 45A(3): 373–398.

Webber, B. L. 1991. Structure and ostension in the interpretation of discourse deixis. *Language and Cognitive Processes* 6: 107–135.

Zelinsky-Wibbelt, C. 2000. *Discourse and the Continuity of Reference: Representing Mental Categorization*. Berlin: de Gruyter.

Zelinsky-Wibbelt, C. 2003. *Text, Context, Concepts*. Berlin: de Gruyter.

Lexical predictability in comprehension: A study of cumulative priming

Arne Zeschel and Alex Deppert[1]

1 Introduction

What's funny about *I wouldn't send a knight out on a dog like this*? How come that we readily pick up on the allusion in "productive quotation phraseology"(Partington, 1998) of the type *the mother of all meteors* (Lamb, 1999)? And how is it that characterizing a woman as "something that rhymes with rich" is tantamount to naming the beast straight away, seeing that the implied meaning cannot be cancelled (Allan, 1992)? Different as they are, all of these examples draw on our amazing capacity for understanding the lexically implicit and playfully obfuscated, which is a crucial prerequisite for certain modes of communication: most humour is based on substituting the predictable with the unexpected, and there would be no poetry if words were not suggestive of specific linguistic and non-linguistic associations that can be played on and exploited for aesthetic effect.[2] On the other hand, it is not at all clear how such commonplace observations tie in with current accounts of linguistic processing and memory for text. Some of the relevant questions here include: how do the lexical patterns and relations tapped in the above examples inform an ongoing comprehension process? Is predictability limited to idiomatic structures, and what exactly do we mean by "idiomatic"? How do qualitatively different (e.g. semantic and collocational/probabilistic)

[1] This research was conducted as part of the DFG-funded research project LexiKurs (reference number ZE 345/5-3) based at the University of Hanover, Germany. We are grateful to Cornelia Zelinsky-Wibbelt, the project leader, for her comments on earlier versions of this paper.

[2] As Roman Jakobson (1960, 366) has put it in his famous account of the "poetic function", "both the warranted and the frustrated expectations"in Hearer's interpretive performance combine to this end.

retrieval cues interact in a complex verbal allusion? And, last not least, how do the above observations integrate with models of language comprehension at large (be they linguistic or psychological in nature), and do they have any implications for questions of lexical representation in memory?

2 Objectives

The present paper seeks to address these issues from an empirical perspective, with special attention devoted to the last question. In other words, we will be concerned with questions of predictability in wording, and how such phenomena can be accounted for in two influential approaches to comprehension from cognitive psychology and linguistic pragmatics, Kintsch's (1998) Construction Integration (CI)-Model and Sperber and Wilson's (1995) Relevance Theory. To this end, we investigated the build-up (and subsequent defeat) of the expectation of the word *zunichte* in the following humorous short poem by Robert Gernhardt (1). The free translation in (2) is somewhat more in keeping with the gist of the original.

(1) *Bekenntnis*
Confession

Ich leide an Versagensangst
I suffer from failure-GEN-fear
Besonders wenn ich dichte
Especially when I write.poems
Die Angst, die machte mir bereits
The fear, it made me-DAT already
Manch schönen Reim zuschanden.
Many beautiful rhyme to.naught

(2) *Confession*
However poetic my temper be
A fear of failure hampers me
Indeed, this fear, I've often thought
Has brought my rhyming skills to zero.

Successful interpretation of this text (i.e., getting its pun) requires anticipating *zunichte* ("to naught") at the end of line 4 as well as additional inferencing relating to the subsequent frustration of this expectation. While this may indeed be a somewhat unusual course of events compared to ordinary discourse processing, a convincing general model of utterance comprehension should nonetheless account for (or, at the very least, must not preclude) the observed effect. Hence, our aims in the present paper are twofold: first, to assess whether our hypotheses about the particulars of the process in question (cf. section 5.1) can be empirically substantiated, and second, to consider in how far these observations can be accounted for within the aforementioned frameworks. Our paper is structured as follows: in order to establish the necessary background, we begin with a short sketch of the significance of "association patterns"in language structure and processing (section 3) and a broad outline of the two theories under consideration (section 4). We then present the experimental design, beginning with our hypotheses as to what actually happens upon successfully interpreting the text (section 5.1). Sections (5.2) and (5.3) are devoted to the methods and results of our investigation. Finally, the discussion in (6) will assess the theories in question with respect to our findings and consider their implications for general issues of lexical representation and retrieval.

3 Guiding assumptions

Memory is associative, and memory for language is memory. It does not come as a surprise, then, that there are pervasive "association patterns" to be uncovered at different levels of linguistic organization. From a "usage-based" perspective on language (Langacker, 2002), linguistic knowledge is inseparably entwined with actual usage events in the form of a permanent feedback loop: hearers categorize their linguistic input by mapping it onto schemas abstracted from previous linguistic experience, and then instantiate these (possibly slightly accommodated) schemas in subsequent production tasks. Even though the process of schematization is thus clearly crucial for both acquiring and restructuring linguistic knowledge, speakers are not in fact expected to always extract (let alone exclusively store) the highest conceivable generalization (i.e. the most abstract schema available). Quite to the contrary, we assume that the bulk of linguistic knowledge consists of rather concrete, i.e. only partly underspecified elements (low-level schemas) which include information about canonical syntagmatic contexts (i.e. conventional collocations and "colligations"). It is thus expected that words retain traces of their variegated usage patterns, a prediction which is strongly supported by the available textual and psychological evidence. In the present section, we will briefly review some of the relevant arguments from both areas of research.

Beginning with evidence from corpora, Sinclair (1987) has drawn attention to the fact that there are two independent structuring principles in naturally occurring language which he refers to as "the open choice principle" and "the idiom principle", respectively. The latter principle is taken to account for the broad range of syntagmatic co-occurrence effects in language that commonly go by the name collocation (Bolinger 1976; Kjellmer 1990, 1991; Altenberg 1991; Sinclair 1987, 1991; Renouf and Sinclair 1991). Sinclair suggests that these effects arise from the fact that fluent speakers of a language have at their disposal a huge stock of virtually prefabricated structures of varying degrees of complexity and formal specification. Fully specified items range from word-level collocations such as *stone deaf* to sentence-level routine formulae (cf. Coulmas, 1981) like *How do you do* or even the considerably complex *You don't want to believe everything you hear.* Underspecified structures include various types of (more or less) schematic idioms such as *lose one's minds/marbles* (cf. Nunberg et al., 1994) and *I haven't the faintest/slightest/remotest/foggiest idea/conception/notion* (cf. Francis, 1993).

Moreover, the fact that speakers have actually committed a large number of such clusters to memory is also taken to account for the existence of yet more abstract patterns like the "semantic prosodies"[3] associated with particular lexical items (Louw, 1993; Sinclair, 1996).

Sinclair's principles can be conceived as endpoints on a continuum of collocational restrictedness, but there is no well-defined cut-off point between the two domains: syntagmatic affinity gradually increases from chance juxtapositions and weak preferences over frequent and then habitual combinations to ever more predictive collocations and finally actual freezes which may at some point culminate in univerbation (e.g. *zu Nichte* > *zunichte*). The phenomenon of lexical chunking thus extends well beyond traditional conceptions of idiomaticity, which commonly build on semantic non-compositionality: as understood here, the elements in question are simply stretches of lexis which are memorized as unified wholes, meaning that they may well have internal syntactic structure and even a fully compositional semantics; what counts is simply that they are stored en bloc and thus have a certain (i.e. more or less strongly entrenched) degree of unit-status as conventionalized expressions of the respective language. In short, contrary to what the dominant view of language in modern linguistics (i.e., a discrete combinatorial system involving largely unrestrained creativity in syntagmatic patterning) might seem to suggest, predictability effects in wording are a phenomenon to be reckoned with in theories of language processing.

Whereas it is easy to see how chunking and collocation should result in partial (i.e. probabilistic) predictability, this cannot be the whole story, though: neither Allan's case of *something that rhymes with rich* nor the poem under consideration here achieve their effect through clippings or other manipulations of some implicit idiom chunk. Instead, Hearer is driven to assume that the actually intended item will be recoverable by rhyme, as suggested by either

3 This term refers to the tendency of certain expressions to be restricted to uses within particular semantic contexts (with no restrictions as to the concrete lexical material encoding the required property). An example would be the semantic prosody of "difficulty" that is associated with the complex lexical item whose core is the collocation *naked eye*, as illustrated by expressions such as *barely/hardly/scarcely/just visible to the naked eye* or *be too faint/small/weak/difficult to discern with the naked eye* (Sinclair 1996).

genre-specific conventions (humorous short poems typically rhyme) or even explicit metalinguistic instruction ("look for a word that rhymes with *rich*"). Seeing that both *rich* and *dichte* in fact have a *set* of rhyme words, rhyme alone is not a sufficient constraint in order to attain a level of concrete predictability in either case: for *something that rhymes with rich*, Allan (1992, 362) suggests that the range of potential candidate items is inferentially narrowed down to "the most dysphemistic member of the set, because the less dysphemistic a remark is, the more likely it is to be made directly". As regards our case, a detailed discussion of the additional cues that support the activation of the intended target item is given in section 5.1. For the moment, suffice it to say that Gernhardt's poem is an example of how logically independent indications can be brought together to jointly yield a strong anticipation of a particular word - strong enough in fact to produce a "leak" in Hearer's lexical processing and fully activate the implicit item so that it will surface to consciousness. This is to say that if Speaker manages to exploit an appropriate array of converging lexical retrieval cues, she may manipulate Hearer's interpretive performance in a way that extends lexical predictability well into the domain of Sinclair's "open-choice principle".

Psychologically, these "cues" manifest in experimentally observable priming effects, i.e. lowered activation threshold values. Such effects have been attested in many different domains, ranging from concepts to phonological representations and even syntactic structures (constructional schemas): in the pioneer study of Meyer and Schvaneveldt (1971), the comprehension of content words was shown to involve the activation of other items from the same semantic domain (e.g., *doctor* - NURSE). Likewise, priming effects were observed to spread across conceptual hierarchies involving hyponymy and meronymy as well as further semantic relations like antonymy - a crucial factor for reference assignment and establishing basic textual coherence in sequences as simple as (33):

(3) (3) *My car*$_i$ *wouldn't start because thebattery*$_i$ *was flat.*

In the initial stages of comprehension (i.e. during an interval of approx. 700 msec. after perception; cf. Zwitserlood 1989), the underlying process of spreading activation affects all senses of the tentatively identified percept, even including contextually inappropriate homonyms (e.g., *bug* - ANT vs. *bug* - SPY; Swinney 1979). Other findings in the phonological domain include priming effects below word-level (e.g., *trombone* - BONE; Shillcock 1990) and across word boundaries (e.g., *he broke all records for the new distance* - NUDIST; Altman cf. 1997, 82). Moreover, lexical items prime frequent collocates as in *rain* - WET (Howard, 1981), and priming effects were also shown to pertain to syntactic constructions (Bock, 1986).[4]

Considering the on-line character of comprehension as an incremental process involving a fair amount of guesswork and (unconscious) anticipatory conjecture, it appears that the various effects described above may in fact serve rather different functions: phonological priming is helpful for identifying the correct percept in the first place, allowing the identification mechanism to successively narrow down the range of conceivable target representations whilst still permitting a switch to other likely candidates if the input appears to have been misinterpreted (Aitchison, 2003). Spreading activation in semantic memory is not only an essential prerequisite of language production (by allowing Speaker to choose between alternate ways of encoding a specific conceptual content), it is also crucial for comprehension as linguistic messages cannot be interpreted without an appropriate backdrop of activated semantic domains. Furthermore, it will also prepare Hearer to expect the occurrence of certain other elements of these domains in the unfolding discourse. Likewise, the coactivation of conventional collocates of the percept serves to further relieve subsequent word identification tasks by providing additional (probabilistic) retrieval cues.

In sum, then, priming effects are attested for a number of different entities involved in language processing (concepts, phonological representations, and syntactic schemata), which means that they oc-

[4] Subjects primed with either double-object or prepositional object sentences of the type *She gave me the book/She gave the book to me* were found to prefer the primed construction when later asked to verbalize visually presented ditransitive scenarios.

cur at different stages and hence contribute to different aspects of the overall comprehension process. This observation provides strong evidence for the assumption that routinized patterns of association between different elements of linguistic knowledge play an important role in comprehension, and we expected the association patterns exploited in our text to manifest in clearly observable priming effects of the kind described in this section.

4 Theoretical prerequisites

Before we discuss the particulars of our investigation, we will offer a brief sketch of the theories under consideration with special reference to their expected contribution to a convincing reconstruction of our case. We do not intend to offer an explicit comparison of Kintsch's CI-model and Sperber and Wilson's Relevance Theory here, as this would not only require substantially more space but is also difficult to envisage on principled grounds - as yet, the bulk of psycholinguistic and pragmatic work on comprehension is rather difficult to reconcile, seeing that researchers in these areas typically focus on entirely different aspects of the overall process. The present issue is a case in point: although Kintsch's model is not in fact limited to early processing stages like lexical access but also covers higher level representations like complex "situation models", it has little to offer in the way of an explicit reconstruction of the inferential chain that leads to Hearer's recovery of the pun. Relevance Theory, by contrast, has nothing to say about the "leakage" effecting the activation of *zunichte* in our experiment, seeing that the whole of lexical processing is taken to be "not so much a part of the comprehension process as something that precedes the real work of understanding" (Sperber and Wilson, 1995, 177), to the effect that there are but some sparse remarks on this supposedly ephemeral topic. Hence, departing from the assumption that Kintsch's model may be useful for a reconstruction of how the crucial word enters into the comprehension process in the first place, whereas Relevance Theory may offer instructive insights as to how and why subsequent assumptions relating to its actual absence from the text surface are formed and then subject to "higher level" inferential processing, we are in fact more interested in how the two theories may *complement* one another in accounting for our observations. The reason for choosing these particular models out of the range of available frameworks is that both Kintsch and Sperber/Wilson claim to offer comparably explicit and rigorous approaches in their respective areas which stand the test of empirical evaluation.

4.1 The Construction-Integration Model of Text Comprehension

Kintsch's Construction-Integration (or shortly CI) model is a two-stage model of comprehension comprising a "construction phase" and an "integration phase". It is framed in connectionist assumptions about knowledge representation and invokes processes of spreading activation as a key mechanism in language comprehension. The model was devised in response to theories centered around notions such as "schemata" (Bartlett, 1932), "frames" (Minsky, 1975) and "scripts" (Schank and Abelson, 1977), according to which the larger knowledge configurations that go by these names are activated in a manner of "all or nothing", i.e. as whole, monolithic entities that supply large chunks of information en bloc. Consequently, comprehension is conceived as an essentially top-down process directed by strong rules on such accounts. As pointed out in Kintsch (1988), however, such models have proven to be very inflexible in several computer simulations: given only minor deviations from the idealized standard course of events which they are supposed to schematize, they either fail or have to be modified until there is a specific "schema", "script" or "frame" for each and every individual situation. The CI-model, by contrast, has a strong bottom-up component: the initial "construction phase" which comprises the activation of concepts related to the linguistic input, the construction of propositions, and the association of the constructed propositions with yet further concepts. The production rules involved in this phase are weak and dumb, to the effect that numerous "wrong" elements which have to be discarded later will receive some tentative activation during construction. In fact, it is only in a second step (the subsequent "integration phase") that context effects are brought to bear on the initial net by boosting the activation values of elements which are strongly interconnected with other activated elements and suppressing the more marginal, i.e. only poorly supported nodes in the current network.

Evidence for Kintsch's distinction between these two phases of the comprehension process comes from experimental studies of lexical access: many results suggest that the early processing stages are context-blind, meaning that e.g. ambiguous stimuli prime conventional collocates and semantically related items for all available readings irrespective of contextual appropriateness.[5] With a longer delay between prime and target word presentation, however, ill-fitting readings do not display increased activation values anymore, whereas their contextually appropriate counterparts receive prolonged priming. Drawing on a wide range of such findings, Kintsch estimates that it takes up to approx. 750 milliseconds to suppress the contextually inappropriate meanings, concluding that "[i]nitial lexical access does appear to be exhaustive and context independent [...] Thus, what appears to be a context effect on lexical access is really an effect of the context on the integration of the word into the discourse subsequent to lexical access" (1998, 129).

Within the CI model, lexical association patterns of the sort discussed in section 3 would be interpreted as elaborations of the initial input manifesting during the construction phase. As indicated above, such effects may arise from different mechanisms and in response to different functional pressures: collocation, for instance, emerges from routinized co-activation and serves to reduce the number of lexical choices; rhyme, by contrast, may be a privileged relation because it supports flexible and failsafe word-recognition in comprehension.

5 Till et al. (1988), for instance, used the sentence "The townspeople were amazed to find that all buildings had collapsed except the *mint*". In line with the results of Swinney (1979) reported in section 1.1, they found that *mint* primed both target words like MONEY (related to the contextually appropriate meaning of *mint*) *and* CANDY (related to the contextually inappropriate meaning of *mint*), even though the ambiguity did not actually surface to consciousness.

However, we have to be a little more specific about which elements are involved in such processes (we are not dealing with either concepts or propositions here, as the above characterization of the construction phase would suggest) and how these elements enter into activation networks. To begin with, it is obvious that the process of "elaborating" a propositional net during construction by means of a largely unconstrained mechanism of context-blind "association" may easily produce inconsistencies or even downright semantic clashes between the various activated elements. In order to handle this in his model, Kintsch posits that links between any two elements in the emerging nets will be either (i) positive, which means there are associations between them; (ii) neutral, which means that there is no link between them, or (iii) negative, which means that only one of the two linked elements can actually be part of an integrated semantic representation of the input. Hence, the different meanings of a homonym for instance will be connected by a negative link because usually only one of them will work in a specific context (except for puns). Within an extended approach, the link strengths are more variable than described above, with starting values provided by Latent Semantic Analysis, or LSA (Landauer and Dumais 1997; Landauer et al. 1998). This method that cannot be described here (but see Deppert 2002), and it does not offer the possibility to calculate values for German so far. At any rate, the CI-model does not appear to be "overly sensitive to the selection of particular parameter values within some reasonable range" (Kintsch, 1998, 266). That is, as long as the type of relation (positive - neutral - negative) is not changed, the model is surprisingly robust regarding the variance of link strength values (or activation values). The links between nodes in a net are not semantically specified in Kintsch's model, i.e. there are no links specifying relations like e.g. causation or hyponymy. Relations like these are expressed by the nodes (i.e., a sentence like *A dog is an animal* would potentially constitute a net with a proposition like BE [DOG, ANIMAL], there would be no *is-a*-link).

As indicated, the propositional net constructed in the construction phase is not coherent - it may even contain overt contradictions. Such inconsistencies are straightened out by the integration process that seeks to resolve all contradictions and render the propositional net coherent. Setting in posterior to construction, its results are currently taken to manifest after approx. 750 msec. Kintsch emphasizes that the joint processes of construction and integration should not be confused with conscious problem-solving activities (which are resorted to when the subconscious CI-routines fail). The essential effect of the integration process consists in the strengthening of nodes that are strongly bound to the currently established propositional net in that they have many positive links to highly activated neighbouring nodes (in fact, these neighbouring nodes should be strongly bound to the propositional net, too - this can be a mutual effect). In this final stage of the spreading activation process, activation spreads from nodes positively linked with each other and strengthens them, whereas nodes which are not strongly bound to the net become suppressed and wither away.

As regards our stimulus text, we may suspect that there are positive links between different elements of the input and the implicit target item *zunichte* which are established during the construction phase (cf. 5.1 for details). Whereas context-blind priming effects of this type usually peter out without ever surfacing to consciousness, the activation of *zunichte* in our experiment is - at least for those subjects achieving full text comprehension - sustained posterior to integration, seeing that it is supported by several such links at the same time. In other words, Kintsch's framework can accommodate the observed "leakage" that introduces *zunichte* into the comprehension process within a general model, and it also makes specific predictions as to the interaction of the involved retrieval cues that can be evaluated empirically: in particular, there should be a difference between unspecific, context-blind priming effects that indicate the respective item's individual association strength in isolation and a cumulative, integrated effect that emerges from the interaction of all hitherto decoded cues - a prediction which can be tested by varying the delay time between prime and target word presentation. Furthermore, Kintsch (1998, 206) explicitly acknowledges that aspects of the textual surface structure (such as rhythm and rhyme) may play an important role in literary text comprehension, meaning that elements bound to the net via such links may figure more importantly in the interpretive process than they would do in ordinary discourse comprehension. Empirical evidence supporting this claim was supplied by Zwaan (1994): in his experiment, subjects reading under a "literary" perspective differed in reading time and memory for surface information from subjects reading the same text under a "news story" perspective.[6] We will come back to a more detailed discussion of the applicability and the specific predictions of Kintsch's model for our case in sections 5 and 6.

4.2 Relevance Theory

Relevance Theory (RT) is a theory of linguistic pragmatics which has grown out of Grice's (1989) groundbreaking work on the way in which interlocutors observe and exploit certain "maxims" of conversation in order to efficiently pursue their communicative goals. Both approaches depart from the observation that natural languages are rather coarse-grained codes which severely underspecify the intended meanings of speakers: even though verbal communication is clearly the most explicit form of communication, linguistic stimuli are nevertheless still vague and usually in many ways ambiguous, to the effect that their interpretation relies heavily on context. As a consequence, both theories emphasize the concomitant central role of inferential reasoning in verbal communication: according to RT, utterance comprehension comprises two essentially different mechanisms ("linguistic decoding" and inference), and it is the inferential component alone which can provide sufficiently sophisticated hypotheses about Speaker's informative intention.

The basic idea of RT is that there is an inescapable trade-off between effort and effect in both cognition and communication, meaning

[6] "In terms of the construction-integration model, news comprehension would entail a radical integration process in which irrelevant or unimportant information is rapidly deactivated. Literary comprehension, on the other hand, would entail a far less drastic integration process so that (seemingly) irrelevant or unimportant information is kept longer in an active state" (Zwaan, 1994, 930)

that the human mind is always geared towards achieving the maximum cognitive effect for the minimum amount of processing load. This hypothesis is formulated in the "first principle of relevance": "Human cognition tends to be geared to the maximisation of relevance" (Sperber and Wilson, 1995, 260). Relevance in turn is characterized as a property of inputs to cognitive processes in terms of a certain cost/benefit-ratio: the greater the cognitive effect of processing the particular input (i.e. either an assumption or a stimulus) in a context, and the lower the effort of establishing this context and its implications in the first place, the greater the relevance. In other words, a piece of new information (e.g., a linguistic message) is called *relevant* to the degree that it yields rich contextual effects when integrated with currently accessible old information (i.e., presently activated knowledge). Relevance is also claimed to play a key role in communication: here, cost and effort are balanced by the "second principle of relevance" which states that "[e]very act of ostensive communication communicates a presumption of its own optimal relevance" (Sperber and Wilson, 1995, 158). This is to say that Hearer can be sure of two things: first, on one of the conceivable interpretations, the perceived stimulus will produce an effect which Speaker considered worth bringing to his attention, and second, the stimulus is presumed to be *optimally relevant* in order to achieve this goal (i.e., the intended effect should be obtainable by processing the message in the most naturally available context). In other words, it is the communicators' mutual adherence to the second principle of relevance which guides Hearer in selecting the appropriate set of background assumptions that will allow him to infer Speaker's intended meaning. To achieve this, he will always process the message in the least effort-consuming manner given what he takes to be common ground between himself and Speaker. Only if the cognitive effects achieved thereby are not sufficient[7] is the initial context expanded in order to

[7] An obvious (and crucial) shortcoming of the theory is its failure to spell out what exactly will count as "sufficient" here. Sperber and Wilson suggest that an interpretation is "consistent with the principle of relevance if and only if a rational communicator might have expected it to be optimally relevant to the addressee" (Sperber and Wilson, 1995, 166). Since mutual knowledge

explore additional implications of the utterance. It has been noted at this point (Pateman, 1986, 750) that the mechanism envisaged by Sperber and Wilson in fact involves the serial application of two separate rationales rather than a single principle that would truly *balance* cost and effort: Hearer's overriding strategy is to minimize processing effort, and it is only in a second step that effects are considered.

Utterance interpretation is divided into three major steps, the last two of which involve inferencing: first, "linguistic decoding", which maps a phonetic signal onto a structured set of concepts and yields as output a highly abstract and semantically incomplete "logical form". Second, the "development" of this representation in terms of various inferential enrichments, involving the processing of the initial representation in an appropriately selected context until the fully-fledged "propositional form" of the utterance is arrived at. Third, "assessing import", which involves the formation and evaluation of assumptions relating to the implications of the propositional form of the utterance in currently accessible contexts; this process is repeated until the first plausible interpretive hypothesis is encountered. It is only these assumptions ("explicatures"[8] and implicatures in Sperber and Wilson's terminology) which are of any use regarding the overall end of utterance comprehension, i.e. the recovery of the addresser's informative intention. Processing the utterance in context comes to a halt as soon

---

is dismissed on their account, however, both Speaker and Hearer can never be quite sure about what would be optimally relevant to one another; in particular, Hearer has no way of knowing in advance exactly what Speaker might have considered "worth his attention", and why. As a consequence, it might well be that the interpretive hypothesis to appear optimally relevant to Hearer is not in fact the interpretation envisaged by Speaker. This might explain the fact that communication indeed often fails, but given the above definition of "consistency with the principle of relevance" *as a criterion for choosing interpretations*, it does not explain how Hearer can actually arrive at an interpretation at all.

8 As opposed to the notion of implicature, Sperber and Wilson refer to the assumptions *explicitly* communicated by an utterance as its "explicatures", with "explicitness" being defined as follows: "An assumption communicated by an utterance *U* is *explicit* if and only if it is a development of a logical form encoded by *U*" (Sperber and Wilson, 1995, 182).

as the first interpretation which is consistent with the principle of relevance is arrived at, thereby making the first spontaneously plausible hypothesis the "output" of the comprehension process. The principle of relevance is claimed to apply at all stages of the comprehension process and hence to govern each of the various subtasks involved. Two of these are of particular interest here: on the one hand, the step identified as "access to lexical entries" (a subtask of "linguistic decoding", this is where the activation of *zunichte* would have to be located in the model), and on the other hand, the identification of propositional attitude (a subtask of "assessing import", the stage at which the pun is reconstructed). In the present section, we will merely outline Sperber and Wilson's general account of the respective processing stages, i.e. the actual application to our data will be postponed to section 5.

As regards the activation issue, RT does not actually address it: Sperber and Wilson remain agnostic on collocation and other lexical priming effects, even though these phenomena have a manifest influence on decoding. In fact, RT is not overly concerned with the early stages of comprehension at all: arguing that "linguistic decoding is not so much a part of the comprehension process as something that precedes the real work of understanding, something that merely provides an input to the main part of the comprehension process" (Sperber and Wilson, 1995, 177), the authors focus on the inferential component straight away. There is one respect, though, in which the principle of relevance is claimed to also impinge on the procedure of linguistic decoding, and this is where issues of predictability and anticipation come into play: Sperber and Wilson assume that the inferential component interacts with the (supposedly dumb) decoding mechanism by imposing grammatical constraints on ongoing word recognition tasks. These restrictions come in the shape of "anticipatory syntactic hypotheses" which serve to predict the lexical category of the immediately following word: by suppressing the grammatically inappropriate items out of the set of present candidates, Sperber and Wilson argue, these constraints serve to reduce processing effort and thus increase relevance. Abstracting away from prosodic differences here, this means that with a sequence such as *these constraints serve?*

being recognized already, the inferential component would "inform" the decoding mechanism that an incoming sound sequence [tu] should at this point be interpreted as *to* (*these constraints serve to?*), rather than *too* (**these constraints serve, too?*), which would disqualify as a grammatically inappropriate homonym (cf. section 6 for discussion). At any rate, since Sperber and Wilson's account of anticipatory effects in lexical processing is limited to syntactic constraints, we must conclude that RT has nothing to offer as to how lexical items which are not directly "decoded" can nevertheless become part of the comprehension process.

As regards the second issue, however, we suspected that Sperber and Wilson's theory of irony might offer a convincing account of the inferential processes that lead to Hearer's recovery of the pun. Their argument proceeds from the idea that ironical utterances are "echoic" in nature: Speaker communicates an assumption from which she implicitly distances herself, in that this assumption is being attributed to someone else. The characterization of irony as an echo-phenomenon in turn goes back to one of the most fundamental tenets of RT - the distinction between "descriptive" and "interpretive" modes of language use. Roughly, the idea is that an utterance can be used either as a *description* of a state of affairs in the world, in which case it is a matter of its propositional form being either true or false of this state; or it can be used as an *interpretation* of some other propositional representation (i.e., another utterance or a thought), in which case its propositional form has to *resemble* the propositional form of this other representation. The essential property of irony (as a case of interpretive language use) is that the propositional attitude involved in this act of mimicry is one of disapproval. In order to grasp the ironical gist of an utterance, therefore, Hearer has to i) identify the utterance in question as echoic; ii) make out the source of the opinion echoed; and iii) recognize that Speaker's attitude to the represented thought or utterance is one of dissociation.

Sometimes, however, these questions are rather difficult to decide. There might be cases in which an utterance appears to be echoic, but the source of the opinion echoed cannot be clearly determined. Such utterances may echo to popular wisdom, fixed phrases and sayings and generally any formulaic chunk or stereotypical assumption which Speaker considers well-established enough to be supplied in order to recognize the echoic nature of her utterance. The second condition is thus not a necessary one: the fact that the element in question cannot be attributed to a specific source need not prevent successful recognition of the ironical nature of the alluding utterance. Then, there are many cases where Speaker's attitude is difficult if not impossible to pin down: between the two extremes of emphatic endorsement and outright rejection, echoic utterances may display a plethora of subtly graded attitudes involving a certain element of either affirmation or dissociation. Sperber and Wilson (1995, 240) hold that these options form "a continuum, with different blends of attitude and emotion giving rise to a whole range of borderline cases which do not fit neatly into any existing scheme". In the case of irony, however, it must be manifestly clear that Speaker is distancing herself from what is being echoed, else Hearer will end up with a positively wrong interpretation. Evidence for the intended attitude can be supplied in the form of prosodic and paralinguistic cues as well as left to Hearer to gather from contextual information. Hence, with an ironical prompt like *Go ahead and ruin my carpet*, Hearer can be safely entrusted to supply the information that the ruin of carpets is generally not considered a desirable state of affairs. Moreover, *Go ahead and ruin my carpet* is echoic in that it refers to a thought which Speaker expects to have occurred to Hearer when he caused whatever mishap it was. We suppose that it is precisely this mechanism (ironically alluding to a presently salient thought of Hearer) that accounts for the pun in our text (see below for details).

5 Empirical assessment

As indicated in section 2, successful comprehension of our stimulus text (repeated here as (4)) requires two things: first, activating the lexical representation of the fully implicit word *zunichte*, which is expected to occur at the end of line 4; and second, assessing the import of its non-occurrence through a particular chain of inferences. Naturally, issues of lexical priming are "more amenable to experimental testing than the recovery of implicatures" (Sperber and Wilson, 1995, 257), but we attempted to devise suitable empirical designs for either component of this process. Before we discuss the methods (5.2) and results (5.3) of these investigations, let us begin with a more detailed consideration of what happens upon comprehending the poem.

(4) *Bekenntnis*
Ich leide an Versagensangst
Besonders, wenn ich dichte.
Die Angst, die machte mir bereits
Manch schönen Reim zuschanden.

5.1 Hypotheses

By choosing the rare and archaic near-synonym *zuschanden* instead of the expected word *zunichte* at the end of line 4, the author frustrates Hearer's expectation and creates a paradoxical pun: the communicated message (which can be paraphrased as: "the author is a bad poet who often fails at rhyming") is reinforced and directly exemplified by the fact that the poem itself indeed does not rhyme. At the same time, it is obvious that the presence of *zuschanden* (and hence, the avoidance of the rhyme) is the product of a deliberate and, as will be realized on the inferential plane, well-calculated choice rather than the outcome of some "fear of failure" which is presented as the reason for the author's seemingly poor performance. The text thus strongly suggests that the author could well have supplied the appropriate rhyme if only he had wanted to. In order to get the pun, Hearer first has to supply the envisaged element and in a second step explore the contextual implications of the fact that it has been spared out with what must be deliberate intent. In other words, the intended propositional attitude (irony) can only be inferred correctly if Hearer has actually expected *zunichte* in the first place, meaning that the corresponding lexical entry must have been activated without the word being actually "decoded" in the sense of Sperber and Wilson. If this account is correct, the theories under consideration will have to account for two separate issues: first, how does *zunichte* become involved in the comprehension process, and second, what happens in reconstructing the pun?

5.1.1 Activation of *zunichte*

As regards the activation of *zunichte*, we expected a cumulative increase in priming with four factors contributing to the overall effect: rhyme expectation, collocation, identical word-onset of *zuschanden* and *zunichte* as well as an interplay of semantic and syntactic constraints on the final slot in the second sentence. First and foremost, Hearer expects the text to rhyme, which would require a match with *dichte* at the end of line 4. Subjects had been informed that they would be presented with short humorous verse, and each of the preceding stimulus texts had confirmed the stererotypical genre expectation that such poems commonly rhyme. Second, there is a syntagmatic lexical relation between *machte* and *zunichte* which form a well-established collocation in German. Incidentally, a weaker relation of the same sort also holds between *machte* and *zuschanden*; the word *zuschanden*, however, is extremely rare and presumably no longer in the active vocabulary of most speakers of contemporary German. Evidence supporting this intuition was obtained from a frequency check of both *zunichte* and *zuschanden* as well as the two collocations *zunichte machen* and *zuschanden machen* in the IdS-corpora of written language (PUBLIC):

Table 1. Total frequency of *zunichte* / *zuschanden machen* in PUBLIC

	raw counts
zunichte	4845
zunichte machen	4727
zuschanden	90
zuschanden machen	18

Seeing that lexical retrieval is more time-consuming for rare words,[9] we expected that other things being equal, the more frequent item *zunichte* should be more readily available than *zuschanden* when collocationally primed by *machte*, especially since *machen* also collocates much more strongly with *zunichte* than with *zuschanden* (irrespective of absolute frequency): whereas 97,56% of all instances of *zunichte* appear in connection with *machen*, this is only true for 20% of the attested instances of *zuschanden*, which is a further reason why *zunichte* should receive higher activation values than its competitor. The same holds for the third factor, i.e. the identical onset of *zunichte* and *zuschanden*: even granted that the very rare *zuschanden* is actually among the initial set of activated candidate representations at all, *zunichte* should still display significantly higher activation values due to its greater degree of entrenchment. The fourth factor emerges from an interaction of semantic and syntactic constraints on plausible fillers of the position in question: on the one hand, the semantics of *Bekenntnis* ("confession"), *leiden* ("to suffer") and *Versagensangst* ("fear of failure") combine to the effect that the consequences of whatever this "fear" has caused are foreshadowed as something presumably negative. On the other hand, by the time Hearer has arrived at the last word of line 4, an "anticipatory syntactic hypothesis" in the sense of Sperber and Wilson will have narrowed the focus of the recognition procedure by informing it that the target item should be an adverb: with both direct object/patient (*manch schönen Reim*) and an additional indirect object/ "maleficiary" argument (*mir*) being identified already, Hearer will know that *machte* is being used as a function verb requiring an additional element in the present context. As laid out in section 3, Hearer's preliminary syntactic analysis of the stimulus should thus prime the grammatical template of the resultative construction. According to Goldberg (1995), the resultative schema (cf. Figure 1) is a

[9] This is the so-called "word-frequency effect" observed in studies of lexical access; cf. Forster (1976, 263): "words with a relatively high frequency of occurrence are classified faster [when presented in a lexical decision task] than words with a low occurrence frequency, e.g. *mildew, perspire, radiate*, although the latter are still perfectly familiar to the subjects of the experiment".

subtype of caused motion constructions that canonically encodes the process of (metaphorically) transferring a patient argument to a new state:

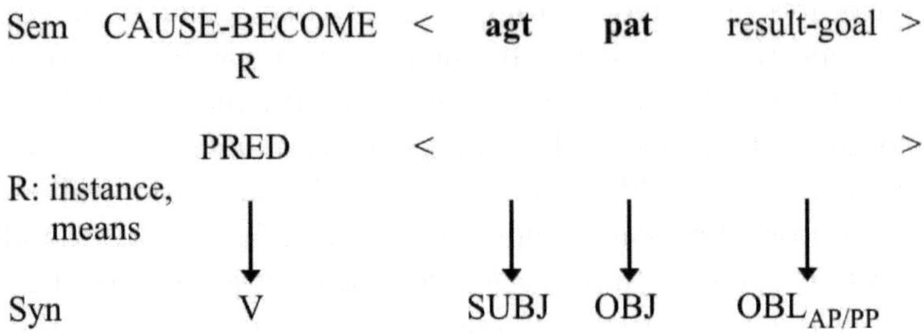

Figure 1. The Resultative Construction (Goldberg, 1995, 189)

In the given context, Hearer will thus be in a position to anticipate that the referent of the direct object is being brought into a new state, and that the expressed change of state is likely to be of a destructive quality, i.e. geared towards some negative outcome. The combination of these cues thus yields a further indication that *zunichte* is highly appropriate for the position in question.

Summing up, we expected both immediate priming effects of differing strengths and an overall cumulation of cues resulting in the ever stronger activation of *zunichte.* We hypothesized that the latter effect should require contextual "integration" in the sense of Kintsch's CI-model, i.e. that delays of target word presentation of more than 750 msec. should lead to a marked increase in priming.

5.1.2 Assessment of propositional attitude

As regards the pun, we have claimed that the anticipation of *zunichte* is a necessary prerequisite for successful comprehension of the poem. However, this is not to say that it is also a necessary corollary of processing the text, in the sense that it will inevitably surface to consciousness and actually occur to each and every subject. It is clearly conceivable that Hearer may fail to consciously acknowledge the allusion or fail to grasp its implications. In both cases, we hold that this will lead to a wrong assessment of propositional attitude resulting in only partly successful comprehension. Hence, we suspected that there should be a clear interdependence between subjects' awareness of their anticipation and positive evaluations of the texts as original, witty etc. Furthermore, we supposed that the peculiar effect of the text could be explained along the lines of Sperber and Wilson's theory of irony: basically, the idea is that the thought underlying the poem is something like "I [i.e., the author] can't rhyme", that this thought is being attributed to Hearer, and that the activation of *zunichte* provides evidence conflicting with this assumption, thereby ridiculing the all too premature above conclusion. This process may be reconstructed as follows: first, the text itself implicates that the author is a bad poet whose "failure" lies in his notorious inability to come up with rhymes. Second, the poem provides direct evidence for this assumption, as an appropriate match for "dichte" is seemingly amiss. In this, the text exploits Hearer's rhyme expectation, and it is precisely this move that allows the attribution of the underlying thought to Hearer himself: having realized that the text indeed does not rhyme, he is tricked into strengthening the implicature that the author is a pathetic poet who cannot come up with appropriate rhyme words - a deduction which is carried out solely on the responsibility of Hearer himself. In the third step, however, this conclusion is yet again refuted by the observation that the rhyme must have been avoided on purpose. Consequently, Hearer is so to speak "caught in the act" of subscribing to the unwarranted implicature which the text has previously forced onto him.

It is only against the backdrop of *zunichte* that the defeat of Hearer's rhyme expectation can be understood as an intended effect that has significant consequences for the immediate implicatures of the poem. Hence, for subjects achieving full text comprehension, the unconscious priming effect was predicted to surface to consciousness at the very moment that their expectation was disconfirmed, and this in turn was predicted to trigger the extra layer of inferences needed in order to reconstruct the pun. By contrast, if it is not understood that the rhyme was avoided *on purpose* (which presupposes the conviction that the particular rhyme must have been at the author's disposal) in order to illustrate the poem's point, we hypothesized that the original implicatures of the text would be retained in the context, to the effect that Hearer would not attain fully successful comprehension. In this case, the wrong assessment of propositional attitude would coincide with a low degree of relevance, thereby prompting evaluations of the text as all in all unsatisfactory, banal and pointless.

5.2 Methods

The activation of *zunichte* was investigated in a cross-modal priming experiment involving a lexical decision task. 72 subjects, mostly students of German or English linguistics at the University of Hanover, were tested individually using a fully automatic experimental programming - that is, they were presented with standardized recordings of the stimulus texts, the target words were presented visually on a computer screen, and both was part of an automatic procedure. Reaction times were measured automatically using ERTS. Subjects were told that they were going to be presented with poems, some of which would be interrupted, i.e. the recordings were only played up to a certain point. Immediately after the presentation, they were told, a string of letters would appear on the screen and they would have to decide as quickly as possible whether the presented letter string is meaningless or if it forms an existing German word.

Subjects were presented with seven poems in total. The texts were taken from the works of several German authors (Joachim Ringelnatz, Christian Morgenstern, Eugen Roth, Ansgar Anders and Alex Dreppec). The stimulus texts were all short (presentable in spoken form within less than 20 seconds), humorous and rhymed.[10] The first six runs merely served as a training, but were not marked as such. During the six training runs, subjects were presented with three existing words and three senseless letter strings as targets. Three of the

[10] This counts for the six training runs. The poem given in the control condition of the seventh run did not rhyme.

six poems that served as a training were interrupted (i.e. not presented in full length), three were not. The choice of the interrupted poems was varied systematically. In the seventh run, all subjects were presented with Gernhardt's poem "Bekenntnis" and the target word *zunichte*. In order to reconstruct the build-up of the anticipatory effect, the presentation of the text was interrupted at one of the following five measure points:

(5) *Bekenntnis*
Ich leide an Versagensangst
Besonders, wenn ich dichte (1)
Die Angst, die machte (2) *mir bereits*
Manch schönen Reim (3) *zu*(4)*schanden* (5)

The first four measure points were chosen in order to investigate the respective contributions of the hypothesized cues detailed in section 5.1. The fifth measure point served to make sure whether *zunichte* was still primed after its competitor *zuschanden* had been perceived. Each of these five conditions was presented to 12 of the subjects. A sixth condition with an alternative seventh poem not priming *zunichte* at all was presented to another 12 subjects. This served as a control condition in order to obtain values for a comparison with the values of the other five conditions where priming effects were expected. The results were evaluated with variance analysis. In the terminology of quantitative statistics, the dependent variable - the variable that was expected to vary depending on the different conditions - was constituted by the reaction times; independent variables were the different options of the final presentation (which amounted to six different conditions: four interrupted versions, the complete presentation and the control condition) and the delay with which the target word was presented (two different options), giving a total of 12 conditions altogether.

Our second investigation was concerned with the expected interdependence between lexical retrieval of *zunichte* and correct assessments of the text's propositional attitude. We constructed a questionnaire consisting of the poem and 16 questions. The 16 questions formed two scales, each consisting of eight questions. The first eight questions were all concerned with the reader's evaluation of the poem - i.e., subjects were asked to comment whether they found the text original, funny, appealing etc. The questions of the second scale asked whether they had noticed a "surprise" of some sort when reading the text, whether there had been an element of unfulfilled expectation or a sudden change of orientation etc. at some point. We expected these two scales to correlate significantly. The participants, 34 students of English, had to choose between 4 standardized answering possibilities ("yes", "rather yes", "rather no" and "no"), later coded from 1 to 4. Moreover, they were also asked to freely formulate reasons for their answers regarding some of the questions. The data were subject to a correlation analysis (Pearson).

5.3 Results

Figure 2 shows the results of the priming experiment. Each of the columns stands for one of the conditions resulting from the combination of the variations and sums up the data of six participants. The priming effect is highly significant with $F\ (5,\ 60) = 4{,}02$, $p < .005$ (Variance Analysis is legitimated by a Levene Test). All conditions with an expected priming effect in fact display this effect compared to the control condition. However, the expected cumulative priming effect regarding conditions 1 to 4 only appears when the target word is presented with 1 sec delay. This result will be discussed below in more detail. It is backed up by another heuristic analysis, that is, a correlation analysis including the data for the delayed presentation (1 sec) of the target word with the control condition coded as "point 0" (no priming effect) and condition 5 not included (a "prolonged" cumulative priming effect was not expected for this condition). The correlation between the reaction times (of six participants per condition) and these five conditions (1, 2, 3, 4 and 6 interpreted as 0) coded from 0 to 4 is highly significant with $r = -.64$, $p < .001$.

The effect of the presentation time of the target is also significant with $F\ (1,\ 60) = 5{,}17$, $p < .05$. Even though this is not reflected by all of the conditions, participants tended to react more slowly when the

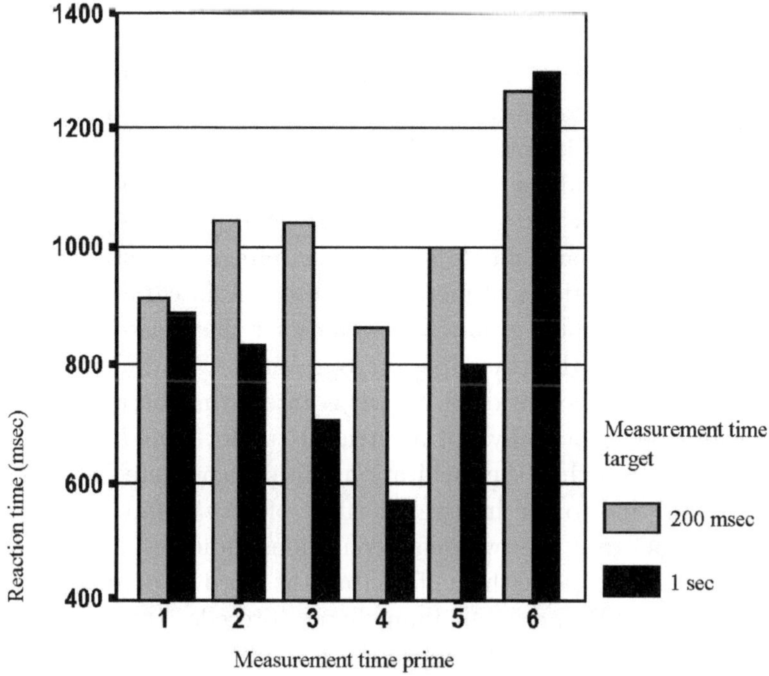

Figure 2. Priming results

target was presented with only 200 msec delay. This is also reflected by the data of the training runs, where it took the participants an average of 107,7 msec longer to react when the target was presented with a delay of 200 msec rather than 1 sec. Apart from this general tendency, there are of course specific differences between the single conditions: first, the delay does not make much difference in conditions 1 and 6. This is in accordance with our expectations: at both points, there is not much to integrate. As regards the control condition 6, we did not expect *any* element of the alternative poem to prime *zunichte*, implying of course that there is no need to integrate more than one element that would do so. As regards condition 1, we see *dichte* as the first cue privileging the activation of *zunichte*, so it is not necessary to integrate it with any preceding indication. Thus, the priming effect of *dichte* stands mostly for itself in both conditions, which is in fact reflected by the small difference between the two delay conditions. The other conditions differ in this respect: in condition two, the collocational effect of *machte* has to be integrated with the effect of its predecessor *dichte*. We interpret the difference between the two delay conditions at this point as follows: with a delay of 1 sec, the integration can be performed, thus, the priming effects of *machte* and *dichte* merge to an integrated retrieval cue for *zunichte*. With a delay of merely 200 msec, no integration is allowed for, meaning that the result here stands for the isolated priming effect of *machte*, with little support from *dichte*. The difference is even more marked in condition 3, which is interesting because the word *Reim* in itself is actually not a retrieval cue for *zunichte* at all; this in turn suggests that the facilitation effect encountered at 200 msec here is still due to the integrated effect of *dichte* and *machte*. The difference between the two delay conditions indicates that this effect is not yet integrated with the fact that the word *Reim* completes the direct object NP and hence immediately precedes the syntactic slot in which the semantically appropriate adverb *zunichte* would have to be located. If this observation can be integrated with the preceding indications, the priming effect is markedly stronger. Regarding condition 4, the strong priming effect observed in the condition with 200 msec delay can be interpreted as resulting from the part-whole relation between *zu-* and *zunichte*: upon perceiving the onset of the poem's last word, the strongly primed item *zunichte* will receive even more activation (this time in a bottom-up fashion). In the condition with 1 sec delay, this effect is again integrated with its predecessors, resulting in the strongest priming effect measured in the experiment.

As regards the questionnaire-based survey, our predictions were borne out, too: not surprisingly, the two scales correlate highly significantly with $r = .47$ ($p < .005$). Participants who expected that the poem would end with *zunichte* did notice an "orientation shift" and evaluated the poem more positively. The opposite is true for those who did not experience such a shift. Figure 3 illustrates the correlation using the original data of the single participants. Two points mark the two scale sums for each of the participants. What matters here is the harmonic "movement" of the two lines connecting all of the scale sums for the two scales separately. This illustrates that, with little exceptions (and these exceptions are natural within quantitative statistics), a high scale sum on one of the two scales goes along with a high scale sum on the other one. The fact that some of the partici-

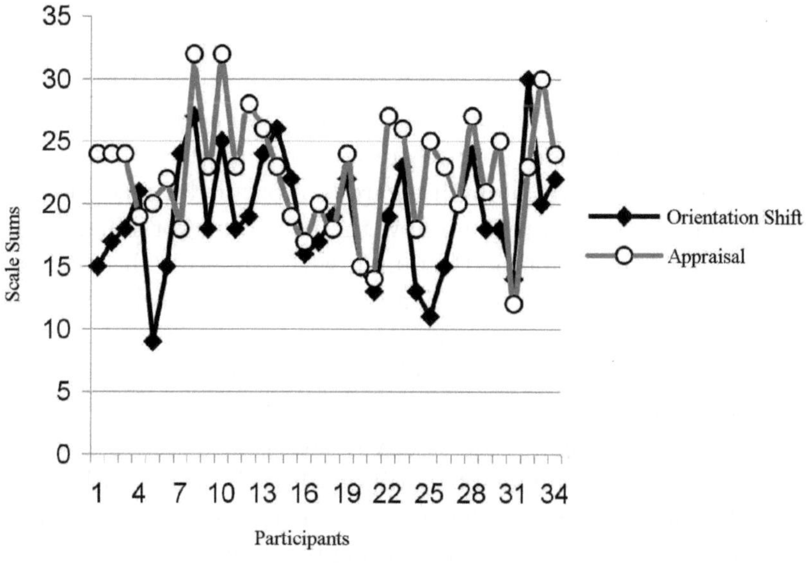

Figure 3. The correlation between anticipation and appreciation

pants did reconstruct the author's intention and some did not can also be illustrated by quoting from the freely formulated reasons for their answers. Subjects who evaluated the text negatively stated reasons such as the following: "Ein Gedicht sollte sich meiner Meinung nach reimen. Das vergrößert die Wirkung um ein Vielfaches" ("I believe that a poem should rhyme. That increases the effect of the poem significantly"). Positive evaluations came along with comments such as "Der Reim wird tatsächlich zuschanden gemacht" ("The rhyme is indeed brought to naught").

Summing up the results in total, we have found that there is a cumulative increase in the activation of *zunichte* if contextual integration is allowed for. Furthermore, consciously acknowledging the fact that lexical retrieval of *zunichte* was actively encouraged by the author leads to a completely revised interpretation of the text (as manifest in subjects' markedly different evaluations of the poem).

6 Discussion

We set out to discuss how effects of predictability in wording (which may be indicative of certain general properties of lexical representations in memory) may be accommodated in two current accounts of language comprehension, and we are now in a position to assess the models under consideration with regard to a particular case and some specific data. Let us first recap how the two frameworks handle the data presented in section 5. Beginning with Kintsch's theory, it can offer a straightforward explanation of the priming results presented in Figure 2: the activation of *zunichte* increases significantly if "integration" in the sense of the CI-model is allowed for. This result, illustrated by the difference between each pair of black and grey columns in Figure 2 (as well as by the steady decrease in reaction time indicated by the black columns of conditions 1-4), is clearly in line with the predictions of the CI-model. Hence, our results can be interpreted as support for Kintsch's basic distinction between "construction" and "integration" phases as well as his claim that interrelated elements strengthen one another within the integration phase: *zunichte* receives priming from several items in the activated net, but the full effect is only observable if the separate cues can be "integrated" in the manner envisioned by Kintsch.

RT in turn can offer a convincing account of what happens next (or, in other words, an explanation of the data in Figure 3): on the one hand, there are several cues which encourage the anticipation of *zunichte* rather than the more effort-consuming retrieval of *zuschanden* (being an archaism, the latter would be improbable anyway, but in the given linguistic context, it is downright inappropriate); on the other hand, Hearer generally expects that he is not incurred with processing effort gratuitously, meaning that greater effort should always be offset with additional intended effects. Seeing that the recovery of the implicit item is strongly encouraged by the text, the principle of relevance will lead Hearer to suspect that there might be some underlying rationale for conning him into anticipating the "wrong" item. Once the assumption that *zunichte* would have been a much more likely and appropriate choice in the position in question is added to the current context and processed together with the "explicatures" and implicatures of the text, the extremely unlikely preference of *zuschanden* will all of a sudden appear consistent and significant: Hearer is now in a position to realize that the author must have avoided the rhyme on purpose in order to provide direct evidence for the poem's literal message ("I [i.e., the author] can't rhyme"), and that this proposition is not actually entertained as a would-be sincere *description*, i.e. that the poem should not be taken to actually assert this proposition. This conclusion in turn gives rise to a whole range of new contextual effects which cancel the text's original implicatures, and as relevance is merely a function of effort and effect, it follows that the ironical interpretation is more relevant than the assertion reading: if *zunichte* has been activated so that the crucial assumption can eventually be formed, contextual effects will be larger than if the original implicatures are simply endorsed and taken at face value. This increase in relevance is reflected in Hearer's realization that the author is actually not failing at all, but rather skillfully playing with his expectations.

On the other hand, just as the strengths of Relevance Theory and the CI-model complement each other in reconstructing our observations, so do their limitations. RT cannot explain how *zunichte* can become part of the comprehension process in the first place. The CI-model does explain that, but it has nothing substantial to say about the inferential processes involved in reconstructing the pun; moreover, it cannot accommodate the fact that *zuschanden* remains highly activated, too (cf. the simulation data in the appendix).[11]

[11] This can be illustrated by means of heuristic computer simulations performed with the CI-simulation-program: because of its weaker connections to the

Therefore, before we move on to discuss whether our case can shed light on more general issues of lexical processing, let us consider the extent to which these observations may point to relevant shortcomings of either model.

As regards Kintsch's paradigm, it provides a general model that can recast lexical association phenomena in terms of spreading activation processes, but it does not explicitly detail how these activation patterns are transformed into specific interpretive assumptions, and it does not cover the full range of elements that will actually co-activate one another in the envisaged manner, either. Let us briefly discuss both issues in turn. First, Kintsch is not very specific about which particular assumptions will in fact be formed during comprehension: to stay with our example, if Hearer arrives at the crucial conclusion that the author of our text must have avoided the rhyme on purpose, this assumption is fairly removed from the actual "text base", i.e. it is the product of a complex chain of inferences which cannot be reduced to merely "constructing" and "integrating" the text's propositional net itself. True, Kintsch maintains that his model is not intended to cover conscious problem solving activities, but the fact remains that many assumptions which are formed during comprehension are *neither* consciously constructed nor immediately entailed by elements of the text base, either. A theory of human utterance comprehension which does not account for these assumptions (meaning that it will predict which ones will and which ones will not be formed, and why this should be so) is not fully satisfactory. Second, our data indicate that the exclusively semantic focus of Kintsch's account of the CI-process may be too limited in scope. Kintsch's model relies on a

---

other nodes, *zuschanden* always receives very little to no activation at all, although it is evidently as important for successful comprehension as *zunichte* (which always gets the highest possible activation). Regarding the values entering the process (link strengths and activation values), this result is very robust given variation "within some reasonable range", to quote Kintsch again. These simulations cannot be described here in full detail, but the activation value vectors and the connectivity matrix for one example can be found in the appendix (as a documentation aimed at readers who are already familiar with the simulation procedure).

priori stipulations of which elements will actually count as "related" and how the "strength" of these relationships should be measured. As indicated, a method for obtaining such independent data as far as semantic relationships are concerned is supposed to be provided by LSA; it is unclear, however, how other lexical relations such as e.g. rhyme should be incorporated into this account, and how the respective strengths of different types of lexical relations in memory should be compared. Apart from predicting that the integrated effect of e.g. phonological and syntactic-semantic priming of *zunichte* should be larger than the respective priming effects in isolation, Kintsch's approach therefore does not offer an exhaustive account of how the individual effects arise and how they interact in processing.

Our problems with RT lie elsewhere. Relevance Theory may not be a theory of linguistic structure in itself, but it nevertheless builds on certain assumptions about what constitutes relevant aspects of linguistic knowledge, and as such it plain ignores the rich fabric of lexical patterning in language that accounts for the phenomenon investigated in this paper. More generally, the fact that RT does not address such issues in the first place is indicative of its essentially modular and "syntactocentric" (Jackendoff, 1997) orientation. We see our findings as evidence that such approaches miss out on relevant facts about speakers' linguistic knowledge: specifically, Sperber and Wilson do not preclude the existence of top-down effects in lexical processing in principle, but arbitrarily limit their scope to those which are *syntactically* motivated (as outlined in section 4.2, Sperber and Wilson's concept of "anticipatory syntactic hypotheses" may constitute *one* aspect of such effects, but it is unclear why this should be a privileged factor, let alone the only one involved). For means of illustration, recall our earlier example of the rather simple sequence *these constraints serve ... to/*too*, where an anticipatory syntactic hypothesis would influence the decoding procedure by suppressing the potential target representation too; still, there are often many additional options to be considered which would escape a purely syntax-based account since *each* of them would be grammatical (consider e.g. the numeral *two*in the present example, as in *these constraints serve two different functions*). The point is that constraints relating to grammatical well-formedness *alone* are probably not enough - they need to be combined with additional indications in order to allow for rapid real-time performance (in computational linguistics, this insight has often led to the incorporation of statistical heuristics into the analysis, seeing that a purely formal "deep analyses" may run into complexities that cannot be handled anymore). While such observations actually provide strong evidence for the importance of economy considerations (and therefore something like Sperber and Wilson's principle of relevance) in utterance comprehension, they also illustrate that it is ill-advised to explicitly exclude certain types of probabilistic cues in processing which could otherwise relieve processing load to a significant extent. In fact, Sperber and Wilson are only drawn to this move because of their commitment to cognitive modularity in the Fodorian sense (Fodor, 1983): they conceive of the linguistic system as an autonomous and dumb "input system" into central cognition and therefore maintain that the putative basic heuristic of the central component (i.e. the principle of relevance) does not affect the operations of the linguistic input module (i.e. "automatic decoding"). To us, however, Sperber and Wilson's account of why "anticipatory syntactic hypotheses" of the type described above should constitute an exception from this rule is not convincing - either the decoding procedure is "informationally encapsulated" or it is not (you can't have your cake and eat it!). At any rate, some probabilistic effects other than syntax-based constraints undoubtedly show up during the initial stages of lexical processing already, i.e. within what would be the "construction phase" in Kintsch's terminology: as reported in section 5, lexical access is less effort-consuming for frequent words, which points to the significance of cognitive entrenchment for lexical processing. Extending the logic of RT to this domain, frequent words are per definitionem more likely to actually occur in discourse and less effort-consuming to retrieve, which is why there is good reason for Hearer to utilize frequency information if indeed his overarching strategy is to minimize processing load.

Applied to our case, this observation indicates the direction in which a jointly CI- and RT-compatible explanation of lexical predictability effects may be sought: they reflect probabilistic conjectures which emerge from an overlap of activation patterns that have arisen from otherwise independent associative processes. In the terminology of RT and the CI-model, considerations of relevance will affect the way in which the initial network will be both constructed and integrated: it is the most strongly entrenched and most frequently co-activated (i.e. least-effort-consuming-to-access) items which will become involved in the construction process first, and it is the most strongly interconnected items (i.e. those with the highest amount of straightforward contextual implications) which will be retained posterior to integration. Hence, the individual priming effects for *zunichte* need not even be particularly strong, as long as the cumulative value is sufficient in order to surpass the item's activation threshold (which should be lower than that of e.g. *zuschanden* from the outset).

Our notion of converging retrieval cues is in fact strongly reminiscent of a key mechanism in yet another psycholinguistic model, namely Allport's (1985) theory of "distributed memory" with its notion of "engram capture": on this account, lexical representations (like any other elements of knowledge) consist of activation patterns spread across larger regions of the brain, and the elements of such an activation pattern (i.e., the various different specifications of the particular word) are associated with each other. This is what Allport calls an auto-associated pattern or "engram". Additionally, the various elements of an engram are associated with elements of other activation patterns - hence, among others, the activation pattern for *zunichte* would be connected to the patterns for *dichte* and *machte* for instance. Associative connections between activation patterns manifest in priming effects and may ultimately serve as retrieval cues given a certain threshold value is surpassed. In that way, we can describe the observed "merger" of retrieval cues for *zunichte* as the result of a "capture" of its activation pattern due to cumulative priming, which would explain why associative (i.e., purely top-down) factors in processing may be as effective for the activation of lexical representations in memory as ordinary bottom-up decoding.

What are the implications of these observations? First of all, modelling lexical items as "auto-associated activation patterns" that synthesize qualitatively different and independently stored information marks a point of departure from the pre-theoretical conception of words as unified wholes (comprising a particular sound sequence and a "convenient capsule of thought"). Metaphorically speaking, our data show that lexical access may in fact proceed through several "backdoors" from "different sides" at the same time, since the different elements of the activation pattern of *zunichte* are independently co-activated by associated elements in their respective domains. In that, our findings support the idea that lexical representations in memory should not be conceived of as reified atomic units stored at some particular "location", and that they need not necessarily be activated at one specific point of lexical access, either.[12] Various psycholinguistic accounts of the lexicon have called the classical Saussurean conception of the sign (as a unified element with inextricable linkage of form and meaning) into question,[13] and if the formal and semantic specifications of lexical items are indeed stored separately, we would have to conclude that the mental representation of a particular word in fact comprises a number of distinct smaller components (i.e., the "elements" of the overall activation pattern in Allport's sense).

Somewhat paradoxically, however, there is also reason to assume that what is stored is actually *larger* structures than the individual word. Evidence in favour of this claim is provided by collocational phenomena: rather than saying that the activation patterns corresponding to words such as *machen* and *zunichte* are somehow "related" (i.e. essentially distinct but connected) in memory, it has also

12 In fact, the very notion of "lexical access" might be somewhat misleading already, seeing that it takes the underlying "lexicon"-metaphor rather literally; cf. Günther (1989, 265): "Gedacht war an einen Vorgang ähnlich dem im Wörterbuch suchenden Zeigefinger. Lexikalischer Zugriff erfolgt genau in dem Moment, in dem der Finger auf den gesuchten Eintrag deutet. Es ist ein magischer Moment: Sobald der Eintrag gefunden ist, werden mit einem Schlag alle Informationen über das gesuchte Wort verfügbar: Bedeutung, Wortart, Register, Reim, Flexionsweise, etc."

13 Aitchison (2003) assumes two independent modules for syntax/semantics and phonology, Levelt (1989) suggests a dichotomy of "lemma lexicon" vs. "form lexicon", and Morton (1979) decomposes the psychological correlate of words into separate phonological and graphological input and output "logogens" which merely serve as evidence collectors for a particular item

been suggested that such collocations are stored as unified chunks, i.e. represented as holistic (albeit analysable) *units* in the lexicon. This would amount to claiming that - contrary to what the term itself suggests - the "lexical entry" of a particular word in memory does not consist of a single schematic representation but rather of a massively redundant *network* of overlapping usage patterns (i.e. memorized occurrences of the respective word within experienced contexts). This is not to suggest that speakers simply "record" their entire linguistic input without analysis and any sorting out - quite to the contrary, it is commonly assumed hat speakers strive for the optimal (i.e. maximally motivated) organization of their individual inventory of words and syntactic constructions. This means that the existing network will only be accommodated if the present input cannot be assimilated to an appropriate sanction structure; furthermore, speakers will attempt to establish mutually supporting links between elements of the network that are categorized as relevantly similar. For this reason, the overlaps and redundancies between different usages of the same word indeed provide ample motivation for extracting one or more schemas that capture the relevant commonalities - still, it would be neither legitimate to equate the lexical entry of the respective word with the topmost schema ultimately emerging from such abstractions, nor indeed plausible to assume that the original instances are "unlearned" once such a schema is extracted. If these latter assumptions are rejected, it is difficult to see how collocation as a manifest distributional fact should be explained at all: if the lexicon really only contained that which cannot be computed (as most mainstream grammatical theories would have it), how can one account for speaker's knowledge of fully compositional collocations such as *zunichte machen*, and where else should such information be stored if not in the lexicon? If one pursues the above assumptions further, by contrast, they may have rather radical implications for the conception of linguistic knowledge at large: according to Barlow (2000, 316), for instance, "the main component of the grammar [?] comprises a large set of redundantly specified schemas, both abstract and lexically-specified, and the role of rules or constraints (or highly abstract schemas) is to provide the glue or mortar to combine these prefabricated chunks".

Even though we cannot go into these issues in the given context, the quote illustrates that questions of lexical association and chunking may in fact have important implications for linguistic and psycholinguistic model-building.

7 Conclusion

We hope to have shown that predictability effects in wording are actually a far less outlandish thing than certain received views of linguistic knowledge and processing would lead to believe. As it stands, however, neither of the two theories invoked for explaining particular aspects of our findings can provide a fully comprehensive account of what happens upon successfully interpreting our stimulus text. Even though the CI-model and Relevance Theory appear to provide very different approaches to the phenomenon in question, we have nevertheless attempted to hint at where there might be interesting points of contact between these influential psychological and linguistic perspectives on comprehension that may merit further consideration. Finally, we hope to have illustrated that the phenomenon in question is not merely less unusual than one might suspect at first glance, but that it may also shed light on general issues of lexical processing and storage.

Appendix

As indicated in footnote 11, we have conducted a series of simulations using the computer implementation of Kintsch's CI-model. In the following example, our target item *zunichte* was given a smaller activation value (0,25) than that of the other nodes (activation value: 1). We hold that it becomes part of the elaborated propositional net within the construction process because of its associative links to several of the nodes that can be directly constructed from the text surface.

As evident from the last table, D has become the node with the strongest activation, while E is much less activated. This result was confirmed in many variations of the present simulation with other input values which are not documented here for reasons of space.

Table 2. Activation Values, Start

A1	Versagensangst	1
B1	dichte	1
C1	machte	1
D1	zunichte	0,25
E1	zuschanden	1

Table 3. Connectivity Matrix

	A	B	C	D	E
A	1	1	0	1	1
B	1	1	0	1	0
C	0	0	1	1	1
D	1	1	1	1	-1
E	1	0	1	-1	1

Table 4. Activation Values, Results

A	Versagensangst	1
B	dichte	0,92
C	machte	0,58
D	zunichte	1
E	zuschanden	0,27

References

Aitchison, Jean. 2003. *Words in the Mind. An Introduction to the Mental Lexicon.* Oxford: Blackwell. (first published 1987).

Allan, Keith. 1992. Something that rhymes with rich. In: A. Lehrer and E. F. Kittay (eds.), *Frames, Fields and Contrasts. New Essays in Semantic and Lexical Organization.* Hillsdale NJ: Lawrence Erlbaum Associates, 355–374.

Allport, D. A. 1985. Distributed memory, modular subsystems and dysphasia. In: S. Newman and R. Epstein (eds.), *Current Perspectives in Dysphasia.* Edinburgh: Churchill Livingstone, 207–244.

Altenberg, Bengt. 1991. Amplifier collocations in spoken English. In: S. Johansson and A.-B. Stenström (eds.), *English Computer Corpora*. Berlin: Mouton de Gruyter, 127–147.

Altman, G. T. M. 1997. *The Ascent of Babel*. Oxford: Oxford University Press.

Barlow, M. 2000. Usage, blends, and grammar. In: S. Kemmer and M. Barlow (eds.), *Usage-based Models of Language*. Stanford: CSLI, 315–345.

Bartlett, F. C. 1932. *Remembering*. Cambridge: Cambridge University Press.

Bock, J. K. 1986. Syntactic persistence in language production. *Cognitive Psychology* 18: 355–387.

Bolinger, Dwight. 1976. Meaning and memory. *Forum Linguisticum* 1: 1–14.

Coulmas, Florian. 1981. Introduction: Conversational routine. In: F. Coulmas (ed.), *Conversational Routine. Explorations in Standardized Communication Situations and Pre-patterned Speech*. The Hague: Mouton, 1–17.

Deppert, Alex. 2002. Comparing apples and pears: Latent semantic analysis. In: Cornelia Zelinsky-Wibbelt (ed.), *Text, Context, Concepts*. Berlin: Mouton de Gruyter, 127–155.

Fodor, Jerry A. 1983. *The Modularity of Mind*. Cambridge, MA: MIT Press.

Forster, Kenneth I. 1976. Accessing the mental lexicon. In: R. J. Wales and E. Walker (eds.), *New Approaches to Language Mechanisms*. Amsterdam: North Holland, 257–287.

Francis, Gill. 1993. A corpus-driven approach to grammar. Principles, methods and examples. In: M. Baker, G. Francis and E. Tognini-Bonelli (eds.), *Text and Technology. In Honour of John Sinclair*. Amsterdam: John Benjamins, 138–156.

Goldberg, Adele. 1995. *Constructions. A Construction Grammar Approach to Argument Structure*. Chicago: University of Chicago Press.

Grice, Herbert P. 1989. Logic and conversation. In: H. P. Grice (ed.), *Studies in the Way of Words*. Cambridge, MA: Harvard University Press, 22–40. (first published 1967).

Günther, H. 1989. Wörter im Kopf? Gedanken zu einem Buch von Jean Aitchison. In: G. Kegel et al. (ed.), *Sprechwissenschaft und Psycholinguistik*, volume 3. Opladen: Westdeutscher Verlag, 257–267.

Howard, D. V. 1981. Semantic priming of lexical decisions in young and old adults. *Journal of Gerontology* 36: 707–714.

Jackendoff, Ray. 1997. *The Architecture of the Language Faculty*. Cambridge, Mass.: MIT Press.

Jakobson, Roman. 1960. Linguistics and poetics. In: T. A. Sebeok (ed.), *Style in Language*. Boston: Technology Press of MIT, 350–377.

Kintsch, Walter. 1988. The use of knowledge in discourse processing: A construction-integration model. *Psychological Review* 95: 163–182.

Kintsch, Walter. 1998. *Comprehension. A Paradigm for Cognition*. Cambridge: Cambridge University Press.

Kjellmer, Göran. 1990. Patterns of collocability. In: J. Aarts and W. Meijs (eds.), *Theory and Practice in Corpus Linguistics*. Amsterdam: Rodopi, 163–178.

Kjellmer, Göran. 1991. A mint of phrases. In: K. Aijmer and B. Altenberg (eds.), *English Corpus Linguistics*. London: Longman, 111–127.

Lamb, Sydney. 1999. *Pathways of the Brain: The Neurocognitive Basis of Language*. Amsterdam: John Benjamins.

Landauer, T. K. and Susan T. Dumais. 1997. A solution to plato's problem: The latent semantic analysis theory of acquisition, induction, and representation of knowledge. *Psychological Review* 104(2): 211–240.

Landauer, T. K., P. W. Foltz and D. Laham. 1998. An introduction to latent semantic analysis. *Discourse Processes* 25(2-3): 259–284.

Langacker, Ronald. W. 2002. *Concept, Image, and Symbol*. Berlin: Mouton de Gruyter. (first published 1991).

Levelt, Willem J. M. 1989. *Speaking: From Intention to Articulation*. Cambridge, MA: MIT Press.

Louw, Bill. 1993. Irony in the text or insincerity in the writer? The diagnostic potential of semantic prosodies. In: Mona Baker, Gill Francis and Elena Tognini-Bonelli (eds.), *Text and Technology. In Honour of John Sinclair*. Amsterdam: John Benjamins, 157–176.

Meyer, D. E. and R. W. Schvaneveldt. 1971. Facilitation in recognizing pairs of words: Evidence of a dependence between retrieval operations. *Journal of Experimental Psychology* 90: 227–234.

Minsky, Marvin A. 1975. A framework for representing knowledge. In: P. Winston (ed.), *The Psychology of Computer Vision*. New York: McGraw-Hill, 211–277.

Morton, J. 1979. Word recognition. In: J. Morton and J. C. Marshall (eds.), *Psycholinguistics: Structures and Processes*, volume 2. London: Elek.

Nunberg, Geoffrey, I. A. Sag and Th. Wasow. 1994. Idioms. *Language* 70: 491–538.

Partington, Alan. 1998. *Patterns and Meanings: Using Corpora for English Language Research and Teaching*. Amsterdam: John Benjamins.

Pateman, Trevor. 1986. Relevance, contextual effects and least effort. *Poetics Today* 7, 4: 745–754.

Renouf, Anette and John Sinclair. 1991. Collocational frameworks in English. In: K. Aijmer and B. Altenberg (eds.), *English Corpus Linguistics*. London: Longman, 128–144.

Schank, R. C. and R. P. Abelson. 1977. *Scripts, Plans, Goals and Understanding*. Hillsdale, NJ: Lawrence Erlbaum Associates.

Shillcock, Richard. 1990. Lexical hypotheses in continuous speech. In: G. T. M. Altmann (ed.), *Cognitive Models of Speech Processing: Psycholinguistic and Computational Perspectives*. Cambridge, MA: MIT Press, 24–49.

Sinclair, John. 1987. Collocation: A progress report. In: Ross Steale and Terry Threadgold (eds.), *Language Topics. Essays in Honour of Michael Halliday*, volume 2. Amsterdam: John Benjamins, 319–332.

Sinclair, John. 1991. *Corpus, Concordance, Collocation*. Oxford: Oxford University Press.

Sinclair, John. 1996. The search for units of meaning. *Textus* 4: 75–106.

Sperber, Dan and Deirdre Wilson. 1995. *Relevance: Communication and Cognition*. Oxford: Blackwell. (first published 1986).

Swinney, David A. 1979. Lexical access during sentence comprehension: (re)consideration of context effects. *Journal of Verbal Learning & Verbal Behavior* 18(6): 645–659.

Till, R. E., E. F. Mross and W. Kintsch. 1988. Time course of priming for associate and inference words in discourse context. *Memory and Cognition* 16: 283–299.

Zwaan, R. A. 1994. Effects of genre expectations on text comprehension. *Journal of Experimental Psychology: Learning, Memory and Cognition* 20, 4: 920–933.

Zwitserlood, P. 1989. The locus of the effects of sentential-semantic context in spoken word processing. *Cognition* 32: 25–64.

Index

Sabest
Saarbrücker Beiträge zur Sprach- und Translationswissenschaft

Fachrichtung Angewandte Sprachwissenschaft
sowie Übersetzen und Dolmetschen
der Universität des Saarlandes

Alberto Gil – Johann Haller – Erich Steiner – Elke Teich
(Hrsg.)

Band 1 Alberto Gil / Johann Haller / Erich Steiner / Heidrun Gerzymisch-Arbogast (Hrsg.): Modelle der Translation. Grundlagen für Methodik, Bewertung, Computermodellierung. 1999.

Band 2 Uwe Reinke: Translation Memories. Systeme – Konzepte – Linguistische Optimierung. 2004.

Band 3 Stella Neumann: Textsorten und Übersetzen. Eine Korpusanalyse englischer und deutscher Reiseführer. 2003.

Band 4 Erich Steiner: Translated Texts: Properties, Variants, Evaluations. 2004.

Band 5 Sisay Fissaha Adafre: Adding Amharic to a Unification-Based Machine Translation System. An Experiment. 2004.

Band 6 Tinka Reichmann: Satzspaltung und Informationsstruktur im Portugiesischen und im Deutschen. Ein Beitrag zur Kontrastiven Linguistik und Übersetzungswissenschaft. 2005.

Band 7 María Jesús Barsanti Vigo: Análisis paremiológico de *El Quijote* de Cervantes en la versión de Ludwig Tieck. 2005.

Band 8 Christoph Rösener: Die Stecknadel im Heuhaufen. Natürlichsprachlicher Zugang zu Volltextdatenbanken. 2005.

Band 9 Fadia Sami Sauerwein: Dolmetschen bei polizeilichen Vernehmungen und grenzpolizeilichen Einreisebefragungen. Eine explorative translationswissenschaftliche Untersuchung zum Community Interpreting. 2006.

Band 10 Rosario Herrero: La metáfora : revisión histórica y descripción lingüística. 2006.

Band 11 Ursula Wienen: Zur Übersetzbarkeit markierter Kohäsionsformen. Eine funktionale Studie zum Kontinuum von Spaltadverbialen und Spaltkonnektoren im Spanischen, Französischen und Deutschen. 2006.

Band 12 María José Corvo Sánchez: Los libros de lenguas de Juan Ángel de Zumaran. La obra de un maestro e intérprete de lenguas español entre los alemanes del siglo XVII. 2007.

Band 13 Vahram Atayan: Makrostrukturen der Argumentation im Deutschen, Französischen und Italienischen. Mit einem Vorwort von Oswald Ducrot. 2006.

Band 14 Alberto Gil / Ursula Wienen (Hrsg.): Multiperspektivische Fragestellungen der Translation in der Romania. Hommage an Wolfram Wilss zu seinem 80. Geburtstag. 2007.

Band 15 Anja Rütten: Informations- und Wissensmanagement im Konferenzdolmetschen. 2007.

Band 16 Valerio Allegranza: The Signs of Determination. Constraint-Based Modelling Across Languages. 2007.

Band 17 Andrea Wurm: Translatorische Wirkung. Ein Beitrag zum Verständnis von Übersetzungsgeschichte als Kulturgeschichte am Beispiel deutscher Übersetzungen französischer Kochbücher in der Frühen Neuzeit. 2008.

Band 18 Ramona Schröpf: Translatorische Dimensionen von Konnektorensequenzen im Spanischen und Französischen. Ein Beitrag zur linguistisch orientierten Übersetzungswissenschaft Romanisch – Deutsch. 2009.

Band 19 Windyam Fidèle Yameogo: Translatorische Fragen der Ambivalenz und Implizitheit bei Mephistopheles. Dargestellt an französischen Übersetzungen von Goethes Faust I. 2010.

Band 20 Manuela Caterina Moroni: Modalpartikeln zwischen Syntax, Prosodie und Informationsstruktur. 2010.

Band 21 Kerstin Anna Kunz: Variation in English and German Nominal Coreference. A Study of Political Essays. 2010.

Band 22 Sandra Strohbach: Die Übersetzungen der chemischen Werke von Stanislao Cannizzaro. Ein Beitrag zur Geschichte der Fachübersetzung im 19. Jahrhundert. 2010.

Band 23 Cornelia Zelinsky-Wibbelt (ed.): Relations between Language and Memory. Organization, Representation, and Processing. 2011.